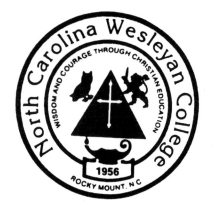

North Carolina Wesleyan College

WISDOM AND COURAGE THROUGH CHRISTIAN EDUCATION

1956

ROCKY MOUNT, N.C.

Exploring Exercise Science

Gregory S. Wilson, PED, FACSM

Associate Professor and Chair of the Department of Exercise and Sport Science
University of Evansville
Evansville, Indiana

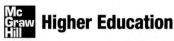 **Higher Education**

Boston   Burr Ridge, IL   Dubuque, IA   New York   San Francisco   St. Louis
Bangkok   Bogotá   Caracas   Kuala Lumpur   Lisbon   London   Madrid   Mexico City
Milan   Montreal   New Delhi   Santiago   Seoul   Singapore   Sydney   Taipei   Toronto

The McGraw·Hill Companies

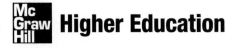 **Higher Education**

Published by McGraw-Hill, an imprint of The McGraw-Hill Companies, Inc., 1221 Avenue of the Americas, New York, NY 10020. Copyright © 2010. All rights reserved. No part of this publication may be reproduced or distributed in any form or by any means, or stored in a database or retrieval system, without the prior written consent of The McGraw-Hill Companies, Inc., including, but not limited to, in any network or other electronic storage or transmission, or broadcast for distance learning..

This book is printed on acid-free paper.

1 2 3 4 5 6 7 8 9 0 QPD/QPD 0 9

ISBN: 978-0-07-352363-7
MHID: 0-07-352363-1

Editor in Chief: *Michael Ryan*
Editorial Director: *William Glass*
Executive Editor: *Christopher Johnson*
Director of Development: *Kathleen Engelberg*
Developmental Editor: *Gary O'Brien, Van Brien Associates*
Development Editor for Technology: *Julia Akpan*
Editorial Coordinator: *Sarah Hill*
Marketing Manager: *Bill Minick*
Production Editor: *Alison Meier*
Media Project Manager: *Ron Nelms*
Design Coordinator: *Andrei Pasternak*
Cover Design: *Andrei Pasternak*
Interior Design: *Linda Robertson*
Illustrator: *Dartmouth Publishing, Inc.*
Photo Research: *Brian J. Pecko*
Production Supervisor: *Richard DeVitto*
Composition: *10/12 Novarese Book by Aptara*
Printing: *45# New Era Matte Plus, Quebecor World*

Cover image: Photograph: Lori Adamski Peek/Stone/Getty Images; Diagram by Susan Hall. Credits: The credits section for this book begins on page 420 and is considered an extension of the copyright page.

Library of Congress Cataloging-in-Publication Data

Exploring exercise science / edited by Gregory Wilson.
    p. cm.
  Includes bibliographical references and index.
  ISBN-13: 978-0-07-352363-7 (alk. paper)
  ISBN-10: 0-07-352363-1 (alk. paper)
  1. Sports—Physiological aspects.   2. Physical education—Training.   3. Exercise.
4. Sports sciences.   5. Sports medicine.   I. Wilson, Gregory S. (Gregory Scott), 1960–
  RC1235.E97 2010
  613.7'1—dc22

                                                                2008042518

The Internet addresses listed in the text were accurate at the time of publication. The inclusion of a Web site does not indicate an endorsement by the authors or McGraw-Hill, and McGraw-Hill does not guarantee the accuracy of the information presented at these sites.

www.mhhe.com

Brief Contents

Contents

PART 3

Exploring the Behavioral 57

PART 4

Exploring the Biomechanical 95

PART 5

Exploring Sports Medicine 113

Preface

The importance of exercise to one's quality of life cannot be overstated. Exercise positively affects both our physical and emotional health. Readers of this text already understand the important role of exercise to both longevity and quality of life but are interested in learning more about the underlying principles involved in bringing about these benefits. In other words, they are interested in the discipline of exercise science.

Exploring Exercise Science will help students acquire current knowledge in this area while providing up-to-date information on career opportunities and professional organizations and credentials. Exercise science is a wide-ranging field of study comprised of distinctive yet intermingling subdisciplines (exercise physiology, nutrition, exercise and sport psychology, motor behavior, biomechanics, athletic training, and social sciences). Upper-level undergraduate classes offer specific details in each of these subdisciplines, but a growing number of colleges offer an exploratory course that introduces the discipline of exercise science to the first-year student. *Exploring Exercise Science* provides an overview of the subdisciplines of exercise science while offering freshmen-level students necessary and practical information concerning societal health trends, physical activity, epidemiology, and professional legal and ethical concerns related to the exercise scientist.

This book is designed for students exploring the discipline of exercise science who have only a general idea of the areas that comprise this field of study. There has been renewed interest in exercise in recent years in the United States; unfortunately, much of this attention has arisen as a result of health problems resulting from a lack of exercise participation. Hence, undergraduate exercise science curriculums must cover an increasing number of topics, ranging from the preventive health aspects of regular exercise participation and exercise adherence for regular exercisers, to performance enhancement of athletes. *Exploring Exercise Science* explains what exercise scientists study, provides informations about career opportunities, and gives students a global understanding of the discipline.

Exploring Exercise Science is divided into seven parts. Part 1 introduces the main themes of the book and provides an introduction into the subdisciplines of exercise science. The components of research are described along with how the exercise scientist uses these components to answer pertinent questions. Part 2 presents detailed information on the physiologic knowledge base of exercise science: namely, exercise physiology and nutrition. Basic concepts central to the study of these two areas are presented along with potential areas of study. Part 3 introduces the behavioral basis of exercise science, exploring the subdisciplines of exercise and sport psychology and motor behavior. Part 4 is devoted to a discussion of the biomechanical knowledge base of exercise science, and Part 5 offers insights into the sports medicine component, providing a comprehensive overview of the field of athletic training. Part 6 explores the sociology of physical activity and the history of exercise and sport, which combine to make up the social science aspect of exercise science. Finally, Part 7 presents a unique discussion of societal, ethical, and legal factors that influence the work of the exercise scientist, focusing on current societal health trends and how these influences affect the health status of the country. This is followed by a detailed discussion of physical activity epidemiology that explores the rates of physical activity and its effect on the population's health status. Legal and ethical discussions are important to any field of study, and an exploration of how these affect the exercise scientist is presented. We conclude with a look into the future. The final chapter explores future trends in exercise science and possible new areas of research and employment.

FEATURES OF THIS TEXTBOOK

An important feature of this book is its practicality. It blends scientific elements such as metabolic responses to exercise or the amount of force needed to generate an overhand throw with professional issues such as legal liability and employment opportunities. Each chapter is written by a leading expert in the field. A distinctive feature of this textbook is the unique format for each chapter. Chapter topics are arranged in the following order (1) history of the subdiscipline, (2) what a specialist in the subdiscipline studies, (3), professional organizations important to the subdiscipline, (4) certifications relevant to the subdiscipline, and (5) employment opportunities in the subdiscipline. Most books only present an overview, but *Exploring Exercise Science* integrates these concepts with practical information concerning types of employment possibilities and the certifications required to work in a specific area. The distinct approach of this textbook bridges the gap between subject material and how that information is used in the workplace. Students interested in employment in specific areas of exercise science have the opportunity to truly understand what is required in pursuit of their long-term goals.

Another unique feature of this book is its focus on important issues such as the legal and ethical responsibilities of the exercise science professional. This information is valuable as students prepare for future internship and practicum experiences in their later college years. In addition, this book offers a detailed look at physical activity epidemiology, which is important to the understanding of the health benefits of exercise. This complements the societal health trends chapter, which explains why exercise is important to the prevention of heart disease and other chronic and debilitating diseases. Designed for students first entering the discipline, *Exploring Exercise Science* provides a building block for future courses while offering insights into the future of exercise science.

Ancillaries

The instructor Web site includes the following resources that will help you teach the class using this book:

- Instructor's Manual
- Test Bank Questions
- PowerPoint Slides

Acknowledgments

It is difficult to adequately acknowledge all the people who make a project like this possible. I have been fortunate to be surrounded by knowledgeable and devoted colleagues and mentors throughout my professional life. To them, I owe a deep debt of gratitude. However, the most important influence has always been my family, who has continued to support me in all things.

Gary O'Brien has been an invaluable asset in the development of this book. His insights and guidance have been remarkable. Of course, this book would not be possible without the tireless efforts and expertise of the chapter authors. They are true champions.

I wish to thank the following individuals for their helpful reviews of this book:

Joseph Andreacci, Bloomsburg University of Pennsylvania

Dawn Castro, Indiana Wesleyan

Mark Clark, University of Wisconsin, Eau Claire

Jared Coburn, California State University, Fullerton

Scott Collier, Syracuse University

Jami Craps, University of South Carolina, Aiken

Margaret Duncan, University of Wisconsin, Milwaukee

Craig Harms, Kansas State University

Pam Kocher Brown, University of North Carolina at Greensboro

Priscilla Macrae, Pepperdine University

John Mercer, University of Nevada, Las Vegas

Tim Michael, Western Michigan University, Kalamazoo

Elizabeth O'Neil, Central Connecticut State University

Jennifer Petit, University of Akron

John Pfau, Pennsylvania State University

Brady Redus, Central OKlahoma University

Laura Richardson, University of Akron

Contributors

Thomas A. Baker III, JD, PhD *The University of Georgia* Thomas Baker has a PhD in Sport Management from the University of Florida and a Juris Doctorate from Loyola University School of Law. His research emphasis is sport law and risk management with a focus on contract and tort-related legal issues. He is a member of the Louisiana Bar Association and specializes in commercial litigation and alternative dispute resolution. Baker lives in Georgia with his wife Susana.

Ray Castle, PhD, ATC, LAT *Department of Kinesiology, Concentration in Athletic Training, Louisiana State University* Ray Castle received his BS degree in Kinesiology from Louisiana State University (1990), and MS (Human Performance–Exercise Science) and PhD (Human Performance–Administration and Teaching) degrees from the University of Southern Mississippi (1993, 2000). He currently serves as assistant professor of professional practice and director of the CAATE-accredited undergraduate Concentration in Athletic Training in the Department of Kinesiology at Louisiana State University (Baton Rouge, LA). Castle has been both a BOC Certified Athletic Trainer (ATC) and Licensed Athletic Trainer (LAT) by the Louisiana State Board of Medical Examiners since 1991. He is highly active in the athletic training profession, having served on the USOC Medical Staff for the 2003 Pan American Games and given numerous professional and research presentations at state, regional, national, and international symposia. In addition, he is highly active within various professional committees, including a current position on the Education Council Executive Committee of the National Athletic Trainers' Association.

Kelly J. Cole, PhD *Department of Integrative Physiology, The University of Iowa* Kelly J. Cole has been teaching motor control, motor learning, and motor development at The University of Iowa for two decades. Many of the undergraduate students in these courses have gone on to careers in the health professions and research. His research has focused on the control of the hand in health, disease, and in old age.

Daniel P. Connaughton, PhD *Associate Professor, Department of Tourism, Recreation & Sport Management, University of Florida* Daniel P. Connaughton is an associate professor at the University of Florida (UF) where he conducts research and teaches in the area of sport law and risk management. He received a bachelor's degree in Exercise and Sport Sciences and a master's degree in Recreational Studies from UF, a master's degree in Physical Education from Bridgewater State College, and a Doctorate in Sport Management from Florida State University. He holds numerous professional certifications including ACSM Health/Fitness Instructor and Certified Strength and Conditioning Specialist. He has several years of experience in the exercise science field as a health/fitness instructor and program director and frequently serves as a consultant and expert witness in health/fitness and sport-related litigation.

Susan J. Hall, PhD *Professor and Chairperson, Department of Health, Nutrition and Exercise Science, University of Delaware* Susan Hall is a Fellow of the American College of Sports Medicine and the AAHPERD Research Consortium. Her research interests have focused on low back pain prevention and the biomechanical aspects of selected sports and exercises, and she has published numerous research papers and book chapters related to these topics. She is President-Elect of the AAHPERD Research Consortium and has served as Chair of the Biomechanics Academy of AAHPERD, Vice President of the American College of Sports Medicine, and member of the Board of Directors of the International Society for Biomechanics in Sport. She has delivered the Amy Morris Homans Lecture and the EDA Research Keynote Address. Hall is also the author of several successful textbooks.

William Harper, PhD *Department of Health and Kinesiology, Purdue University* William Harper teaches at Purdue University and has published journal articles and essays in the areas of the history and philosophy of sport, play, and leisure/recreation. He has also published a lengthy biography of the American sportswriter Grantland Rice (1880–1954). Currently he is head of the Department of Health and Kinesiology.

Gregory W. Heath, DHSc, MPH *Guerry Professor and Head, Department of Health and Human Performance, University of Tennessee, Chattanooga* Gregory W. Heath is former Lead Health Scientist with the Division of Nutrition and Physical Activity at the Centers for Disease Control and Prevention (CDC). His training is in physiology, nutrition, and epidemiology. His master's of Public Health and doctorate of Health Science degrees are from Loma Linda University in California. He completed his postdoctoral training in applied physiology at the Washington University School of Medicine in St. Louis. A former Epidemic Intelligence Service Officer (EISO), he worked at CDC for over 20 years. He has devoted most of his professional career to understanding and promoting physical activity and exercise for the enhancement of health and the prevention and treatment of chronic diseases. He has published widely in the scientific literature and is a Fellow in the American College of Sports Medicine, and American Heart Association's Councils on Epidemiology and Prevention and Nutrition, Physical Activity, and Metabolism.

Jennifer E. Ketterly MS, RD *Director of Sports Nutrition, University of North Carolina at Chapel Hill* Jennifer E. Ketterly oversees the sports nutrition needs for UNC's 28 varsity sports, including nutrition education, counseling, training tables, body composition analysis, and supplement evaluation. In addition to working with Tar Heel teams, she collaborates with the UNC-based Center for Study of Retired Athletes as their Sports Dietitian. She also serves as a speaker and writer for various professional organizations and publications. Ketterly has a bachelor's degree from the Department of Nutritional Sciences at Cornell University, where she was also a member of the Big Red women's basketball team. She completed her dietetic internship training and earned her master's degree in Clinical Nutrition from the University of Kentucky.

Anthony D. Mahon, PhD *Human Performance Laboratory, Ball State University* Anthony D. Mahon is a professor of Physical Education at Ball State University. He has been a member of the Human Performance Laboratory since 1990 where he teaches undergraduate and graduate courses in exercise physiology. His research area is in pediatric exercise physiology.

Mary McElroy, PhD *Department of Kinesiology, Kansas State University* Mary McElroy is a professor of Kinesiology and American Ethnic Studies at Kansas State University. She is author of numerous articles and several books focusing on the sociological aspects of physical activity and public health. She is a past president of the North American Society for Sport Sociology.

Lynn R. Penland, PhD *Dean, College of Education and Health Sciences, University of Evansville* Lynn R. Penland has a PhD in health education from The Ohio State University. She has experience teaching at three different institutions in the areas of health, wellness, and fitness as well as in health professions programs. She also worked for a state department of health. She is currently at the University of Evansville where she serves as dean of a unit which includes exercise and sport science, education, physical therapy, and nursing and health sciences.

Matthew J. Robinson, PhD *Associate Professor of Sport Management, University of Delaware* Matthew J. Robinson is associate professor and the director of the Sport Management Program at the University of Delaware. He is also a member of the legal studies faculty and has a secondary appointment with the School of Education at the University and serves as director of the International Coaching Enrichment Certificate Program (ICECP) funded by the United States Olympic Committee and the International Olympic Committee's Olympic Solidarity fund. He also serves as Director of Management Education for the National Soccer Coaches Association of America (NSCAA) and is the author of the highly successful sport management text, *Profiles of Sport Industry Professionals: The People Who Make the Games Happen*. In addition, he has authored over 25 articles and made over 100 national and international scholarly and professional presentations.

Michelle S. Rockwell MS, RD, CSSD *Sports Nutrition Consultant, RK Team Nutrition* Michelle S. Rockwell is a sports dietitian based in Durham, North Carolina. She consults with individual athletes and athletic teams locally and nationwide on issues related to enhancing performance and health status through nutrition intervention. Her clients range from recreational exercisers to professional athletes. She also serves as a speaker, writer, and consultant for a number of college and university athletic departments, sports clubs and teams, and professional organizations. She recently cofounded RK Team Nutrition, a sports nutrition consulting service providing sports nutrition education to students and health professionals throughout the United States Previously, she served as the Director of Sports Nutrition for the University of Florida Athletic Association (1999–2005). Rockwell holds master of science and bachelor of science degrees from the Human Nutrition, Foods, & Exercise department at Virginia Tech, where she was captain and five-time conference champion for the Hokies' track and field team. She completed her dietetics internship training at the National Institutes of Health.

Tonya R. Skalon, MS *Ball State University* Tonya R. Skalon obtained her bachelor of science in Kinesiology with an emphasis in Exercise Science in 1997 and her master's of science in Kinesiology with an emphasis in Clinical Exercise Physiology in 1999, both from Indiana University. In 1999 she became an instructor at Ball State University, teaching various classes including fitness and wellness, exercise assessment, and foundations of exercise science, and she assisted with the clinical exercise physiology program. In 2003 she assumed the role of Exercise Science internship coordinator, and in 2004 she began advising all exercise science majors.

Beverly J. Warren, PhD, EdD, FACSM *Virginia Commonwealth University* Beverly J. Warren is Dean of the School of Education at Virginia Commonwealth University. Previously, she served as Professor and Chair of the Department of Health, Physical Education, and Recreation at VCU as well as at Auburn University, Appalachian State University, and Lander University. She received her BS degree from the University of North Carolina–Greensboro, an MS degree from Southern Illinois University, an EdD from the University of Alabama, and a PhD in exercise physiology from Auburn University. She has numerous publications in the areas of treatment of childhood obesity and the physiological parameters of youth fitness. She is a Fellow of the American College of Sports Medicine and the Research Consortium of the American Alliance of Health, Physical Education, Recreation, and Dance. She was elected to the Board of Trustees of the American College of Sports Medicine in 2004 and is a former president of the Southeast Chapter of ACSM. Her research currently involves issues in urban education.

Gregory S. Wilson, PED, FACSM *Department of Exercise and Sport Science, University of Evansville* Gregory S. Wilson is an associate professor and chair of the Department of Exercise and Sport Science at the University of Evansville. He has numerous publications in the area of exercise and sport psychology and has coauthored chapters for various textbooks on subjects ranging from anxiety and sport performance to overtraining and staleness in athletes. Recently, he has coedited a textbook titled *Applying Sport Psychology: Four Perspectives*. He is a Fellow of the American College of Sports Medicine and has received several awards for teaching at UE.

Introduction

CHAPTER 1
Introduction to Exploring Exercise Science
Gregory Wilson, PED, FACSM, University of Evansville

What is exercise science? It is the study of the physiological and behavioral changes that occur in the body in response to exercise and sport training. Exercise science is an exciting and dynamic discipline made up of the subdisciplines of exercise physiology, nutrition, exercise and sport psychology, motor behavior, biomechanics, and sports medicine. The purpose of Part 1 is to introduce you to the multifaceted and diverse study of exercise science and some of the issues commonly dealt with by the exercise scientist in research settings.

Introduction to Exploring Exercise Science

Gregory Wilson, PED, FACSM, University of Evansville

■ Chapter Objectives

After reading this chapter, you should be able to:

1. Describe what is meant by the term *exercise science*.
2. Explain what is meant by a discipline and subdiscipline and list the subdisciplines of exercise science.
3. Identify the four knowledge bases that define the subdisciplines of exercise science.
4. Explain the differences between "exercise and health promotion" and "sport performance enhancement" aspects of exercise science.
5. Describe the differences between applied research and basic research.
6. Explain what is meant by the statement "exercise science is an integrative discipline."

■ Key Terms

athletic training
applied research
basic research
biomechanics
discipline

exercise physiology
exercise science
exercise and sport psychology
motor behavior
sociology of physical activity

sport history
sport nutrition
subdiscipline

BRIEF HISTORY OF EXERCISE SCIENCE

In 1954 a track athlete named Roger Bannister believed something that many people in his day thought impossible—that humans could run a mile in under 4 minutes. To find out what was needed to accomplish this feat, Bannister, who was also a medical student, began a series of physiological tests measuring variables such as the amount of oxygen consumed and energy used when running. In doing so, Bannister was among the first modern-day athletes/researchers to utilize "science" as a way to enhance physical performance.

However, Bannister was not the first person to be interested in the effects of exercise on the human body or the athletic feats that the body could perform. In fact, the Olympics in ancient Greece provided the foundation for much of our modern day search for the ultimate answers concerning health, fitness, and sport performance.

Despite this early interest in human physical capabilities, it was not until the late 18th century that most people acknowledge the actual beginnings of scientific research into how the body functions during exercise. It was at this time that two young French researchers named Seguin and Lavoiser investigated the differences in oxygen consumption at rest and during exercise (Robergs & Keteyian, 2003; Wilmore, Costill, & Kenney, 2008). Although they were the first to investigate these differences, they incorrectly concluded that a complicated process of oxygen utilization and carbon dioxide production in the lungs was involved in this process, a notion that was later disproved. In 1889 a very speculative textbook focusing on the effects of exercise appeared titled *Physiology of Bodily Exercise* by Fernand LaGrange. Although this is sometimes called the first textbook devoted solely to the question of how the human body responds to exercise and physical activity, much of its content was based on the little available research of the day, and it was not always correct in its conclusions.

What we today call exercise science had its beginnings in physical education. Much of the renewed interest in the United States in this area occurred during the early part of the 20th century as people developed an increasing awareness of physical fitness and bodily responses to exercise. In part this renewed interest was the result of the two World Wars (Robergs & Keteyian, 2003). Because of the immediate need for information concerning optimal training regimens for soldiers preparing to go off to combat, physical rehabilitation of wounded soldiers, and environmental factors such as heat and cold stress, research in the area of exercise science became important. Hence, to a great extent, the field of exercise science derived its beginnings from physical education. However, physical education is an educational process designed to promote fitness and the development of physical skills through physical activity, whereas exercise science utilizes the scientific method to understand the effects of exercise upon the body (Wuest & Bucher, 2009).

Perhaps no other research facility influenced the growing interest in exercise science more than the Harvard Fatigue Laboratory (HFL). Founded in 1927 by David B. Dill (1891–1986), the HFL greatly increased our knowledge in such key areas of exercise physiology as the physiology of endurance performance and environmental physiology. So vast was the amount of research conducted at the HFL that approximately 330 scientific papers were published before its closing in 1947 (Wilmore, Costill, & Kenney, 2008). An important researcher at the HFL during this time was a student of Dr. Dill's named Sid Robinson (1903–1981), who eventually established the Human Physiology Laboratory at Indiana University. Robinson went on to fame as a leading early investigator of the effects of aging on the heart and lungs. The HFL was a very important milestone in the history of exercise science, and its influence cannot be overestimated. (See a complete description of its development and importance in Chapter 2.)

During the 1960s, exercise science took another step forward as research moved into the area of biochemical approaches to the study of exercise. A leading scientist in this area was Phil Gollnick of Washington State University who looked at muscle metabolism and its relationship to exercise fatigue in animal studies, contributing greatly to our knowledge of how energy depletion affects muscle fatigue. Moreover, during this decade, the USA space program also made significant contributions to our understanding of how the human body responds to environmental stresses.

Another important milestone in exercise science occurred with the work of Kenneth Cooper. The popularity of the term *aerobics* can be traced to the work of Dr. Cooper (1931–) and the Cooper Institute. Studies conducted there in the 1970s examined the healthy benefits of jogging and greatly popularized the need for aerobic fitness in this country. Today the Cooper Institute continues to conduct and publish vital research in this area while serving as a leading proponent for the importance of an active lifestyle.

The American College of Sports Medicine (ACSM) was founded in 1954 and helped to solidify the importance of exercise to a healthy life. Today, the ACSM is the major voice in the area of exercise and sport performance, speaking for thousands of exercise scientists around the world. So important is this organization that many of the chapters in this textbook talk of its influence in the specific areas that make up exercise science.

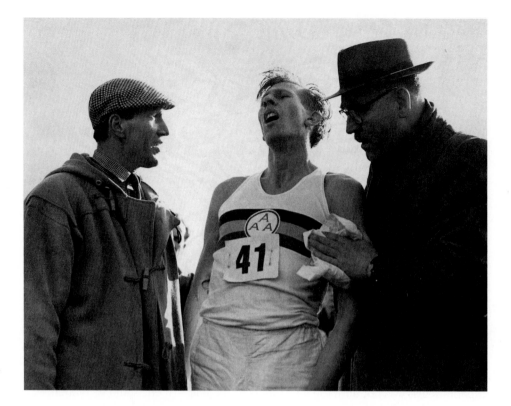

Roger Bannister was the first person to break the 4-minute mile barrier on May 6, 1954, in front of a crowd of 3,000 spectators at Oxford University, when he crossed the finish line in 3:59.4 despite the windy and rainy conditions.

It was also in 1954 on a rain-swept day in Oxford, England, that Roger Bannister finally decided it was time to put the training and knowledge he had compiled to the ultimate test—breaking the 4-minute mile. Four laps later, pushing himself to near total exhaustion, he became the first person in history to run a sub-4-minute mile, with a time of 3:59.4.

However, even with his science-based training, there were many things that Roger Bannister still did not understand. For instance, such factors as the differences in the types of muscle fibers and the many different cardiovascular adaptations that occur because of exercise were unknown in 1954 (Bascomb, 2004). In fact, questions such as these and others continue to be answered today through the discipline known as exercise science.

WHAT IS EXERCISE SCIENCE

Defining Exercise Science

We can define *exercise* as the participation in some quantified form of physical activity with the intended purpose of improving or maintaining health (see Chapter 2). Exercise is usually measured by its intensity, duration, mode (e.g., type), and frequency. *Science*, on the other hand, is a structured inquiry of study with the goal of explanation (Berg & Latin, 2004). In other words, science represents a systematic, empirically based search for knowledge. Hence, **exercise science** is the *study of how the human body responds to exercise or physical activity*. Those that study the relationship of exercise to physical health and sport performance are known as exercise scientists. An exercise scientist may study the role of exercise in relation to health promotion or in the area of sport performance enhancement for athletes.

What Is a Discipline?

When most people think of exercise science, they tend to think of exercise physiology or possibly sport psychology. However, these are actually subdisciplines within the major discipline of exercise science. A **discipline** is a field of study that has a central focus with its own body of knowledge. In the sciences, we often think of the classical disciplines of biology, chemistry, or physics. Exercise science, with its origin in physical education, is a relatively new scientific discipline that emerged in the latter part of the 20th century.

Typically, a discipline is made up of many integrated **subdisciplines.** For example, a biologist may decide to specialize in one particular area of interest and select the field of molecular biology as her topic of specialization. In the same way, many subdisciplines make up the study of exercise science. Because human movement is such a complicated area of study, many integrated subdisciplines exist to study how the body responds to exercise and physical activity.

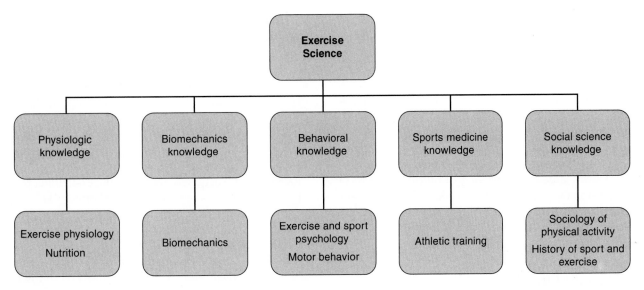

Figure 1.1 The knowledge areas of exercise science.

SUBDISCIPLINES OF EXERCISE SCIENCE

The subdisciplines of exercise science can be categorized into five integrated bases of knowledge: physiological (*exercise physiology*; *sport nutrition*), behavioral (*exercise and sport psychology*; *motor behavior*), sports medicine (*athletic training*), biomechanical (*biomechanics*), and social science (*sport sociology*; *sport history*). Working in tandem with investigators from different subdisciplines, the exercise scientist is able to answer many questions concerning the relationship of physical activity to health and improvements in sport performance (see Figure 1.1).

Physiologic Knowledge

Exercise physiology represents the cornerstone of the exercise science curriculum and is probably the most readily recognized of the subdisciplines. Exercise physiology encompasses areas of study that include physiology, anatomy, biochemistry, and biology. It is the study of how the human body functions and how it responds or changes when exposed to bouts of exercise.

A typical course in exercise physiology includes a survey of the effects of both acute and chronic exercise on the different systems and structures of the body. Moreover, the effects of exercise intensity, duration, frequency, and mode are important to understanding the consequences of exercise training. Chapter 2 introduces these concepts and illustrates how these exercise components influence changes in various physiological systems of the body, including the metabolic (energy), nervous, endocrine, skeletal muscle, cardiovascular, and respiratory systems. The

exercise physiologist may work in a number of professional settings, including clinical settings such as cardiac rehabilitation and pulmonary rehabilitation. Another important role of the exercise physiologist is that of clinical exercise testing and prescribing an exercise program based on the results obtained. This chapter will discuss these and other career opportunities, as well as prominent professional organizations such as the American College of Sports Medicine (ACSM) and the National Strength and Conditioning Association (NSCA).

Sport nutrition is a fairly young and rapidly growing subdiscipline in exercise science. Nutrition and exercise physiology share a common bond because proper nutrition forms the building blocks for all forms of physical activity (McArdle, Katch, & Katch, 2001). The study of sport nutrition looks at how what we eat affects human health and fitness and, when applied to athletes, how this information can improve sport performance. Together with information gleaned by the exercise physiologist, the exercise nutritionist can assist in developing nutritional programs that will foster improvements in physical health and in sport performance through an understanding of how the body's metabolic system works and what types of foods are most efficiently used as fuel. Chapter 3 discusses the typical areas covered in an undergraduate sports nutrition curriculum, including such topics as macronutrients and micronutrients, fluids and electrolytes, how athletic performance may be enhanced through nutrition, weight control and body composition, eating disorders and the female athlete triad, and dietary supplements and erogenic aids.

Nutritionists often work within a health care facility performing such duties as nutritional screening and counseling. They also may work in conjunction with doctors in patient recovery following illness or injury by utilizing proper nutrition as a means to facilitate recovery. Nutritionists also work in college and university settings, teaching classes and providing nutritional information for students. *Exercise* or *sport nutritionists* are primarily employed in college or university settings and work directly with sport teams or with professional teams. In addition, they may work in corporate wellness or fitness centers or private health clubs.

The most prominent professional organization in sports nutrition is the American Dietetic Association (ADA), the largest organization of nutrition and food professionals in the United States. Other important organizations include the International Society of Sports Nutrition (ISSN) and the American College of Sports Medicine (ACSM).

Behavioral Knowledge

The subdiscipline of **exercise and sport psychology** is another rapidly growing field that covers a wide assortment of issues relating to the psychological aspects of exercise participation and sport performance. As with the other subdisciplines of exercise science, the field of exercise and sport psychology encompasses a wide variety of clinical, research, educational, and applied activities related to health and sport performance enhancement. For example, *sport psychology* is the study of cognitive factors that influence sport performance, such as confidence, motivation, and anxiety. For instance, Roger Bannister believed that breaking the 4-minute mile was not just a physiological challenge but a psychological one as well. The *sport psychologist* helps athletes achieve their physiologic potential through mental preparation and interventions. Many sport psychologists work in applied settings within a university athletic department, and a growing number of professional sport teams hire sport psychologists. Conversely, *exercise psychology* examines such issues as behavioral factors associated with exercise adherence and the relationship between positive mental health and exercise.

In the exercise science curriculum, it is difficult to separate physiological and mental aspects of human responses. Hence, knowledge of cognitive factors related to both exercise participation and sport performance is important to understanding exercise participation and sport success. Often, exercise and sport psychology courses are taught as upper-level classes in the junior or senior year of study, and advanced classes are typically required of most exercise science graduate programs as well. Chapter 4 covers the salient issues of both exercise and sport psychology and provides information concerning major professional organizations in the subdiscipline such as the American Psychological Association (APA), the Association for the Advancement of Applied Sport Psychology (AAASP), and the American College of Sports Medicine (ACSM).

Motor behavior can be defined as the study of the neural mechanisms that influence the learning of movement. As a field of research, motor behavior has focused on two broad, overlapping areas: motor control and motor learning. *Motor control* focuses on the processes that underlie the production of movement, including neural, physical, and behavioral aspects of the human nervous system. These areas provide the basic laws that skilled movements appear to obey. *Motor learning* focuses on the mechanisms by which skilled movements are acquired, including understanding the optimal conditions for learning new motor skills. A third area is *motor development*, which looks at changes in both motor control and learning over the lifetime.

An understanding of both motor control and motor learning are important for the exercise science student as we attempt to understand how human motor behaviors develop, how we as humans best learn and modify new motor skills, and how we recover motor function after disease and injury. Chapter 5 provides an overview of the material covered in an introductory motor behavior curriculum important to the dual areas of motor learning and control. This discussion includes sensory integration, brain plasticity, postural control, conditions for optimal learning, and the principles of skill learning.

In the clinic, physical therapists, occupational therapists, speech/language pathologists, and athletic trainers apply their knowledge of motor control and motor learning on a daily basis as they determine how best to help their clients establish, modify, or regain motor function. Career opportunities in these and other areas are discussed in Chapter 5, along with relevant professional organizations such as the National Athletic Training Association (NATA), the American Physical Therapy Association (APTA), the Society for Neuroscience, and the Biomedical Engineering Society (BES).

Biomechanical Knowledge

Biomechanics is a multidisciplinary approach involving the application of mechanical principles in the study of living organisms (Hall, 2003). Chapter 6 discusses how information from such diverse fields as anatomy, physiology, mathematics, engineering, and physics is used in biomechanics to explain how forces such as inertia, acceleration, and reaction act upon the body to shape human movement. For example, Roger Bannister examined how efficiency of movement was related to energy expenditure in running. Knowing that the more efficient his biomechanics were the less energy he would use while running, much of his training focused on proper form and mechanics.

Although biomechanics involves the study of human movement, biomechanists may also have an academic background in zoology, medicine, engineering, or physical therapy, with the common factor being an interest in the biomechanical aspects of the structure and function of living things. Biomechanics is a key course in the undergraduate exercise science program and is most often an upper-level course (junior or senior year of study) with prerequisite courses (often anatomy, physics, and mathematics). Important areas covered in the curriculum include kinematics (linear and angular), kinetics, and fluid mechanics. These forces exert powerful influences on the human body, and an understanding of biomechanics promotes a comprehensive understanding of human body function.

Often, the biomechanist finds employment working for a sport shoe company, designing sport-specific shoes. Other sport equipment products are also biomechanically designed. In addition, those interested in biomechanics may find teaching opportunities at the college or university level or work in a variety of hospital and clinical settings. Important professional organizations in biomechanics include the American College of Sports Medicine (ACSM), the American Society for Biomechanics (ASB), the International Society for Biomechanics (ISB), and the Biomechanics Academy of the NASPE.

Sports Medicine Knowledge

Athletic training is a specialization within sports medicine that is primarily concerned with the health and safety of athletes. It combines an interdisciplinary approach including such specialties as medicine, anatomy, exercise physiology, psychology, biomechanics, and nutrition in the prevention and treatment of athletic injuries. The role of the certified athletic trainer involves not only the prevention of athletic injuries but also the recognition and evaluation of athletic injuries when they do occur, along with the rehabilitation and reconditioning of the injured athlete (Arnheim & Prentice, 1997). This professional field continues to grow, and current statistics show that athletic training is ranked as the 16th fastest growing profession (projected growth 2004–2014) among all professions requiring a minimum of a bachelor's degree in the United States.

Athletic trainers must complete an extensive and diverse medical education program that is accredited by the Commission on Accreditation of Athletic Training Education (CAATE), and then pass a national medical board examination administered by the Board of Certification, Inc. (BOC) to practice as a certified athletic trainer (ATC). *Certified athletic trainers* are employed in a wide array of professional settings. These can include working with high school, collegiate, or professional sport teams, recreational sports, the military, industrial settings, clinical settings, or the local YMCA or similar fitness center. The governing body for athletic trainers is the National

Athletic Training Association (NATA). Chapter 7 discusses the ever-growing role of the athletic trainer and the knowledge and skills needed to become certified through the NATA.

Social Science Knowledge

The subdiscipline of **sociology of physical activity** uses a variety of social frameworks to evaluate the role of organized sport and physical activity in today's society. The sport and physical activity patterns of individuals are determined to a great extent by their larger social environment. Numerous social variables such as social stratification, race, gender, ethnicity, and education play a role in understanding sport and physical activity in our society (McElroy, 2002). The *sport sociologist* seeks to understand the potential role of organized sport and physical activity in promoting social change in the area of health and wellness for the betterment of society.

Chapter 8 examines the sociological consequences of both *physical activity* (health-related physical activities) and *sport* (organized, competitive physical activity). Traditional areas in an introductory sport sociology class typically include topics such as sport and social class, sport and social institutions (family, education, corporate sport, religion), professional sports, gender and sport, race/ethnicity in sport, politics in sports, the economics of sport, the Olympic Games, sport and social problems (crime, violence, deviance, drugs), and issues surrounding youth sport programs. Sport sociologists often work in a college or university setting as teachers or researchers, but they also find employment opportunities in professional health care roles, identifying sociological variables related to exercise and sport participation and structuring positive sport and exercise opportunities. Relevant professional organizations include the North American Society for the Sociology of Sport (NASSS), the American Public Health Association (APHA), the American College of Sports Medicine (ACSM), and the International Society for Sociology of Sport (ISSS).

Sport history is another branch of social science that examines how such variables as religion, social attitudes, politics, economics, and tradition have influenced the formation and growth of sport and physical activity. The sport historian views sport and physical activity as both a powerfully divisive and cooperative component of our global society that attracts literally millions of adherents.

Shortly after Bannister ran the first sub-4-minute mile, another runner from Australia, John Landy, bettered his record by running the distance in 3:58. This set up the most famous race in sport history several months later, termed the "Race of the Century" (which was won by Bannister). Many sport historians and sociologists view this as a turning point in sport.

Socially, sports would be viewed increasingly as a professional pursuit, with greater media attention and social significance. Historically, this marked the end of the self-coached athlete and the beginning of the scientific pursuit of athletic excellence.

Chapter 9 examines potential careers for the sport historian, which include work as a college or university professor, archivist in a museum or Hall of Fame, sport broadcaster, or sports writer/editor. The major professional organization for the sport historian is the North American Society for Sports History (NASSH).

THE SCOPE OF EXERCISE SCIENCE

Health Promotion Versus Sport Performance

The work of the exercise scientist can be further divided into two additional categories: *exercise and health promotion* and *enhancing sport performance*. Physiological components of health include variables such as cardiorespiratory endurance, muscular strength and endurance, flexibility, and body composition (Fahey, Insel, & Roth, 2005). Exercise scientists interested in health promotion seek to combine the five bases of knowledge to improve both individual and societal levels of fitness.

Physiologic variables related to sport performance include speed, strength, power, agility, and quickness (Wilmore et al., 2008). Although these are important to performance, they are typically unrelated to health and fitness. Exercise scientists who are interested in improving athletic performance look for ways to utilize information from the five bases of knowledge to assist athletes.

Basic Research Versus Applied Research

One last way to categorize exercise science is by the type of research performed (see Figure 1.2). The primary purpose of research is to gather information and then to make quality decisions based on this new knowledge (Berg & Latin, 2004). **Basic research** attempts to answer a specific research question. Typically, basic research examines a theoretical concept and is not concerned with its immediate application (Berg & Latin, 2004). An example of a basic research problem would be answering the question, "How does anxiety affect sport performance in elite athletes?" To answer this question, the researcher might measure levels of anxiety prior to a series of athletic competitions and then record the athlete's performance for each competition. At the end of the season, the researcher could compare levels of anxiety to good, average, and poor performances and determine at which level of anxiety

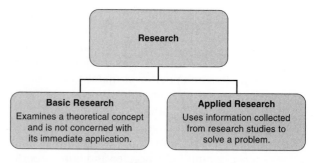

Figure 1.2 Types of research.

an athlete performed optimally. The goal of basic research is to acquire new knowledge and advance the knowledge base of exercise science.

Applied research typically revolves around a specific question with the intention of "applying" the new information to solve a problem (Berg & Latin, 2004). One of the main questions faced by the exercise scientist is how to improve athletic performance. For instance, once the exercise scientist has determined the appropriate level of anxiety for an athlete to achieve optimal performance, the question becomes, "How do we help the athlete attain the appropriate level of anxiety?" Applied research involves working directly with the athlete using techniques or interventions that will raise or lower anxiety to the desired level. Basic research supplies the cornerstone for knowledge in an area, and applied research uses this knowledge in efforts to improve performance.

The Integrative Nature of Exercise Science

In 1954 when Roger Bannister ran 3:59.4 for the mile, he barely trained 30 miles a week. Today it is not uncommon for runners to train as much as 3 times this distance. However, with such increases in training, certain athletes are experiencing a phenomenon known as *staleness*, which leads to a variety of psychobiological problems that can hinder and prevent an athlete from training. As a result, the important question for the exercise scientist becomes, "How much training can an athlete tolerate before she becomes stale and can no longer train?"

Because staleness is characterized by a host of physiological, psychological, neurological, motor behavior, and nutritional changes within the athlete (Raglin & Wilson, 2000), it presents an interdisciplinary problem for the subdisciplines of exercise science. For example, in attempting to identify markers that might predict staleness in athletes, exercise scientists have teamed together to measure physiological (Costill et al., 1988), neuromuscular (Raglin, Koceja, Stager, & Harms, 1996), nutritional (Kuipers & Keizer, 1988), and psychological (O'Connor, Morgan, & Raglin, 1991) changes during intense training. Moreover, the athletic trainer is often the first health professional to notice negative changes in an athlete, such as the weight loss and fatigue that often accompany impending staleness.

The study of staleness represents an important example of the integrative nature of exercise science and how professionals in a variety of subdisciplines have attempted to solve a common research question. Although at present there are no definitive physiological markers that can successfully predict staleness in athletes, exercise scientists continue working to define and predict the occurrence of this psychobiological phenomenon.

BOOK STRUCTURE AND ORGANIZATION

Exploring Exercise Science is organized into seven parts. The first six parts provide an introduction and a comprehensive review of each of the knowledge areas that make up exercise science: physiologic, behavioral, biomechanical, sports medicine, social science. Each chapter provides a history of the subdiscipline illustrating how the specific area of study has evolved. Following this, a discussion of the concepts and knowledge base important to the subdiscipline is presented. Next, each chapter offers an overview of relevant professional organizations within a specific subdiscipline along with the various certifications offered through these bodies. Finally, employment opportunities and future directions within each subdiscipline are presented.

Part 7, Exploring the Context and Future of Exercise Science, provides an overview of issues important to the exercise scientist, including societal health trends (Chapter 10), physical activity epidemiology (Chapter 11), legal considerations in exercise science (Chapter 12), and ethics in exercise science (Chapter 13). Although not often considered true components of exercise science, each of these areas contributes in many important ways to the manner in which the exercise scientist conducts research, makes decisions, and uses research findings to broaden our knowledge of health and wellness. The book concludes with a look into the future. The future trends in exercise science discussed in (Chapter 14) include potential professional opportunities in health and wellness as the field of exercise science continues to grow. Part 7 provides a unique and much needed view of these important areas that shape the work of the exercise scientist.

SUMMARY

Exercise science is a relatively new and fast-growing discipline made up of five integrated bases of knowledge that can be categorized into physiological, behavioral, biomechanical, sports medicine, and social science areas of study. Each of these knowledge bases makes up a subdiscipline of exercise science. Most research questions in exercise science rely on an interdisciplinary approach, so students need a solid foundation in each of these integrated knowledge bases. Researchers in exercise science approach questions from either a basic or applied research perspective. Knowledge gained from new findings in these subdisciplines is used to enhance individual health and fitness levels and to facilitate improved sport performance in athletes.

■ Key Points

- Exercise science consists of the subdisciplines of athletic training, biomechanics, exercise physiology, exercise and sport psychology, sport history, sport nutrition, and sport sociology.
- The subdisciplines of exercise science can be categorized into four integrated bases of knowledge: physiological, behavioral, sports medicine and kinesiology, and social science.
- Exercise scientists typically work in one of two distinct areas of health and fitness: exercise and health promotion or enhancing sport performance.

- Basic research attempts to answer a specific research question, whereas applied research typically involves applying the new information to solve a specific problem.
- The subdisciplines of exercise science form an integrative body of knowledge that allows the exercise scientist to study many different aspects of physical performance.

■ Review Questions

1. Define exercise science as a field of study.
2. How are the subdisciplines of exercise science interrelated?
3. What is the difference between exercise physiology and sport physiology?
4. Explain the difference between a "health promotion" and a "performance enhancement" approach to the study of exercise science.

5. Provide a hypothetical example of a basic research question and explain how that same question would be addressed in applied research.
6. Exercise science is an interdisciplinary approach. Give an example of an interdisciplinary research question that could be studied by three or more subdisciplines in exercise science.

■ References

Arnheim, D. D., & Prentice, W. E. (1997). *Principles of athletic training* (9th ed.). Madison, WI: Brown & Benchmark.

Bascomb. N. (2004). *The perfect mile*. Boston: Houghton Mifflin.

Berg, K. E., & Latin, R. W. (2004). *Essentials of research methods in health, physical education, exercise science, and recreation* (2nd ed.). Philadelphia: Lipppincott Williams & Wilkins.

Costill, D. L., Flynn, M. G., Kirwan, J. P., Houmard, J. A., Mitchell, J. B., Thomas, R., & Park, S. H. (1988). Effects of repeated days of intensified training on muscle glycogen and swimming performance. *Medicine and Science in Sports and Exercise, 20*, 249–254.

Fahey, T. D., Insel, P. M., & Roth, W. T. (2005). *Fit & well* (6th ed.). Boston: McGraw-Hill.

Hall, S. J. (2003). *Basic biomechanics* (4th ed.). Boston: McGraw-Hill.

Kuipers, H., & Keizer, H. A. (1988). Overtraining in elite athletes: Review and directions for the future. *Sports Medicine, 6*, 79–92.

LaGrange, F. (1889). *Physiology of bodily exercise*. London; Kegan Paul International.

McArdle, W. D., Katch, F. I., & Katch, V. L. (2001). *Exercise physiology: Energy, nutrition, and human performance* (5th ed.). Philadelphia: Lippincott Williams & Wilkins.

McElroy, M. (2002). *Resistance to exercise: A social analysis of inactivity*. Champaign, IL: Human Kinetics.

O'Connor, P. J., Morgan, W. P., & Raglin, J. S. (1991). Psychobiological effects of 3 days of increased training in female and male swimmers. *Medicine and Science in Sports and Exercise, 23*, 1055–1061.

Raglin, J. S., Koceja, D. M., Stager, J. M., & Harms, C. A. (1996). Mood, neuromuscular function, and performance during training in female swimmers. *Medicine and Science in Sports and Exercise, 28*, 372–377.

Raglin, J. S., & Wilson, G. S. (2000). Overtraining in athletes. In Y. L. Hanin (Ed.), *Emotions in sport*. Champaign, IL: Human Kinetics.

Robergs, R. A., & Keteyian, S. J. (2003). *Fundamentals of exercise physiology: For fitness, performance and health* (2nd ed.). Boston: McGraw-Hill.

Wilmore, J. H., Costill, D. L., & Kenney, W. L. (2008). *Physiology of sport and exercise* (4th ed.). Champaign, IL: Human Kinetics.

Wuest, D. A., & Bucher, C. A. (2009). *Foundations of physical education, exercise science, and sport* (16th ed.). Boston: McGraw-Hill.

Exploring the Physiologic

Part 2 examines the two cornerstone components of exercise science that make up the physiologic knowledge base of the discipline: exercise physiology and nutrition. Nutrition and exercise physiology are interrelated components because all physical activity begins with metabolic responses. These two chapters show how the two areas contribute to the physiological aspect of exercise participation. Chapter 2 provides an overview of how energy is used for exercise and describes how the various physiological systems of the body (nervous, endocrine, skeletal muscle, cardiovascular, and respiratory) function in response to the demands of exercise participation. Chapter 3 follows with a nutritional look at how the body uses food to create energy and the importance of fluids and electrolytes in exercise performance. Other important areas such as body composition, weight control, the female-athlete triad, and nutritional supplements are also examined. The physiologic knowledge components provide the basic building blocks of exercise science.

CHAPTER 2

Exercise Physiology

Anthony Mahon, PhD, Ball State University
Tonya Skalon, MS, Ball State University

■ Chapter Objectives

After reading this chapter, you should be able to:

1. Define the term *exercise physiology* and relate its significance in the exercise science curriculum.
2. Provide a brief overview of the history of exercise physiology including the key events in the late 1800s and the early 1900s that served as the impetus for the evolution of exercise physiology as an academic discipline.
3. Describe the typical course content taught in most exercise physiology classes.
4. Recognize some of the scientific research journals that publish findings in exercise physiology.
5. Identify the various professional scientific and fitness organizations and the certification programs offered through these organizations.
6. Explain the various career options for students with training in exercise physiology.

■ Key Terms

acute response
adenosine triphosphate
aerobic training
anaerobic training
cardiovascular system
certification

chronic adaptation
endocrine system
energy systems
exercise physiology
Harvard Fatigue Laboratory
hormone

muscle fiber types
nervous system
oxygen uptake
respiratory system

Exercise physiology can be defined by examining the individual definitions of the two words that make up the term. First, *physiology* is the study of human function. Function can be studied from the molecular level to the whole organism level. *Exercise* is a form of physical exertion that can be carefully quantified and results in an improvement in physical fitness (Caspersen, 1989). Quantification usually is in the form of the duration of exercise, the intensity of exercise, type or mode of exercise, and the frequency with which exercise is performed. Although all exercise is a form of physical activity, not all physical activity is considered exercise. The main difference is that exercise is quantifiable with respect to duration, intensity, type, and frequency. This is an important point because, as a field of study, exercise physiology is concerned with understanding the role of exercise in health, fitness, and sport performance. To better understand how exercise affects the body as well as to be able to develop guidelines and recommendations for the appropriate amount of exercise for fitness and performance, it is important to be able to carefully match the amount of exercise performed with a physiological outcome. Thus, **exercise physiology** can be defined as the study of how the body functions during physical exertion that is carefully quantified.

In the exercise science curriculum, exercise physiology is a cornerstone course because most programs of study are designed around the science of fitness assessments and exercise prescription. Therefore, knowledge of the physiological responses to exercise becomes an important aspect of the program of study. Often, exercise physiology is taught as an upper-level course (junior or senior year of study) and is sequenced in a manner that allows the student to take classes in biology, chemistry, anatomy, and physiology prior to enrolling in exercise physiology. Indeed classes in these other areas provide the foundation from which learning and understanding exercise physiology is enhanced.

BRIEF HISTORY OF EXERCISE PHYSIOLOGY

From an academic standpoint, exercise physiology has evolved from a number of different disciplines including anatomy and physiology, biochemistry, biology, and, of course, physical education. The roots in anatomy and physiology can be traced to the fact that in exercise physiology the function of the body is being studied. A strong background in basic anatomy and physiology prepares the student to understand how the function is affected during a single bout of exercise, referred to as an **acute response,** as well as how it changes in response to regularly performed exercise, which is referred to as a **chronic adaptation**

(Wilmore, Costill, & Kenney, 2008). The biology influence stems from the realization that exercise physiology is the study of how a living system responds to the physiological stress imposed by exercise. Biochemical aspects are apparent in the intricate chemical pathways that regulate cell function. The events involving the use of oxygen and nutrients in the production of cellular energy are an excellent example of the biochemical influence in exercise physiology.

It is difficult to precisely define the birth of exercise physiology, but one important event in the evolution of the discipline was Antoine Lavoisier's discovery in the late 1700s that **oxygen uptake** increased with physical exertion (McArdle, Katch, & Katch, 2007). In the mid- to late-1800s emphasis was placed on the development of physical fitness for healthy and productive living (deVries, 2000; Powers & Howley, 2007). At about the same time, one of the first textbooks of exercise physiology, *The Physiology of Bodily Exercise* by Fernand LaGrange, was published (Wilmore et al., 2008).

Two other important events in the evolution of exercise physiology also occurred during this time period. In 1879 Dudley Sargent, a Yale-educated MD, developed a physical fitness program at Harvard University (deVreis, 2000). This program focused on developing physical fitness programs on an individual basis (Powers & Howley, 2007), a practice that is very much in place today. In 1891 an exercise physiology laboratory was created in the Department of Anatomy, Physiology, and Physical Training at Harvard under the leadership of George Fitz, MD. Fitz taught courses in exercise physiology, directed the research laboratory, and carried out his research program. The combination of lecture and laboratory classes used by Fitz is a model that continues today (McArdle et al., 2007).

The transition from the 19th to the 20th century brought more knowledge in the field of exercise physiology. One important discovery very early in the 20th century was that muscle activity is powered by carbohydrates and not heat as previously believed. The basis for this conclusion was evidence that lactic acid, which is formed in the breakdown of carbohydrates for energy, accumulated in fatigued muscles (Wilmore et al., 2008). Many of the contributions to the field of exercise physiology in the early 1900s can be traced to Europe. Among the prominent researchers in the field during this time were Danish physiologist August Krogh, who studied muscle activity and blood flow (Powers & Howley, 2007) and was awarded the Nobel Prize in physiology/medicine for 1920 (deVries, 2000), and Archibald Vivian (A. V.) Hill, a British physiologist and fellow Nobel Prize recipient in the 1920s who was instrumental in studying muscle force at different lengths and different movement speeds (deVries, 2000). He also was a pioneer in studying oxygen uptake (VO_2) responses during and after exercise in runners (Wilmore et al., 2008). Other notable European physiologists included John Haldane, who was influential in the development of a respiratory gas analyzer and studied the influence of carbon dioxide on the regulation of breathing, and Otto Meyerhof, a German physiologist who shared the Nobel Prize with Hill and conducted studies on energy metabolism (deVries, 2000; Powers & Howley, 2007; Wilmore et al., 2008).

Although exercise physiology emerged prior to 1900 in the United States, the field did not begin to flourish until the late 1920s. The development was due largely to the scientific contributions of the **Harvard Fatigue Laboratory**, which opened in 1927. David B. (D. B.) Dill, a biochemist from Stanford, was the director of the laboratory (Dill, 1985). Initially, the laboratory studied the physiological, psychological, and sociological factors associated with manual labor—the form of work that predominated in the United States at that time (Tipton, 1998). The research conducted at the Harvard Fatigue Laboratory is legendary and covered a variety of topics including metabolic responses to exercise, environmental stress, aging-induced changes in exercise responses, and blood-gas and acid-base chemistry (Powers & Howley, 2007). In existence for only 20 years, research at the Harvard Fatigue Laboratory resulted in more than 300 scientific publications, spawned the development of young scientists who went on become prominent researchers in exercise physiology, and provided an opportunity for collaboration with foreign scholars (McArdle et al., 2007; Wilber, 1985). After leaving Harvard, Dill carried on his research at several other institutions and, amazingly, continued to be a prolific researcher into his 90s (Wilber, 1985).

At about the same time the Harvard Fatigue Laboratory was coming into existence, a number of prominent European researchers, including Erik Howhu-Christensen, Ehrling Asmussen, and Marius Nielsen, began to make an impact on the field. Christensen was one of the first researchers to examine fuel use patterns during exercise and went on to become a faculty member in physiology at the Gymnastik-och Idrottshogskolan in Stockholm. Christensen mentored Per-Olof Astrand, who went on to write one of the most recognized textbooks in exercise physiology, *The Textbook of Work Physiology*, and whose name is attached to a popular submaximal exercise test known as the Astrand-Rhyming Submaximal Exercise Test. Christensen also mentored Bengt Saltin, one of leading contemporary exercise physiologists. Asmussen and Nielsen joined the faculty at the University of Copenhagen. Asmussen's contributions included work in the area of exercise and muscle function, and Nielsen studied temperature regulation during exercise in hot and cold temperatures (Wilmore et al., 2008).

In the 1950s two important events further fueled the evolution of exercise physiology. First, the American College of Sports Medicine (ACSM) came into existence in 1954 and held its first scientific meeting (under the name of Federation of Sports Medicine), and in 1955 the organization officially adopted its current name (ACSM) and became incorporated. At its inception, the goal of the ACSM founders was to expand the knowledge of the exercise responses in healthy individuals and in highly trained athletes (Berryman, 2004).

A second major event in the 1950s was the evidence obtained from Korean War casualties that young adult males displayed evidence of atherosclerosis and coronary artery disease. Prior to this time, these cardiovascular problems were viewed as maladies of aging, but this information provided evidence that the roots of cardiovascular disease begin to develop very early in life (Powers & Howley, 2007). Moreover, exercise is now recognized as an important component in lowering one's risk for coronary artery disease.

Today there are many exercise physiology laboratories around the United States and worldwide. The research being conducted in these laboratories ranges from the study of cell function at the molecular level to whole body responses and how these responses, in turn, are associated with health and human performance. Many of the laboratories in operation today exist in part because of the pioneering research conducted years ago and the subsequent establishment of exercise physiology as a recognized academic discipline.

COURSE CONTENT

Most courses in exercise physiology model the content around the effects of exercise on the various physiological systems in the body:

- Energy
- Nervous
- Endocrine
- Skeletal muscle
- Cardiovascular
- Respiratory

Other topics usually covered in an exercise physiology class include temperature regulation, the effects of altitude on physiological responses during exercise, body composition, the exercise response in unique populations, fitness assessment techniques, principles of exercise training and prescription, and ergogenic and nutritional strategies to enhance performance.

Typically, exercise responses that are described and explained within these different content areas include a description of the acute response to a single bout of exercise and the chronic adaptations that occur when exercise is performed on a regular basis. A simple example of an acute response to exercise is the increase in heart rate and breathing rate that occur when one goes from rest to exercise. The elevated heart rate and breathing rate is a temporary change in physiological function associated with the stress brought on by exercise; it is short lived and essentially restricted to the duration of the exercise, and perhaps a short time after (Wilmore et al., 2008). In contrast, a chronic adaptation is defined as a change in structure or function that results from regular bouts of exercise. An example of a chronic adaptation is the reduction in resting heart rate that accompanies endurance training. Over time, endurance training will lower resting heart rate in part because of changes in the way the nervous system regulates heart rate (Wilmore et al., 2008).

Most textbooks organize a portion of their content around the physiological effects of exercise in the different systems in the body. In the subsequent paragraphs a brief overview of the content that is usually covered in these areas is presented.

Energy Systems

Energy required for exercise and activity is derived from the breakdown of stored resources (Gollnick, 1988), as very little usable energy is stored. The stored resources are comprised principally of fat and carbohydrates; protein is not a primary energy source. To access the energy found in the stored nutrients, a series of chemical reactions transfer this potential energy into the formation of **adenosine triphosphate** (ATP), the body's usable form of energy. Interestingly, almost as fast as ATP is produced, it is degraded to adenosine diphosphate (ADP) and inorganic phosphate (Pi), a process that liberates energy for cellular work and heat (Gollnick, 1988). Muscle cells use three different **energy systems** to make ATP—phosphagen, glycolytic, and oxidative pathways.

Two of the pathways (phosphagen and glycolytic) are anaerobic; that is, they do not require oxygen. In the phosphagen pathway, a phosphate molecule is transferred to ADP to make ATP. The brevity of the phosphagen pathway allows ATP to be produced quickly; however, phosphocreatine stores are limited and can be depleted in less than 30 seconds (Houston, 2001). Glycolysis requires more steps to produce ATP and involves the breakdown of glucose (a simple form of carbohydrate) to produce ATP (Houston, 2001). Glucose from the blood or glucose liberated from stored glycogen in the muscle can enter the glycolytic pathway. Glycolysis involves a series of chemical reactions that results in the formation of ATP and pyruvate. If pyruvate does not enter the mitochondria,

it is converted to lactate in the final step of glycolysis. Because of the anaerobic nature of the glycolytic pathway, it is not proficient in maintaining energy production during prolonged exercise (Gollnick, 1988; Houston, 2001).

A third energy pathway in skeletal muscle is the oxidative pathway. Unlike the phosphagen and glycolytic pathways, which take place in the cell's cytoplasm, oxidation occurs in the mitochondria and requires oxygen (Houston, 2001). Glucose, derived from carbohydrates, and fatty acids, derived from the breakdown of stored fat, can be oxidized. The oxidation of glucose begins with the entry of pyruvate, from glycolysis, into the mitochondria where it subsequently oxidized in the Krebs cycle; the electron transport chain completes the process of oxidation by producing ATP. Fatty acids undergo a similar fate in the production of ATP from this source. Muscle cells with a high oxidative ability have good endurance (Lieber, 2002).

IMPACT OF EXERCISE TRAINING Both aerobic (endurance) training and anaerobic (sprint) training enhance the specific energy pathways in the muscle. **Anaerobic training** increases the cell's ability to produce energy from the phosphagen and glycolytic pathways (Abernethy, Thayer, & Taylor, 1990). **Aerobic training** increases the ability to synthesize ATP via oxidation. In fact, the aerobic training adaptations in the oxidative capacity may be the single most important determinant of improved endurance with this type of training (Holloszy & Coyle, 1984). In addition, aerobic training increases muscle glycogen concentration, further enhancing the ability of the muscle to resist fatigue during prolonged exercise such as marathon running (Wilmore et al., 2008).

Nervous System

The **nervous system** is a primary control system for physiological function and is comprised of the brain, the spinal cord, and all the peripheral nerves. The brain and spinal cord are collectively referred to as the *central nervous system*. Key parts of the brain associated with movement include the motor and sensory cortexes, the hypothalamus, the cerebellum, and the brain stem. The peripheral nervous system includes all the neurons that transmit information to (sensory branch) and from (motor branch) the spinal cord. Sensory information that is consciously sensed such as light, taste, touch, and sound and voluntary motor transmission occur via somatic nerves (nerves regulating voluntary functions). Skeletal muscles are under the control of the somatic nerves. In contrast, sensory input and motor output that is not consciously controlled, such as pressure and chemical changes in the blood, occur via the autonomic nerves (Wilmore et al., 2008). The heart, airways in the lung, blood vessels, and the organs of digestion are under the control of autonomic nerves (Tortora & Grabowski, 2003).

Autonomic nerves can be subdivided into a parasympathetic and sympathetic branch. *Parasympathetic nerves* tend to dominate the degree of autonomic regulation at rest, whereas *sympathetic nerves* tend to be activated during stress such as exercise (Tortora & Grabowski, 2003). An example of autonomic function is illustrated by what happens to heart rate when one goes from rest to exercise. At rest the parasympathetic effect keeps the heart rate low; however, as exercise intensity increases, the rise in heart rate is mediated by parasympathetic withdrawal and an increase in sympathetic activity (Rowell, 1993).

IMPACT OF EXERCISE TRAINING Exercise training can alter nervous system function with respect to both the somatic and autonomic nerves. For instance, strength training results not only in adaptations in the skeletal muscles that lead to an increase in strength but also in the manner in which the nervous system activates the muscle fibers (Lieber, 2002; Sale, 1988). Endurance training has been shown to reduce the degree of sympathetic activation at a submaximal level of exercise because this type of training reduces the overall stress on the body at a given level of exercise (Clausen, 1977).

Endocrine System

The **endocrine system** is another control system in the body and is comprised of the hormones and all the glands in the body that secrete hormones. This system works in tandem with the nervous system to regulate physiological function, although the nervous system initiates changes in physiological function within seconds whereas the endocrine system is relatively slow acting (minutes to days). The glands that make up the endocrine system secrete chemicals into the blood called **hormones** (Tortora & Grabowski, 2003). All hormones travel through circulation to get to their target organ. Hormones affect cells by binding to receptors and initiating a series of events inside the cell (Bunt, 1986). Broadly speaking, hormones can be categorized as fat or water soluble. *Fat-soluble hormones* cross the cell membrane and bind to an intracellular receptor to carry out its effect on a cell, whereas *water-soluble hormones* bind to a surface receptor. The hormone–receptor combination then initiates a series of intracellular events compatible with the hormone's effect on the cell (Totora & Grabowski, 2003).

A thorough discussion of all the endocrine glands and hormones is beyond the scope of this chapter; however, several glands directly affect physiological responses to exercise and are briefly discussed here. Exercise activates the pituitary gland to secrete growth hormone (GH; anterior pituitary) and antidiuretic hormone (ADH; posterior pituitary). GH, among many of its effects, influences fuel use during exercise, and ADH increases water conservation during exercise (Bunt, 1986; Kjaer, 1992).

Another gland that is important to physiological function during exercise is the adrenal gland. The adrenal gland is comprised of the cortex, which secretes cortisol and alodosterone, and the medulla, which secretes epinephrine (adrenaline) and norepinephrine (noradrenaline). Cortisol, like GH, affects fuel use during exercise, and aldosterone stimulates the reabsorption of sodium and water from the kidney (Bunt, 1986). The adrenal medulla is activated by the sympathetic nervous system and amplifies the sympathetic response to stress (Kjaer, 1992).

The pancreas secretes the hormones insulin and glucagon. Insulin is released in response to an increase in blood glucose level. This occurs after a meal, especially one high in carbohydrates. In contrast, exercise causes insulin levels to decline. A decrease in blood glucose level, which occurs during fasting or prolonged exercise, stimulates the release of glucagon, which then increases the amount of glucose formed and released by the liver into circulation (Bunt, 1986; Kjaer, 1992). Many other important hormones not described in this section play important roles during exercise; these hormones are usually covered in more detail in physiology and exercise physiology courses.

IMPACT OF EXERCISE TRAINING Exercise training can have an impact on the body's hormonal responses. Endurance training reduces the release of epinephrine and norepinephrine during submaximal exercise. This adaptation is consistent with the notion that in the trained state a given exercise workload is less stressful (Kjaer, 1992). Insulin levels are usually higher during exercise when it is performed in the trained state (Wilmore & Costill, 2004). Resistance training may influence the body's response to the hormones testosterone, insulinlike growth factor-I, and cortisol. These responses are related to the increase in muscle mass that accompanies this type of training (Hakkinen & Pakarinen, 1995; Kraemer, 1988).

Skeletal Muscle System

Skeletal muscle mass comprises approximately 40% of total body mass (weight) and, in concert with the nervous system, generates movement. Although whole muscle generates the movement, the functional unit of the muscle is at the muscle fiber or muscle cell level. A single muscle fiber is comprised of repeating units called sarcomeres. Within the sarcomeres are the contractile elements actin and myosin. In response to neural stimulation, the myosin attaches to the actin and pulls the actin toward the center of the sarcomere. As

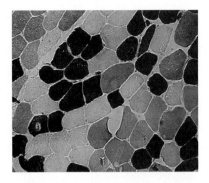

Figure 2.1 Cross-Sectional View of Muscle Fibers Stained for Fiber Type (Type I are black: Type IIa are white; and Type IIb are gray).

Photo courtesy of Dr. David L. Costill, Human Performance Laboratory Ball State University.

this is repeated along the length of a given muscle fiber, the fiber shortens and generates force (Leiber, 2002).

Human skeletal muscle is comprised of three different **muscle fiber types:** slow twitch, Type I; fast twitch a, Type IIa; and fast twitch b, Type IIb (see Figure 2.1). The slow twitch versus fast twitch terminology is based on the observation that Type I muscle fibers shorten more slowly in response to a single stimulus—referred to as a twitch response—than Type IIa or Type IIb fibers; hence the Type I and Type IIa/Type IIb terminology (Saltin & Gollnick, 1983). The various names that have been given to the different muscle fiber types are outlined in Table 2.1.

Functionally, Type I fibers have good endurance because of their high reliance on oxidative metabolism to produce ATP. Type IIa fibers have a combination of good endurance and good power; Type IIb fibers are the most powerful fibers but have very poor endurance (Houston, 2001; Saltin & Gollnick, 1983).

Muscle fiber types are organized into motor units. Motor units are comprised of a single motor neuron and all the muscle fibers that are attached. A unique feature of motor units is that the muscle fibers within a given motor unit are comprised of the same fiber type. When a particular motor neuron is activated, all its muscle fibers will be activated in a process referred to as excitation-contraction coupling (Lieber, 2002). This term is based on the fact that the motor neuron activates (excitation) the muscle fibers, which then shorten (contraction) and generate force and movement. Motor units made of up of Type I fibers tend to be activated at the lowest levels of force and are used during low-intensity exercise like jogging or running and for carrying out many daily activities. Type IIa and Type IIb fibers usually are part of larger motor units (more muscle fibers make up large motor units compared to small motor units). These motor units and muscle fibers are activated at levels of force in the moderate to high range (Saltin & Gollnick, 1983).

IMPACT OF EXERCISE TRAINING Exercise training can have a big impact on skeletal muscle function. Aerobic training will increase the endurance capacity of all three fiber types by virtue of the effect this type of training has on the oxidative energy system (Abernethy et al., 1990; Hawley, 2002; Holloszy & Coyle, 1984). Strength training, on the other hand, usually does not enhance the energetic profile of the muscle fiber but will result in an increase in strength, which is in part attributed to an increase in muscle mass (Sale, 1988; Tesch, 1988), although adaptations in the nervous system (previously described) also make an important contribution to the overall increase in muscle strength (Sale, 1988).

Cardiovascular System

The **cardiovascular system** consists of the heart, blood vessels, and blood. The principle function of this system is to deliver oxygen and nutrients to tissues and carry away carbon dioxide and other substances from the tissues. Exercise will affect each component of the cardiovascular system. Heart rate (HR) and stroke volume (SV) increase from rest to exercise. SV is the amount of blood pumped out of the heart on each beat. The product of HR and SV is the cardiac output (Q); thus exercise increases Q. The increase in Q and HR is directly proportional to the exercise intensity (Bevegard & Shepherd, 1967). These changes increase blood flow throughout the body, but a very high percentage of the blood flow is directed to the exercising muscle (Green, O'Driscoll, Blanksby, & Taylor, 1996).

TABLE 2.1   Skeletal Muscle Fiber Type Classification Schemes

Twitch Term	Energetic Term	Color Term	Generic Term
Slow twitch (ST)	Slow, oxidative (SO)	Red	Type I
Fast twitch a (FTa)	Fast, oxidative, glycolytic (FOG)	Intermediate	Type IIa
Fast twitch b (Type FTb)	Fast glycolytic (FG)	White	Type IIb

Chapter Two Exercise Physiology   **17**

Changes in the blood vessels also have a dramatic effect on blood flow patterns. Arterial blood vessels in the viscera (gut area) will vasoconstrict; that is, they will narrow, reducing blood flow to this area of the body. In contrast, the blood vessels leading to exercising muscle will vasodilate, or enlarge, allowing for more blood and oxygen to be directed to this part of the body (Shepherd & Vanhoutte, 1979). The increase in Q increases blood pressure, which is the primary driving force moving blood through circulation.

Blood is comprised of plasma (the watery part of the blood and cells) and the solid component in the blood, and is affected by exercise. Approximately 55 to 60% of the blood is plasma, and the remaining 40 to 45% is cells with nearly all the cellular component being comprised of red blood cells. The red blood cells contain hemoglobin, which is the oxygen carrying compound in the cell. When an individual starts to exercise, plasma volume declines, and the percentage of red blood cells (but not the amount) increases. The reduction in plasma volume is mostly attributed to an increase in blood pressure, which serves to push water through the capillary vessels. As exercise continues, an increase in sweat rate can cause the plasma volume to decline further (Costill & Fink, 1974).

IMPACT OF EXERCISE TRAINING The long-term effects of exercise training, specifically aerobic training, have a profound effect on the cardiovascular system. Heart size increases, making it a bigger and stronger pump (Wilmore et al., 2008). Blood volume expands due to increases in plasma and red blood cell volumes (Sawka, Convertino, Eichner, Schneider, & Young, 2000). Capillaries surrounding the muscles that were used in training increase in number (Saltin & Gollnick, 1983). At a submaximal level of exercise, HR decreases and SV increases compared to the responses to the same level of exercise in the untrained state. The changes in HR and SV are reciprocal, which results in no change in submaximal Q (Wilmore et al., 2008). At maximal exercise, HR is either unchanged or decreases slightly with aerobic training (Zavorsky, 2000); however, SV increases as does Q. The increase in SV and Q increases muscle blood flow at maximal exercise and may be one of the most important determinants of the increase in maximal oxygen uptake, VO_2max (Rowell, 1986).

Respiratory System

The **respiratory system** is comprised of the lungs and the airways that conduct air flow into the lungs. Two primary functions of the lungs are ventilation and diffusion. *Ventilation* is the process of drawing air into the lungs, and *diffusion* is the process whereby oxygen and carbon dioxide are exchanged between the blood and the alveoli, the inner-most region of the lungs (West, 1985). Exercise induces changes in respiratory function to increase the delivery of oxygen to the lungs and the removal of carbon dioxide from the body. Both tidal volume, the amount of air in one breath, and respiratory rate increase during exercise and serve to increase ventilation. Airways that conduct air in and out of the lungs dilate, which reduces the resistance to air flow. In addition, more airways open up, allowing air to flow to a larger fraction of the lungs. Collectively, these changes increase ventilation (West, 1985).

Diffusion of gases occurs between the alveoli, or air sacks in the lung, and the capillary blood vessels that envelope the alveoli. Blood entering these capillaries is low in oxygen because the oxygen was extracted by cells in the body, whereas the blood entering these capillaries is high in carbon dioxide, a by-product of energy metabolism. As the blood passes through the capillaries, oxygen diffuses into the blood and binds to hemoglobin. At the same time, carbon dioxide is diffusing from the blood into the alveoli and is eventually eliminated in the expired air sample. The diffusion of gases is possible because of pressure differences between the capillary and the alveoli. Alveolar air has a high oxygen pressure and low carbon dioxide pressure. Capillary blood has a low oxygen pressure and high carbon dioxide pressure. Each gas moves from the area of high pressure to the area of low pressure. Under normal conditions, blood leaving the pulmonary capillary is fully loaded with oxygen. This oxygen-rich blood is then circulated to the cells throughout the body to deliver oxygen and carry away carbon dioxide. The transfer of the gases between the blood and cell is similar to what happens in the lung—only in a reverse direction. Oxygen diffuses out of the blood and into the cell, and carbon dioxide diffuses out of the cell and into the blood (Wilmore et al., 2008).

IMPACT OF EXERCISE TRAINING Aerobic training increases the maximal capacity of the lungs to breathe in air (Wilmore et al., 2008). This adaptation is mediated in part by an increase in the capacity for the respiratory muscles to elevate the tidal volume and the respiratory rate (Powers, Coombs, & Demirel, 1997) and not due to an increase in lung size (Wilmore et al., 2008). The rate of oxygen diffusion out of the lungs and into the blood is enhanced by endurance training. This allows the respiratory system to keep pace with the increased capacity of the cardiovascular system at this level of exercise (Wilmore et al., 2008).

Other Topics

A variety of other topics often are included in most exercise physiology textbooks. These topics include

TABLE 2.2 Current Exercise Physiology Textbooks

Title	Authors	Edition/Year	Publisher
Clinical Exercise Physiology	LeMura & von Duvillard	1st ed./2004	Lippincott Williams and Wilkins
Exercise Physiology: Energy, Nutrition and Human Performance	McArdle, Katch, & Katch	6th ed./2007	Lippincott Williams and Wilkins
Exercise Physiology: Exercise. Performance and Clinical Application	Robergs & Roberts	1st ed./1997	Mosby-Year Book
Exercise Physiology for Health, Fitness and Performance	Plowman & Smith	2nd ed./2003	Benjamin Cummings
Exercise Physiology: Human Bioenergetics and Its Application	Brooks, White, & Baldwin	4th ed./2005	McGraw-Hill
Exercise Physiology: Theory and Application to Fitness and Performance	Powers & Howley	6th ed./2007	McGraw-Hill
Physiology of Sport and Exercise	Wilmore, Costill, & Kenney	4th ed./2008	Human Kinetics

nutritional considerations for health and performance, body composition assessment techniques, physiological responses to environmental stress (heat, cold, altitude, microgravity, and underwater), exercise testing protocols and prescription models, and exercise responses in special populations (older adults, children, people with disabilities, and pregnancy). A partial list of current textbooks on exercise physiology is displayed in Table 2.2. It is important to appreciate that the knowledge synthesized in these textbooks is the result of many years of research, research that was subjected to a rigorous review process and originally published in scientific journals. A list of selected journals that publish exercise physiology research is presented at the end of the chapter. Current research topics in exercise physiology include exercise and aging, pediatric exercise responses, the effects of microgravity (spaceflight) on muscle, sports training and performance, exercise effects on risk factors for cardiovascular disease and metabolic disorders such as Type II diabetes, physical activity assessment and determination of healthful amounts, exercise and bone health, genetic factors affecting exercise training adaptations, and how environmental stresses such as heat, cold, and altitude exposure affect performance.

PROFESSIONAL ORGANIZATIONS AND CERTIFICATIONS

Numerous exercise physiology organizations are open for student membership. Often, however, students are unaware of the existence of these organizations and how membership fits in with professional development. Membership benefits usually include access to journals and other publications in the field, discounted fees to attend meetings and workshops, access to professional employment resources and graduate school opportunities, and the occasion to network with like-minded professionals. Moreover, some organizations have certification programs that complement the student's academic training. **Certification** and education guide employers in identifying individuals who are competent and can demonstrate knowledge and skills within exercise physiology. Due to the increasing awareness of health, exercise, and fitness, the need for competent individuals in exercise physiology has grown. The field of health and fitness is flooded with individuals who "like to exercise"; however, many of these individuals lack the knowledge and skills to appropriately assess and prescribe exercise programs. Many employers seek future employees who already possess certification and are members of professional organizations.

Before choosing a certification, an individual should look at the criteria needed: education level, organization's status, career goals, and cost, which should not be the only factor but may play a role on the deciding factor. Realize also that one certification may be more appropriate than another. In the following section, selected professional scientific organizations, including those with certification programs, and several professional fitness organizations that have certification programs are highlighted. A list of these organizations and their Web sites can be found at the end of the chapter.

Scientific Organizations With Certification Programs

AMERICAN COLLEGE OF SPORTS MEDICINE (ACSM)

The ACSM, formerly known as the Federation of Sports Medicine, was founded in the spring of 1954 in New York City during the American Association for Health, Physical Education, and Recreation (AAHPER) meeting. In January 1955 the name American College of Sports Medicine was adopted and in 1961 the first permanent office was established in Philadelphia and subsequently moved to the University of Wisconsin. Today, ACSM has its national headquarters in Indianapolis (Berryman, 2004). The mission statement can be found at their Web site, **www.acsm.org.**

ACSM has more than 20,000 international, national, and regional members. Members are from various specialties including medical doctors, allied health professionals, fitness professionals, exercise physiologists, biomechanists, sport psychologists, and athletic trainers. ACSM provides educational opportunities to its members through an annual national conference, regional conferences, and their official journals, *Medicine and Science in Sports and Exercise*, monthly, and *Exercise and Sport Sciences Reviews*, quarterly. Both journals provide the latest research in exercise science. For health and fitness professionals, ACSM publishes a third journal, *Health & Fitness Journal*, relaying the most recent practical information from fitness, exercise, and nutrition to management and self-marketing (Robinson, 2004). ACSM has a student membership category that comes with a discounted membership fee to the organization (ACSM, 2008).

ACSM CERTIFICATIONS

ACSM currently provides four certifications for members and nonmembers for a 3-year period (ACSM, 2005). The certifications are split into two tracks. The health fitness track is geared to work with apparently healthy people, and the clinical track is aimed at professionals working in the rehabilitative setting with individuals who are at increased or high risk for disease. Each track has two different certification programs.

The ACSM Certified Personal Trainer (cPT) and the ACSM Certified Health Fitness Specialist (HFS) are two certifications in health fitness. In the clinical track certification options are the ACSM Certified Clinical Exercise Specialist (CES) and the ACSM Registered Clinical Exercise Physiologist (RCEP; ACSM, 2005). All four certification examinations are computer based and can be taken throughout the United States and world with instantaneous results (ACSM, 2006a). All certification programs require recertification through continuing education credits. Some ways of obtaining credits include taking self-tests provided by ACSM, attending the national and regional meetings, participating in workshops, and taking or teaching a class at an accredited college or university (ACSM, 2008).

Certified Personal Trainer: The cPT is designed for professionals who work one-on-one with healthy individuals or with individuals who have medical clearance to exercise. The cPT certification is designed for individuals who are responsible for delivering safe and effective methods of training, and they must be knowledgeable in a variety of areas related to fitness training. Unlike other ACSM certifications, the cPT does not have an educational degree requirement. It is designed for individuals who have the knowledge, skills, and experience. CPR certification is required (ACSM, 2005).

The examination content includes exercise physiology and related exercise science; exercise prescription and programming; human behavior; health appraisal and fitness/exercise testing; safety, injury prevention, and emergency procedures; nutrition and weight management; program administration, quality assurance, and outcome assessment; and clinical and medical considerations (ACSM, 2006a).

Certified Health Fitness Specialist: The HFS certification focuses on the apparently healthy population. It is designed for persons in the health fitness field such as personal training or fitness consulting. Individuals with this certification assess, design, and implement group exercise and fitness programs. Eligibility for the HFS certification examination includes an associate's or bachelor's degree in a health-related field such as, but not limited to, exercise science, kinesiology, physical and occupational therapy, human performance, biology, physical education, athletic training, or nutrition from an accredited college or university, or be in the last semester of their senior year. CPR certification also is required.

The 10 content areas on the examination are exercise physiology and related exercise science; exercise prescription and programming; human behavior; health appraisal and fitness testing; safety, injury prevention, and emergency procedures; nutrition and weight management; program administration, quality assurance, and outcome assessment; risk factors and pathophysiology; electrocardiography and diagnostic

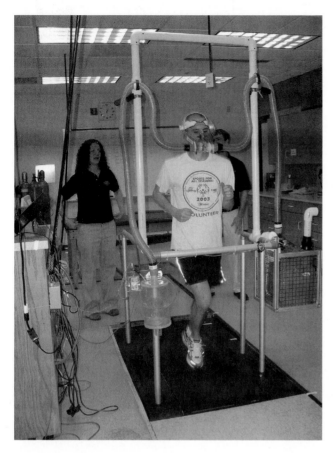

A subject performing a graded exercise test on the treadmill for the determination of VO$_2$max.

techniques; and medical and surgical management (ACSM, 2006b).

Certified Clinical Exercise Specialist: The CES certification is for health care professionals working with cardiovascular, pulmonary, and metabolic rehabilitation programs, exercise testing, physician offices, and medically based fitness facilities. CES certified individuals provide exercise consulting for research and public health, in nonclinical and clinical settings. To qualify for CES certification, candidates must hold a bachelor's degree in an allied health field from an accredited college or university or be in their last semester of study and hold a current CPR certification. In addition to this, candidates need a minimum of 600 hours of practical experience in areas such as cardiopulmonary rehabilitation, exercise testing and prescription, electrocardiography, patient education and counseling, cardiopulmonary and metabolic disease management, and emergency management (ACSM, 2006b). Students taking the CES certification examination need to be knowledgeable in the same 10 content areas of the Certified HFS examination and one additional content area, patient management and medications (ACSM, 2006b).

Registered Clinical Exercise Physiologist: The RCEP certification is for individuals who work in clinical settings where exercise and physical activity have revealed therapeutic or functional benefits to individuals who have cardiovascular, pulmonary, metabolic, orthopedic, immunological, inflammatory, or neuromuscular diseases and conditions. The RCEP works with the high-risk group but also teaches exercise and fitness in special populations such as geriatrics, pediatrics, and obstetrics as well as works in preventive health and fitness. The main objectives of an RCEP include exercise evaluations and prescriptions, exercise supervision, exercise education, and outcome evaluations. Requirements to take the RCEP are more advanced than the cPT, Certified HFS, or Certified CES. Similar to the Certified HFS and Certified CES, all candidates must be CPR certified; however, the educational level is a master's degree in exercise physiology or a related field. In addition, RCEP candidates must either have ES certification or have acquired 600 hours of clinical experience (ACSM, 2006b, 2008). The RCEP examination includes many of the same content areas as the cPT, Certified HFS, and Certified CES (ACSM, 2006b).

NATIONAL STRENGTH AND CONDITIONING ASSOCIATION (NSCA) What is now known as the National Strength and Conditioning Association (NSCA) was organized in 1978 as the National Strength Coaches Association. Due to the growing number of members outside the coaching arena, the NSCA name was adopted in 1981. Today, the nearly 30,000 members include strength coaches, sport coaches, sport scientists, researchers, educators, sport medicine professionals (physicians and athletic trainers), allied health professionals (physical therapists), students in training, business owners, exercise instructors, and personal trainers. NSCA has four publications: *Strength and Conditioning Journal, Journal of Strength and Conditioning Research,* the NSCA *Bulletin,* and NSCA's *Performance Training Journal.* These resources provide the latest research and techniques on strength and conditioning. In addition, NSCA holds an annual scientific conference along with a Sport Specific Training Conference, Personal Trainer's Conference, and NSCS Performance Symposia series. The NSCA's National Office is in Colorado Springs, CO. NSCA also has a student membership category (NSCA, 2008). See Box 2.1 for the NSCA mission statement.

EXPLORE MORE **BOX 2.1**

NSCA Mission Statement

"As the worldwide authority on strength and conditioning, we support and disseminate research-based knowledge and its practical application, to improve athletic performance and fitness" (NSCA, 2008).

NSCA CERTIFICATIONS NSCA certifications are endorsed by the National Commission for Certifying Agencies (NCCA), a nongovernmental body that endorses certifying organizations. To meet NCCA criteria for accreditation, NSCA developed the NSCA Certification Commission (NSCA-CC) and offers two certifications. These certifications are the Certified Strength and Conditioning Specialist (CSCS) and the NSCA-Certified Personal Trainer (NSCA-CPT). Recertification is completed on 3-year cycles, and all certified individuals have the same recertification date. Continuing education units are required for both certifications (NSCA, 2008).

Certified Strength and Conditioning Specialist: The CSCS was created in 1985 and is designed to certify that individuals are capable of developing sport-specific strength and conditioning programs for athletes. The CSCS individual is able to plan and implement a training program that is both safe and effective and is knowledgeable about sports injuries and basic nutrition. The requirements for taking the examination include a bachelor's degree, senior-level status at an accredited college or university, or a degree in chiropractic medicine and maintain current CPR and AED certification (NSCA, 2007). This is a written examination and evaluates knowledge in two primary content areas. The first part tests scientific foundations with respect to knowledge in exercise science and nutrition. The second part focuses on practice and includes content regarding training program design, evaluation of facilities, lifting and other training techniques, and strength and conditioning assessment methods (NSCA, 2007).

Certified Personal Trainer: The CPT was developed in 1993 and is for individual work with clients. Individuals who have this certification work in a variety of settings such as YMCAs, fitness clubs, personal training studios, schools, and clients' homes. They are professionals who put a personal touch to assessing, motivating, educating, and training healthy, elderly, and obese clients for their specific needs. Prerequisites for taking the certification test include being 18 years of age with a high school diploma or equivalent and currently CPR certified. Secondary education is not required; however, knowledge in anatomy, exercise physiology, biomechanics, training adaptations, program design, and special populations is necessary. The examination format is similar to the CSCS examination format (NSCA, 2007).

AMERICAN SOCIETY OF EXERCISE PHYSIOLOGY (ASEP) ASEP was founded in 1997 for exercise physiologists to discuss important topics in the field, disseminate research findings, and provide a platform for collaboration. In addition to a national organization, ASEP maintains regional and state affiliates. Research by ASEP members is presented at an annual meeting and is published in two journals and a newsletter: The *Journal of Exercise Physiology* (online) is a peer-reviewed journal that publishes research findings; the *Professionalization of Exercise Physiology* (online) publishes aspects related to professional development; and the ASEP *Newsletter* (ASEP, 2008).

The membership of ASEP is relatively small compared to other organizations. However, ASEP is specifically for exercise physiologists who have a minimum of a bachelor's degree in exercise physiology. Individuals who do not hold a bachelor's degree in exercise physiology but actively engage in the health, fitness, physical/cardiopulmonary rehabilitation, or sports medicine field can join as affiliated members. Student memberships are encouraged from approved programs (ASEP, 2008). See Box 2.2 for the ASEP mission statement.

EXPLORE MORE **BOX 2.2**

ASEP Mission Statement

"The American Society of Exercise Physiologists, the professional organization representing and promoting the profession of exercise physiology, is committed to the professional development of exercise physiology, its advancement, and the credibility of exercise physiologist" (ASEP, 2008).

ASEP CERTIFICATION Currently, ASEP has one certification program, which is called Exercise Physiologist Certified (EPC). This certification is designed to recognize the exercise physiologist as a certified profession. The certification examination is comprised of both a written and a practical component. The content areas in the examination include exercise physiology, cardiac rehabilitation, exercise metabolism, biomechanics, environmental stress, sports nutrition, research, exercise testing and interpretation, blood pressure assessment, exercise prescription, body composition assessment, flexibility, and contraindications for exercise (ASEP, 2008).

Scientific Organizations Without Certification

AMERICAN ALLIANCE OF HEALTH, PHYSICAL EDUCATION, RECREATION AND DANCE (AAHPERD) AAHPERD came into existence in 1885 as a professional organization for individuals teaching in the area of physical training. Since that time it has expanded to include health, recreation, and dance disciplines. There are six associations under the umbrella of AAHPERD: National Association for Sport and Physical Education (NASPE), American Association for Health Education (AAHE), National Dance Association (NDA), American Association for Physical Activity and Recreation (AAPAR), National Association for Girls and Women in Sports (NAGWS), and the Research Consortium (RC). AAHPERD holds an annual convention and publishes several journals including *Research Quarterly for Sport and Exercise*. Today, AAHPERD has over 25,000 members across the disciplines it serves. AAHPERD has its national headquarters in Reston, VA (AAHPERD, 2008). See Box 2.3 for AAHPERD's mission statement.

EXPLORE MORE **BOX 2.3**

AAHPERD Mission Statement

"AAHPERD's mission is to promote and support leadership, research, education, and best practices in the professions that support creative, healthy, and active lifestyles. AAHPERD's national associations have the following purposes: (1) to develop and disseminate professional guidelines, standards, and ethics; (2) to enhance professional practice by providing opportunities for professional growth and development; (3) to advance the body of knowledge in the fields of study and in the professional practice of the fields by initiating, facilitating, and disseminating research; (4) to facilitate and nurture communication and activities with other associations and other related professional groups; (5) to serve as their own spokespersons; (6) to promote public understanding and improve government relations in their fields of study; (7) to engage in future planning; and (8) to establish and fulfill other purposes which are consistent with the purposes of the Alliance" (AAHPERD, 2008).

AMERICAN ASSOCIATION OF CARDIOVASCULAR AND PULMONARY REHABILITATION (AACVPR)

The AACVPR was founded in 1985 and serves as a professional organization for those who are involved with the cardiopulmonary rehabilitation field. The AACVPR is closely related to clinical exercise physiology, and its members include a variety of professionals working within this field such as nurses, physicians, and other professionals in cardiac and pulmonary rehabilitation. There is also a membership category for students. AACVPR has annual meetings and publishes electronic newsletters and the *Journal of Cardiopulmonary Rehabilitation*. The AACVPR does not have a certification program for individuals working

in clinical practice. However, the organization has a program certification process for institutions and facilities that deal with cardiac and pulmonary rehabilitation patients (AACVPR, 2008). AACVPR's mission statement can be found in Box 2.4.

EXPLORE MORE **BOX 2.4**

AACVPR Mission Statement

The mission of the AACVPR is "to reduce morbidity, mortality, and disability from cardiovascular and pulmonary diseases through education, prevention, rehabilitation, research, and aggressive disease management" (AACVPR, 2008).

AMERICAN PHYSIOLOGICAL SOCIETY (APS)

The APS, founded in 1887, serves as the premier physiological science organization in the world. Members are generally PhD-trained scientists or medical doctors who carry out research in the physiological, medical, and allied health sciences. Today over 10,000 scientists are members of the APS. The organization publishes the latest research in physiology in 16 different journals including the *Journal of Applied Physiology* and the *American Journal of Physiology*. There are several different membership categories including a student membership option for students engaged in physiological research who have the support of two APS members with regular membership status. APS is also a member of the Federation of American Societies for Experimental Biology (FASEB), which is a group of scientific organizations (APS, 2008). FASEB holds an annual meeting where APS members (along with other FASEB-affiliated organizations) present their research (APS, 2008).

NORTH AMERICAN SOCIETY FOR PEDIATRIC EXERCISE MEDICINE (NASPEM)

NASPEM was created in 1985 by a group of physicians who applied exercise as a form of testing and therapy in children with cardiopulmonary disorders. Today, NASPEM has a membership of approximately 200 professionals and students who study the acute responses and chronic adaptations in healthy children and children with diseases and disorders. Members include exercise physiologists, pediatricians, pediatric cardiologists and pulmonologists, and physical therapists. NASPEM holds a scientific conference every 2 years. *Pediatric Exercise Science* is the official journal of NASPEM. NASPEM does not have a certification program (NASPEM, 2008). See Box 2.5 for NASPEM's mission statement.

Fitness-Related Organizations With Certification Programs

AMERICAN COUNCIL ON EXERCISE (ACE)

ACE was established in 1985 and may be the largest certifying nonprofit organization with more than 40,000 certified health and fitness professionals. In 2003 ACE's four certifications were accredited by the NCCA (see NSCA for further information on NCCA). The certification examinations are a written test only; there are no practical sections (ACE, 2008). See Box 2.6 for the ACE mission statement.

ACE CERTIFICATIONS ACE offers four different certification programs: ACE Personal Trainer, ACE Group Fitness Instructor, Lifestyle and Weight Management Consultant, and Advanced Health and Fitness Specialist.

ACE Personal Trainer: This certification is for individuals who work one-on-one with individuals providing fitness instruction and guidance. Individuals receiving the ACE Personal Training Certification work in health and fitness clubs, YMCAs, personal training studios, and clients' homes. Individuals passing the examination show competencies in exercise science, nutrition, fitness assessment, exercise programming, and instructional and spotting techniques. There is no education requirement for this certification; however, a candidate must be 18 years of age and hold a current adult CPR certification (ACE, 2008).

ACE Group Fitness Instructor: Individuals wanting to teach in a group setting should consider this certification. The examination covers exercise science (anatomy, kinesiology, and exercise physiology), exercise programming, instructional techniques, and professional responsibility. The eligibility requirements are the same as the ACE personal trainer (ACE, 2008).

Lifestyle and Weight Management Consultant: This certification is for individuals who have the knowledge and skills to develop sound weight management programs that focus on nutrition, exercise programming, and behavior modification. To be eligible for this certification, a person must be certified as an ACE Personal Trainer or Group Fitness Instructor or Advanced Health and Fitness Specialist (described next) or hold a bachelor's degree in exercise science or the equivalent before completing the certification (ACE, 2008).

Advanced Health and Fitness Specialist: This certification is designed for individuals working in the clinical exercise setting with clients who may suffer from cardiovascular disease, skeletal-muscle problems, hypertension, pulmonary disorders, and metabolic diseases. The focus in this certification is on both prevention and postrehabilitation needs. A bachelor's degree in exercise science or a related field is required; however, certification as an ACE Personal Trainer or other NCCA accredited certifications such as ACSM, NSCA, or National Academy of Sports Medicine merit eligibility. Other eligibility requirements for the Advanced Health and Fitness Specialist are similar to the Personal Trainer and Group Fitness Instructor with the additional requirement that the candidate must have 300 practical hours in designing and implementing training programs for either apparently healthy or high-risk clients (ACE, 2008).

AEROBICS AND FITNESS ASSOCIATION OF AMERICA (AFAA)

The AFAA was established in 1983 and has certified more than 250,000 instructors. Educational materials include textbooks, reference manuals, videos, and American Fitness Magazine. The certifications include a course throughout the multi-day certification process. AFAA does provide a challenge examination opportunity. It is recommended that anyone wishing to challenge an examination attend the workshops prior to the examination. Certification is good for 2 years and continuing education credits must be completed throughout the 2 years to maintain board certification (AFAA, 2008). See Box 2.7 for the AFAA mission statement.

AFAA CERTIFICATIONS AFAA offers several different certifications. Two of these certifications, Personal Trainer and Primary Group Exercise, are designed for work with individuals or in group settings.

Personal Trainer Certification: This certification is designed for individuals who want to work one-on-one with individuals. Candidates are tested on fitness assessment, anatomy and kinesiology, nutrition and weight control, special populations, programming and screening, and leadership and motivational skills (AFAA, 2008).

Primary Group Exercise Certification: This certification is for individuals who wish to instruct clients in a group exercise setting. The content includes basic anatomy, exercise science, exercise standards, and guidelines. The certification has a practical portion and a written portion (AFAA, 2008).

CAREERS IN EXERCISE PHYSIOLOGY

The career path for exercise physiology is very broad in nature. Many students who choose to study exercise physiology have been actively involved in athletics and club sports, "like to exercise," enjoy studying about the body, or need prerequisites for further education. A question often posed by prospective students and parents deals with the employment options upon graduation; there is not necessarily one employment option but, in fact, many choices. Exercise physiology allows the student to consider a variety of options when it comes to employment opportunities or postgraduate study. Some of these options can be obtained with just a bachelor's degree, others require a master's or doctorate degree in exercise physiology. Many careers start in exercise physiology but require further education and specialized degrees. A number a career paths and their degree requirements are shown in Table 2.3.

TABLE 2.3 Career Options in Exercise Physiology

Career	Brief Description	Degree(s) Required
Personal trainer	Prescribes exercise programs, consults with clients; works with individuals one-on-one or in small groups.	Bachelor's
Fitness instructor	Teaches exercise classes, conducts seminars; organizes exercise programs for fitness facilities.	Bachelor's, master's
Sports consultant	Consults with coaches and athletes on psychological issues, nutrition, exercise programming; researches ergonomics of sports equipment.	Bachelor's, master's, doctorate
Exercise physiologist	Researcher, university and private sector.	Master's, doctorate
Clinical exercise physiologist	Works in cardiopulmonary, oncology, rehabilitation, with individuals with metabolic disorders; researcher in university and private sectors.	Bachelor's, master's, doctorate
Exercise technologist or stress testing technician	Conducts diagnostic and functional treadmill tests on clients; hospital or research facility and some fitness facilities.	Bachelor's, master's
Fitness center director	Supervise daily operations of facility; creates and manages budget.	Bachelor's, master's
Fitness center manager	Organizes and manages day-to-day operations in fitness facilities; creates and manages budget.	Master's

(Continued)

TABLE 2.3 Career Options in Exercise Physiology (Continued)

Career	Brief Description	Degree(s) Required
Corporate fitness director	Develops incentive programs,, instructs classes, develops exercise prescriptions for employees of corporations; creates and manages budget.	Bachelor's, master's
Exercise specialist	Prescribes exercise prescriptions; delivers presentations and seminars; trains clients.	Bachelor's, master's
Wellness counselor	Organizes health fairs, gives presentations and seminars, risk factor screening.	Bachelor's, master's
Health promotions director	Organizes health fairs, gives presentations and seminars, risk factor screening; creates and manages budget.	Bachelor's, master's
Older adult exercise specialist	Prescribes exercise program; delivers presentations and seminars; trains clients.	Bachelor's, master's
Strength coach	Designs and implements weight training programs for sport teams.	Bachelor's, master's
Sport enhancement specialist	Designs special exercise and weight training programs for athletes of all ages.	Bachelor's, master's
Professor	Teaches at a college/university setting; conducts research.	Doctorate
Physical therapist	Rehabilitates gross motor skills.	Bachelor's, master's, doctorate in physical therapy
Occupational therapist	Rehabilitates fine motor skills.	Bachelor's, master's in occupational therapy
Medical doctor	Family practice to specialties.	Bachelor's and medical degree
Chiropractor	Facilitates back maneuvers to correct spinal abnormalities.	Chiropractic degree
Nursing	Patient care, cardiopulmonary rehabilitation.	Bachelor's plus degree in nursing

SUMMARY

Exercise physiology is defined as the study of human function during physical exertion or activity. Although the exact origin of exercise physiology is difficult to define, the field became prominent in the mid- to late-1800s and was firmly established as an academic discipline by the mid-1900s. The typical course content taught in most beginning exercise physiology classes includes the effect of acute and chronic exercise on the different systems in the body as well as special topics such as nutritional and ergogenic supplements, environmental stress, exercise in special populations, body composition assessment, and fitness and prescription methods. A number of professional scientific organizations serve the exercise physiologist. These include ACSM, NSCA, AACVPR, APS, NASPEM, and AAHPERD. Some of the organizations such as ACSM and NSCA have certification programs, which serve to enhance the student's academic credentials. There are also fitness organizations such as ACE and AFAA, which do not publish scientific research but have certification programs. Career choices for the exercise physiologist include employment in a variety of settings such as personal training, fitness centers, strength and conditioning, clinical exercise, directing and managing health and fitness facilities, corporate fitness, research, and a variety of allied health settings.

■ Key People

Ehrling Asmussen
Per-Olof Astrand
David Bruce Dill
George Fritz

John Haldane
Archibald Vivian Hill
Eric Hohwu-Christensen
August Krogh

Otto Myerhoff
Marius Nielsen
Dudley Sargent

■ Key Resources

Key Organizations

Aerobics and Fitness Association of America (www.afaa.com)

American Alliance of Health, Physical Education, Recreation and Dance (www.aahperd.org)

American Association of Cardiovascular and Pulmonary Rehabilitation (www.aacvpr.org)

American College of Sports Medicine (www.acsm.org)

American Council on Exercise (www.acefitness.org)

American Physiological Society (www.the-aps.org)

American Society of Exercise Physiology (www.asep.org)

National Strength and Conditioning Association (www.nsca-lift.org)

North American Society for Pediatric Exercise Medicine (www.naspem.org)

Key Journals

Acta Physiological Scandinavica
American Journal of Physiology
Canadian Journal of Applied Physiology
European Journal of Applied Physiology
European Journal of Sport Science
Exercise and Sport Sciences Reviews
International Journal of Sports Medicine
International Journal of Sport Nutrition and Exercise Metabolism

Journal of Applied Physiology
Journal of Cardiopulmonary Rehabilitation
Journal of Sports Medicine and Physical Fitness
Medicine and Science in Sports and Exercise
Pediatric Exercise Science
Research Quarterly in Exercise and Sport
Sports Medicine

■ Review Questions

1. What is the definition of exercise physiology?
2. Who were some of the early European scientists that contributed to the evolution of the field of exercise physiology?
3. What were some of the significant contributions of the Harvard Fatigue Laboratory?
4. What are the different energy systems that produce ATP?
5. How does the central nervous system differ from the peripheral nervous system?
6. Identify three endocrine glands and the hormones that are secreted.
7. What are the three basic muscle fiber types and the various terms used to identify the fiber types?
8. What are the changes in heart function, blood vessel size, and the composition of the blood as one goes from rest to exercise?
9. What is the difference between pulmonary ventilation and diffusion?
10. What are contemporary areas of research in exercise physiology?
11. What are some of the scientific organizations that provide certification for individuals?
12. Which certification programs require a 4-year college degree in exercise science/physiology or a related field?
13. Identify key research journals in exercise physiology.
14. Which professional organizations require a choice of either a fitness or clinical track for certification? What are the certifications for each track?
15. Who would want to become certified through the NSCA as a CSCS versus the NSCA as a CPT?
16. What is the one eligibility criterion that is common across most fitness certifications? Which certifications require multiple criteria for eligibility?

■ References

Abernethy, P. J., Thayer, R., & Taylor, A. W. (1990). Acute and chronic responses of skeletal muscle to endurance and sprint exercise. *Sports Medicine*, 10, 365–389.

Aerobics and Fitness Association of America. (2008). Retrieved from http://www.afaa.com

American Alliance of Health, Physical Education, Recreation and Dance. (2008). Retrieved from http://www.aahperd.org.

American Association of Cardiovascular and Pulmonary Rehabilitation. (2008). Retrieved from http://www.aacvpr.org

American College of Sports Medicine. (2006a). Certification updates. ACSM's *Certified News*, 16(1), 1–11.

American College of Sports Medicine. (2006b). ACSM *certification resource center 2006 catalog*. Baltimore, MD: Lippincott Williams, and Wilkins.

American College of Sports Medicine. (2005). Certification updates. ACSM's *Certified News*, 15(1), 1–12.

American College of Sports Medicine. (2008). Retrieved from http://www.acsm.org

American Council on Exercise. (2008). Retrieved from http://www.acefitness.org

American Physiological Society. (2008). Retrieved from http://www.the-aps.org

American Society for Exercise Physiology. (2008). Retrieved from http://www.asep.org

Berryman, J. W. (2004). ACSM: 50 years of progress and service 1954–2004. In *Advances in sports medicine and exercise science: 50 years of ACSM* (pp. 21–33, 166–168). Tampa, FL: Faircount.

Bevegard, B. S., & Shepherd, J. T. (1967). Regulation of circulation during exercise in man. *Physiological Reviews*, 47, 178–213.

Bunt, J. C. (1986). Hormonal alterations during exercise. *Sports Medicine*, 3, 331–345.

Caspersen, C. J. (1989). Physical activity epidemiology: Concepts, methods and applications to exercise science. *Exercise and Sport Sciences Reviews*, 17, 423–473.

Clausen, J. P. (1977). Effect of physical training on cardiovascular adjustments to exercise in man. *Physiological Reviews*, 57, 779–816.

Costill, D. L., & Fink, W. J. (1974). Plasma volume changes following exercise and thermal dehydration. *Journal of Applied Physiology*, 37, 521–525.

deVries, H. A. (2000). History of exercise science. In T. J. Housh., & D. J. Housh (Eds.), *Introduction to exercise science*, (pp. 12–35). Boston: Allyn & Bacon.

Dill, D. B. (1985). *The hot life of man and beast*. Springfield, IL: Charles C Thomas.

Green, D. J., O'Driscoll, G., Blanksby, B. A., & Taylor, R. R. (1996). Control of skeletal muscle blood flow during dynamic exercise: Contribution of endothelium-derived nitric oxide. *Sports Medicine*, 21, 119–146.

Gollnick, P. D. (1988). Energy metabolism and prolonged exercise. In D. R. Lamb & R. Murray.(Eds.), *Perspectives in exercise science and sports medicine, Vol. 1: Prolonged exercise.* (pp. 1–42). Indianapolis, IN: Benchmark Press.

Hakkinen, K., & Pakarinen, A. (1995). Acute hormonal responses to heavy resistance training in men and women at different ages. *International Journal of Sport Medicine*, 16, 507–513.

Hawley, J. A. (2002). Adaptations of skeletal muscle to prolonged intense endurance training. *Clinical and Experimental Pharmacology and Physiology*, 29, 218–222.

Holloszy, J. O., & Coyle, E. F. (1984). Adaptations of skeletal muscle to endurance exercise and their metabolic consequences. *Journal of Applied Physiology: Respiratory, Environmental, Exercise Physiology*, 56, 831–838.

Houston, M. E. (2001). *Biochemistry primer for exercise science.* Champaign, IL: Human Kinetics.

Kjaer, M. (1992). Regulation of hormonal and metabolic responses during exercise in humans. *Exercise and Sport Sciences Reviews*, 20, 161–184.

Kraemer, W. J. (1988). Endocrine responses to resistance exercise. *Medicine and Science in Sports and Exercise*, 20, S152–S157.

Lieber, R. L. (2002). *Skeletal muscle structure, function and plasticity: The physiological basis for rehabilitation.* Philadelphia: Lippincott Williams and Wilkins.

McArdle, W. D., Katch, F. I., & Katch, V. L. (2007). *Exercise physiology: Energy, nutrition and human performance.* Philadelphia: Lippincott Williams and Wilkins.

National Strength and Conditioning Association. (2007). Retrieved from http://www.nsca-cc.org

National Strength and Conditioning Association. (2008). Retrieved from http://www.nsca-lift.org

North American Society for Pediatric Exercise Medicine. (2008). Retrieved from http://www.naspem.org

Powers, S. K., Coombs, J., & Demirel, H. (1997). Exercise training-induced changes in respiratory muscles. *Sports Medicine*, 24, 120–131.

Powers, S. K., & Howley, E. T. (2007). *Physiology of exercise: Theory and application to fitness and performance.* New York: McGraw-Hill.

Robinson, M. A. (2004). ACSM helps professionals improve their careers. In *Advances in sports medicine and exercise science: 50 years of ACSM.* Tampa, FL: Faircount.

Rowell, L. B. (1986). *Human circulation during physical stress.* New York: Oxford University Press.

Rowell, L. B. (1993). *Human cardiovascular control.* New York: Oxford University Press.

Sale, D. G. (1988). Neural adaptations to resistance training. *Medicine and Science in Sports and Exercise*, 20, S135–S145.

Saltin, B., & Gollnick, P. D. (1983). Skeletal muscle adaptability: Significance for metabolism and performance. In L. Peachy, R.Adrian, & S. Geiger (Eds.), *Handbook of physiology* (pp. 555–631). Bethesda, MD: American Physiological Society.

Sawka, M. N., Convertino, V. A., Eichner, E. R., Schneider, S. M., & Young, A. J. (2000). Blood volume: Importance and adaptations to exercise training, environmental stresses, and trauma/sickness. *Medicine and Science in Sports and Exercise*, 31, 332–348.

Shepherd, J. T., & Vanhoutte, P. M. (1979). *The human cardiovascular system: Facts and concepts.* New York: Raven Press.

Tesch, P. A. (1988). Skeletal muscle adaptations consequent to long-term heavy resistance training. *Medicine and Science in Sports and Exercise*, 20, S132–S144.

Tipton, C. M. (1998). Contemporary exercise physiology: Fifty years after the closing of the Harvard Fatigue Laboratory. *Exercise and Sport Sciences Reviews*, 26, 315–339.

Tortora, G. J., & Grabowski, S. R. (2003). *Principles of human anatomy and physiology* (pp. 388, 572–588). Hoboken, NJ: Wiley.

West, J. B. (1985). *Respiratory physiology: The essentials.* Baltimore, MD: Williams and Wilkins.

Wilber, C. G. (1985). Foreword. In D. B. Dill, *The hot life of man and beast* (pp. vii–viii). Springfield, IL: Charles C Thomas.

Wilmore, J. H., & Costill, D. L. (2004). *Physiology of sport and exercise* (3rd ed.). Champaign, IL: Human Kinetics.

Wilmore, J. H., Costill, D. L., & Kenney, W. L. (2008). *Physiology of sport and exercise.* Champaign, IL: Human Kinetics.

Zavorsky, G. S. (2000). Evidence and possible mechanisms of altered maximum heart rate with endurance training and tapering. *Sports Medicine*, 29, 13–26.

CHAPTER 3

Nutrition for Sports and Exercise

Michelle Rockwell, MS, RD, CSSD,, University of North Carolina
Jennifer Ketterly, MS, RD, University of North Carolina

■ Chapter Objectives

After reading this chapter, you should be able to:

1. Briefly explain how the field of nutrition for sports and exercise evolved.

2. Understand general content information related to the field of nutrition for sports and exercise.

3. Recognize perspectives, challenges, and job responsibilities of sports dietitians and other sports nutrition professionals.

4. Further explore sports nutrition-related organizations, certifications, and careers.

■ Key Terms

amino acid
anorexia nervosa
antioxidant
binge eating disorder
body composition
bulimia nervosa
calorie (kilocalorie)
carbohydrate
dietary reference intake (DRI)
Dietary Supplement and Health
  Education Act (DSHEA)

eating disorder
electrolyte
energy
energy balance
fat
female athlete triad
glycemic index
iron deficiency
iron deficiency anemia
lean body mass (LBM)
macronutrient

medical nutrition therapy
micronutrient
protein
resting metabolic rate (RMR)
saturated fat
thermic effect of exercise (TEE)
thermic effect of food (TEF)
trans fat
unsaturated fat

Human nutrition can be defined as the study of the processes by which people take in, absorb, and utilize food and fluids. Sports nutrition is a specialization in nutrition that deals with the role these nutrients play in the performance, health, and well-being of athletes. When people think of "athletes," they often think of high-level competitors in the Olympic Games and on Monday Night Football. Although working with elite athletes is a fascinating aspect of sports nutrition, in actuality they are just a small segment of the population. For the purpose of this chapter, an *athlete* is any individual who takes part in regular exercise or physical activity.

In many cases, athletes become interested in nutrition as a means of enhancing their physical activity or athletic performance. Improved performance, of course, means different things to different athletes. For example, a collegiate distance runner may use nutritional manipulations to improve his best 5K time, or a middle-aged woman may change her eating habits to keep up better in her aerobics classes. Athletes are often surprised to learn that proper nutrition and hydration habits can not only better fuel their physical performance but also play a role in mental performance, concentration, mood, energy level, and recovery. Nutrition recommendations are also designed to enhance immunity, prevent injuries, support injury rehabilitation, and to delay or treat chronic diseases.

Sports nutrition research and recommendations can be applied to youth and master's competitors, "weekend warriors," and individuals with many different disease states. In fact, the United States Surgeon General, National Institutes of Health, and the American College of Sports Medicine all recommend that all Americans get at least 30 minutes of moderate exercise almost every day, so it is clear that sports nutrition can apply to many, many different individuals in a variety of different settings. Furthermore, incorporating exercise-based nutrition strategies into physical activity programs and general nutrition guidelines is an excellent strategy for improving exercise adherence and overall health and well-being.

BRIEF HISTORY OF NUTRITION FOR SPORTS AND EXERCISE

Although there are stories dating back to the ancient Olympics of athletes using special diets and magical foods to gain a performance edge, the science of sports nutrition is actually quite new and is still developing. It wasn't until the 1960s that significant breakthroughs in sports nutrition research and applications came about. Some of this work started in the lab of Dr. David Costill at Ball State University. Costill and his co-investigators were among the first to research the effects of different diets on running and cycling performance. He perfected the muscle biopsy procedure, which allowed him and many future researchers to identify exactly what effects nutrition and exercise have on the muscle itself. Costill also led some important research about gastric emptying during exercise; perhaps his greatest accomplishment was finding subjects to participate in these studies! For an interesting and light-hearted history of Ball State University's nutrition and exercise physiology research, go to **http://www.bsu.edu/hpl/media/pdf/labhistory.pdf**

It was also in the 1960s that Gatorade was invented by Dr. Robert Cade and colleagues at the University of Florida. Cade wanted to help the Gators' football players handle the intense Gainesville heat and gain an edge over their competitors. At first, critics thought it was ridiculous to feed athletes salt and sugar during games, but benefits were shown so quickly that it took only 3 years for Gatorade to be seen on the sidelines of college and NFL teams all over the country.

Now, of course, hundreds of laboratories do sports nutrition research, and the sports food and beverage industry is booming. Nutrition recommendations for athletes have become more specific and beneficial, and as they continue to evolve, more and more athletes seek out nutrition advice, and more and more sports nutrition job opportunities are available. It's an exciting time for the field of sports nutrition.

Clinicians who are qualified to provide nutrition counseling and make specific dietary recommendations are Registered Dietitians (RD). Those RDs with expertise in sports and activity are known as Sports Nutritionists or Sports Dietitians. A specific board certification in sports dietetics was created in 2006. Individuals who have this certification have CSSD listed among their credentials. Although RDs are the only professionals trained and legally permitted to provide specific nutritional counseling, many other exercise and health professionals provide general nutrition education. Some professions such as athletic training, personal training, strength and conditioning, and nursing include nutrition education in their scope of practice.

CONTENT AREAS OF STUDY IN NUTRITION FOR SPORTS AND EXERCISE

The following sections provide an introduction to both the science and applications of nutrition for sports and exercise.

Energy

Energy is defined as the capacity to do work and is commonly expressed as **kilocalories** (calories). In common practice, the term *calorie* is interchangeable with kilocalorie. Internationally, calories are more often expressed as kilojoules (kJ). One calorie equals 4.184 kJ. Specifically, a **calorie** is the amount of work required to raise the temperature of 1 kilogram (kg) of water 1 degree Celcius (°C) from 15°C to 16°C at one atmosphere.

An athlete is considered in **energy balance** when the amount of energy or calories consumed through foods and beverages (*energy intake*) is equal to the amount of calories expended (*energy expenditure*). Thus, it is important to understand methods for calculating or at least estimating the energy intake and energy expenditure. Manipulating energy balance is a key component of weight gain and weight loss (reviewed later in the chapter). In many cases, the state of energy balance is desirable for supporting exercise, athletic train-

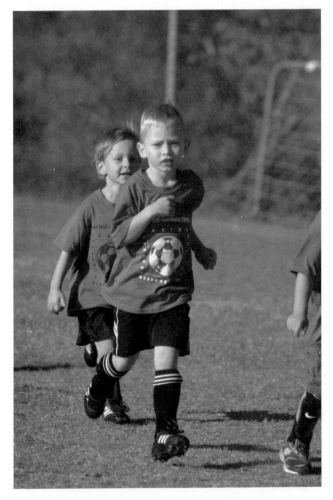

Youth athletes have enhanced calorie and protein needs compared to inactive children, to compensate for physical activity and growth. Children also need more fluids than adults because they sweat less efficiently.

EXPLORE MORE BOX 3.1

Energy (calories) in Spaghetti

1 cup of cooked spaghetti = 140 grams

Contains:
43 grams *carbohydrates* × 4 calories/gram = 172 calories
8 grams *protein* × 4 calories/gram = 32 calories
1.5 grams *fat* × 9 calories/gram = 13.5 calories

Total = 217.5 calories in 1 cup cooked spaghetti

---

ing, and sports performance. Consider that high-level athletes or those training for endurance events can have extremely high energy expenditures. For example, one study showed that professional male soccer players burned over 3,500 calories on game days (Ebine et al., 2002). Young female swimmers training at the U.S. Olympic Training Center were shown to expend over 5,500 calories/day during their heavy training period (Trappe et al., 1997). Finally, in an extreme exercise scenario, one cyclist in the Race Across AMerica (RAAM) bike race expended between 15,000 and 23,000 calories each day of the race (Knechtle, Enggist, & Jehle, 2005). In contrast, casual or infrequent exercisers may only burn a minimal amount of calories above and beyond that of their sedentary counterparts. Matching energy expenditure with sufficient caloric intake is often a challenge for athletes. Working with a sports dietitian to design specific individualized strategies can be very helpful in achieving energy balance.

ENERGY INTAKE Scientists can calculate the amount of calories in foods and beverages through several different laboratory techniques. However, food composition tables are available through the United States Department of Agriculture (USDA). In general, the following conversions are used as standards (see Box 3.1):

- 1 gram of carbohydrate = 4 calories
- 1 gram of protein = 4 calories
- 1 gram of fat = 9 calories
- 1 gram of alcohol = 7 calories

The United States Food and Drug Administration (FDA) requires food and beverage companies to accurately represent calorie content on food labels and has the right to test products to confirm accuracy. Many accurate nutrient databases are available in book and online form; a particularly useful database was

TABLE 3.1 Estimate of Daily Energy Expenditure (expressed as calories/pound of body weight)		
	Males	**Females**
Sedentary	14	11
Moderately active	16	13
Very active	20	17
Elite athletic training*	22+	20+

*especially for endurance or team sports
Source: Dunford (2006).

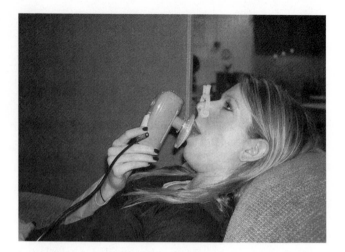

The MedGem (Microlife USA, Inc.) is one of several new portable devices used for measuring resting metabolic rate (RMR). These devices can be much less expensive, invasive, and time-consuming than traditional assessments using metabolic carts.

established by USDA and can be accessed at **http://www.nal.usda.gov/fnic/foodcomp/search/**. By entering a food and reference amount, users can obtain the number of calories in that food in addition to other nutritional information.

Perhaps the most challenging part of determining energy intake is not food composition but getting an accurate record of what an individual has consumed. In controlled research settings, it is possible to weigh and record exactly what is consumed. In practical or clinical settings, it is necessary to rely on methods such as interviews (e.g., a 24-hour recall of foods consumed) and diet records kept by athletes. Many people struggle to precisely describe their energy intake due to forgetting to include certain items (e.g., beverages, toppings, and snacks are commonly omitted), intentionally altering the type or amount of food eaten, or inaccurately representing portion sizes. Researchers have shown that people may underestimate their portions of foods by as much as 20 to 50%. It is critical to provide clear and complete instructions for record-keeping (Berning & Steen, 1998).

ENERGY EXPENDITURE Energy expenditure can be directly assessed using laboratory methods such as *indirect calorimetry* or *doubly-labeled water*. These procedures are performed in the clinical setting, and most individuals do not have access to them. Therefore, estimating energy expenditure is commonplace. A rough "ballpark" estimate of the calories an individual expends each day can be determined using Table 3.1.

Alternately, a more accurate representation of energy expenditure can be computed by either directly measuring or estimating the three primary components of energy expenditure:

- Resting metabolic rate (RMR)
- Thermic effect of exercise (TEE)
- Thermic effect of food (TEF)

Resting Metabolic Rate: The **resting metabolic rate** (RMR) is the number of calories expended to maintain the body's life-sustaining processes during 24 hours. Although they are calculated slightly differently, the terms *basal metabolic rate* (BMR) and *resting energy expenditure* (REE) are commonly considered synonymous with RMR. Athletes are often surprised to learn that they would burn a significant number of calories even if they remained at rest all day long; typically, RMR ranges between 1,000 and 2,200 calories/day. In nonexercising individuals, RMR accounts for 60 to 80% of total energy expenditure (Ravussin & Bogardus, 1989). In athletes burning a high number of calories through exercise training, the contribution of RMR could be significantly lower. RMR is affected by a variety of factors including age, sex (males generally have higher RMR), amount of muscle mass, health status (fever and infection increase RMR), training status, and hormonal imbalances.

RMR can be calculated via measurement of gas exchange (oxygen consumption and carbon dioxide production) using a metabolic cart, a time-consuming but accurate laboratory technique. In recent years, portable handheld devices have been developed for assessing RMR. Although reliability needs to be confirmed with more research, especially in athletes, they offer a promising and relatively inexpensive option for measuring RMR.

Due to the complexity of direct measurements, RMR is often estimated. Several mathematical equations can be used to estimate RMR, with the most common being the Mifflin-St. Jeor equation. Some researchers report that the Cunningham Equation (1980) is more accurate for athletes (Thompson & Manore, 1996). For a quick and easy estimation, the

TABLE 3.2 Resting Metabolic Rate (RMR) Prediction Equations

Equation	Males	Females
Mifflin-St. Jeor	RMR = $(9.99 \times wt) + (6.25 \times ht) - (4.92 \times age) + 5$	RMR = $(9.99 \times wt) + (6.25 \times ht) - (4.92 \times age) - 161$
Cunningham	RMR = $500 + 22(\text{lean body mass})*$	Same as males
WHO	RMR = Ages 18–30: $(15.3 \times wt) + 679$ Ages 30–60: $(11.6 \times wt) + 879$ Ages > 60: $(13.5 \times wt) + 487$	RMR = Ages 18–30: $(14.7 \times wt) + 496$ Ages 30–60: $(8.7 \times wt) + 829$ Ages > 60: $(10.5 \times wt) + 596$

*It is necessary to have body composition data to use the Cunningham Equation.

World Health Organization (WHO) Equation (1985) can be used. For all of these equations, weight is expressed in kilograms (kg) (1 lb = 2.2 kg) and height is expressed in centimeters (cm) (1 in = 2.54 cm). (See Table 3.2.)

Thermic Effect of Exercise: Exercise, activities of general living (i.e.,showering, driving, cooking, etc.), and unplanned movements (e.g., fidgeting) compose the **thermic effect of exercise** (TEE). The TEE depends on the type, duration, and intensity of the work being done and the weight and other characteristics of the person doing the work. Several comprehensive tables are available for use in estimating calories expended through various activities. Table 3.3 shows just

a few activities and their estimated energy expenditure. An estimated rule of thumb is that walking or running a mile at any pace burns approximately 100 calories. Using such a table requires that the athlete keep a very detailed activity record that accounts for what he or she is doing every minute of the day (e.g., 8:00–8:10 a.m., watching television seated; 8:11–8:18 a.m., stretching; 8:19–8:52 a.m., jogging at a rate of 5 miles/hour; etc.). Clearly, this is a tedious and imprecise task. However, it can be useful in some cases.

Thermic Effect of Food: The **thermic effect of food** (TEF) is the energy the body expends to digest, absorb, metabolize, and store food consumed throughout the day. This value varies based on

TABLE 3.3 Energy Expended in Various Activities (above RMR)

Activity	Calories/Pound/Minute	Calories Expended by a 175-lb. Person When Doing Activity for 1 Hour
Sleeping	0 (RMR only)	0 (RMR only)
Sitting quietly	.003	32
Light cleaning	.014	147
Heavy housework	.021	221
Fast dancing	.051	534
Walking (15 min/mile)	.041	431
Running (9 min/mile)	.069	725
Running (5.5 min/mile)	.112	1,176
Golf	.030	315
Soccer	.089	935

Source: Williams (2006).

individual characteristics of the person and the food consumed. Typically, TEF accounts for about 6 to 10% of energy expenditure. In other words, the body expends about 100–300 calories/day above the RMR to process food consumed.

Macronutrients

There are three primary **macronutrients** (*macro* means nutrients the body requires in large quantities): carbohydrates, protein, and fat. Each macronutrient varies in the way it is digested, processed, and stored by the body and the role it plays in exercise and health. The following section reviews primary concepts regarding each macronutrient and how it applies to athletes. It is notable that basic macronutrient recommendations for most athletes actually differ very little from guidelines designed for the general population: 55 to 65% of calories from carbohydrates, 10 to 15% of calories from protein, and 20 to 25% of calories from fat. However, since many athletes require significantly more calories than less active individuals, their *absolute* nutrient requirements (total grams of carbohydrates, protein, and fat) may differ even if *relative* (% of calories) requirements do not. In addition, athletes' macronutrient requirements fluctuate at different points during their training cycles and seasons.

The USDA created a tool known as the Food Guide Pyramid to help guide individuals in macronutrient selection. It was not designed specifically for athletes, but it does take exercise level into consideration in calculating needs. An interactive version of the Food Guide Pyramid can be accessed at **http://www.mypyramid.gov/.**

CARBOHYDRATES: FUELING ACTIVITY

Carbohydrates serve as the primary fuel for most types of exercise and athletic performance, especially high-intensity exercise performance, because the body can convert carbohydrates to energy much more rapidly than other fuels. (One exception is creatine phosphate, which can be converted to energy faster than carbohydrates.) Carbohydrates also provide fuel for lower-intensity exercise (brisk walking, jogging, light swimming, etc.), especially when the duration of exercise is long. The body uses fat for fuel during low-intensity exercise, but carbohydrates are required for the body to transfer fat into energy. In the case of long exercise, carbohydrates are considered the *limiting* fuel because carbohydrate stores in the muscles and liver (known as *glycogen*) eventually deplete. Stores of fat, on the other hand, are plentiful in almost every athlete. Carbohydrates are the primary fuel for the brain and nervous system, and they also play a role in metabolizing protein.

Clearly, it's difficult for athletes to meet many of their goals without consuming appropriate levels of carbohydrates.

Carbohydrates are found in a wide array of food sources including the following:

- Breads, cereals, rice, pasta, grains, flour (bagels, muffins, crackers, pancakes, waffles, etc.)
- Fruits and fruit juices
- Vegetables
- Milk and dairy products
- Desserts, sweets, syrups, and candy
- Sodas and sweetened beverages
- Sports products such as sports drinks, gels, and bars

In addition to providing energy, some carbohydrates contain high amounts of vitamins and minerals. For example, an average orange would contain 140% of daily Vitamin C recommendations in addition to some potassium, folate, and Vitamin A (among others). Each large orange contains about 20 grams of carbohydrates. Oranges contain virtually no fat or protein, so the calorie content of the orange is approximately 80 calories (20 grams × 4 calories/gram). Contrast the 80 calorie orange with 80 calories worth of jelly beans (8 jelly beans). Although the carbohydrate and calorie content are nearly identical, the amount of vitamins and minerals varies drastically. Jelly beans are almost entirely simple sugars, and they do not contain vitamins and minerals. Thus, it can be said that the orange has a higher *nutrient density* than jelly beans because it provides more vitamins and minerals for the same number of calories. In other words, the orange provides "more bang for your buck." In general, it is beneficial to include foods of high nutrient density in the diet whenever possible; this allows for vitamin and mineral needs to be addressed while also meeting macronutrient needs.

In addition to choosing carbohydrates high in nutrient density, including carbohydrates high in fiber is also recommended. Examples of foods high in fiber include whole grains (wheat, oat, rye, bran), fruits, vegetables, nuts, and beans. Diets high in fiber can have a positive effect on lowering blood cholesterol, preventing certain types of cancers, and on improving general bowel health and regular functioning. High-fiber foods can play a role in weight control because individuals report greater satiety (feeling of fullness) after eating high-fiber foods as compared to the same amount of low-fiber foods (Koh-Banerjee & Rimm, 2003). It may be beneficial for an athlete who is trying to lose weight to increase the fiber content of his or her diet.

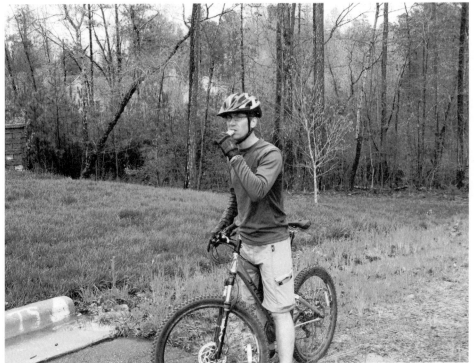

Research has shown that most athletes can oxidize carbohydrates at a rate of 1 gram per minute during continuous, intense exercise. This cyclist eats a sports bar to supply carbohydrates during his ride.

Another strategy athletes can use for selecting which carbohydrates to consume is based on the glycemic index. The **glycemic index** of a food evaluates the increase in blood sugar and insulin levels induced in response to eating the food. Researchers have established glycemic index levels for many different foods (Foster-Powell, Holt, & Brand Miller, 2002). High glycemic index foods such as sodas, candy, honey, potatoes, carrots, and sports drinks raise blood sugar higher and are digested and absorbed faster than low glycemic index foods such as apples, nuts, yogurt, pasta, and lentils. Prior to activity, athletes may be advised to select low glycemic index foods in an effort to provide energy to last throughout their exercise session. Eating lower glycemic index foods throughout the day can also keep energy levels more constant and may help control appetite. During and after activity,

however, higher glycemic index foods may be preferred as a method of providing a quick burst of energy and/or fast-absorbing sugars that can rapidly be converted to glycogen stores during recovery. Diabetic athletes may achieve better blood sugar control by paying attention to the glycemic index of foods they eat.

The amount of carbohydrates an athlete should consume each day is based on a few factors, but mostly on activity level (see Table 3.4). The recommendations discussed here are based on body weight and activity level and likely average out to 55 to 65% of calories (may be higher for athletes training intensely or for long periods of time).

Many athletes are familiar with the carbohydrate content of food, so actively reading food labels and paying attention to serving sizes is important. Other athletes have far less nutrition knowledge and benefit

TABLE 3.4   Summary of Carbohydrate Needs for Athletes

Activity Level	Daily Carbohydrate Recommendation	Daily Needs for a 175-lb. (80 kg) Male
None	4 grams/kg body weight	320 grams
Moderate exercise or general training	5 to 7 grams/kg body weight	400 to 560 grams
Endurance athletes	7 to 10 grams/kg body weight	560 to 800 grams
Ultraendurance athletes	>11 grams/kg body weight	880 grams

from one-on-one work with a sports nutrition professional for education, planning, and counseling purposes. In some cases, meeting the high-carbohydrate needs of training is a challenge. An athlete who is training for an ironman triathlon needs 800 g of carbohydrates per day—that is equivalent to 11.5 large bagels! To meet these needs any athletes need to divide their food intake into multiple small or moderate-sized meals per day rather than just a few large meals. Furthermore, to reduce the quantity of foods eaten, selecting high-carbohydrate beverages can help meet extremely high carbohydrate needs without causing the athlete to feel over-full.

The popularity of several low-carbohydrate diets (e.g., Atkins, South Beach, Zone) has played a role in creating the image that carbohydrates are "fattening" or "bad for you." Many athletes require education that they are likely to require more carbohydrates than their nonathletic counterparts or family members. A training diet insufficient in carbohydrates can result in impaired exercise performance (physical and mental aspects) and recovery due to limited glycogen stores. Inadequate carbohydrate intake can also affect immune function and may even increase the risk of injury. Often, athletes suffering from overtraining syndrome are chronically glycogen depleted.

On the flip side, excess fat storage is likely in an athlete who regularly exceeds his or her carbohydrate needs. Because carbohydrate intake should so closely match training level, athletes must reduce their carbohydrate intake in the off-season, when injured, or when training levels are low (such as during a "taper" period in swimming).

PROTEIN: REGULATION, BUILDING, AND REPAIR Protein plays an important role in many regulatory processes in human metabolism. Enzymes, hormones, and neurotransmitters (responsible for sending nerve impulses) are all made up of protein. Some proteins act as nutrient carriers. For example, hemoglobin is a protein that carries oxygen in the blood to tissues throughout the body. Athletes are often most familiar with the structural role of protein: it is a component of every cell, including, of course, muscle cells. Protein is required in adequate amounts for the growth of muscle and development of **lean body mass** (LBM). It also plays a role in the postexercise recovery and repair process. Protein contains approximately 4 calories per gram and can contribute to energy production during exercise, but it is rare. However, when exercise is extremely long or when an athlete has low glycogen stores (poor carbohydrate intake, dieting, disordered eating, etc.), protein can be utilized as fuel.

Proteins are made up of different combinations of some or all of the 20 **amino acids.** Some amino acids are considered *essential amino acids* because they

cannot be synthesized by the body and must therefore be consumed in the diet. *Nonessential amino acids* are also found in dietary sources, but the body has the ability to produce them as well. (See Box 3.2).

EXPLORE MORE **BOX 3.2**

AMINO ACIDS

Essential Amino Acids

Histidine
Isoleucine
Leucine
Lysine
Methionine
Phenylalanine
Threonine
Tryptophan
Valine

Nonessential Amino Acids

Alanine
Arginine
Asparagine
Aspartic acid
Cysteine
Glutamic acid
Glutamine
Glycine
Proline
Serine
Tyrosine

Most proteins do not contain every amino acid. In fact, a protein can be classified as *high quality* or *low quality* based on the number of amino acids it contains and in what proportion. Eggs and cow's milk are often considered the highest quality protein sources for humans. Other sources of protein include meat, poultry, fish, and seafood; dairy products; beans and lentils; nuts, seeds, and nut butters; soy products; tofu; some vegetables and grains; and sports products such as shakes, powders, and bars. To attain the best combination of all the different amino acids, it is recommended that a variety of different protein sources be consumed each day. This is emphasized particularly for vegetarians because plant-based sources of protein are typically of the lowest quality.

The recommended daily allowance (RDA) for protein for the general population is .8 g/kg body weight. At the RDA level, a 175-pound person would need about 65 grams of protein each day. This amount is easily attainable through dietary sources. A 10-ounce steak has enough protein to meet the 65-gram goal

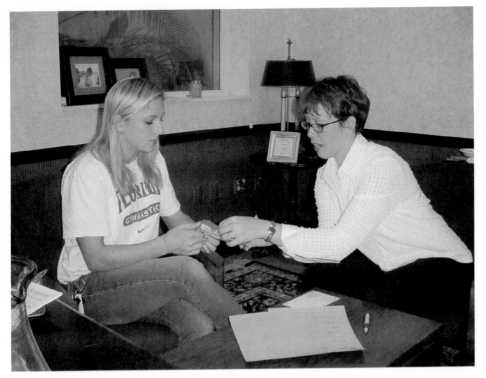

A sports dietitian counsels former University of Florida gymnast (All-American Savannah Evans) on a nutrition plan to enhance her performance. To counsel athletes on specific diet needs, certification as a Registered Dietitian (RD) is required. Many sports nutrition experts become Certified Specialists in Sports Dietetics. Other health and sports professionals may provide general nutrition education to athletes and active individuals.

(not that getting protein exclusively from steak is recommended), and many Americans, especially heavy meat and dairy eaters, consistently consume excessive protein in their diets.

A great deal of research has investigated whether or not athletes need additional protein to compensate for the demands of training, muscle breakdown and repair, and muscle protein synthesis. At this time, the American Dietetic Association recommends that athletes consume about twice the RDA of .8 g/kg body weight. Specifically, guidelines for endurance athletes are 1.2 to 1.4 g/kg body weight per day and 1.6 to 1.7 g/kg body weight per day for strength-trained athletes (Position of the American Dietetic Association, 2000). So, if the 175-pound example person was participating in endurance training, he would require up to 111 grams of protein per day, and if he were strength training, he would need up to 135 grams per day.

In reality, many athletes are eating far more than the recommendations suggest. It is not uncommon for sports dietitians to encounter athletes eating protein at a level of 3–5 g/kg body weight per day. Sometimes this is an intentional strategy for trying to "bulk up" or get stronger. Other times it is simply a consequence of a high-calorie diet. Chronic excessive dietary protein intake can have negative performance and health effects.

Contrary to popular athlete belief, more protein consumed does not necessarily equate to greater muscle mass. A study by Mark Tarnopolsky et al. (1992) compared the effects of three different levels of dietary protein on muscle protein synthesis in weight lifters. The research group compared a .8 g/kg body weight per day diet (current RDA) to 1.4 and 2.4 g/kg body weight per day diets. Results showed enhanced protein synthesis with both higher levels of protein compared to the RDA level, but there was no difference between the 1.4 and 2.4 g/kg body weight per day diets, indicating that the higher level of protein was not used for increasing muscle mass and could be considered unnecessary and even problematic to the athlete. Specific situations may increase athletes' needs for dietary protein, including stages of growth, injury, surgery, or initiating a new strength training program.

Although it is a less common issue, some athletes struggle to meet their protein needs. This is most likely to occur in vegetarians, females, older athletes, those strictly limiting caloric intake, those on extremely high-carbohydrate diets, or individuals with disordered eating patterns. Consuming inadequate protein over an extended period of time can result in poor recovery, loss of body weight or muscle tissue, decreased strength and power, and increased susceptibility to infection.

FAT: HEALTH AND PROTECTION The role of **fat** in the body includes serving as an energy source, a component of cell membranes and other important structures, and aiding in the absorption of fat-soluble vitamins (vitamins A, D, E, K). Despite these functional roles, excess levels of dietary fat can negatively affect health and athletic performance. High-fat diets are associated with the development of chronic diseases such as cardiovascular disease and some cancers. Because fat contains 9 calories per gram, it is a dense energy source and can therefore contribute to excessive caloric intake and obesity. In terms of exercise, high-dietary fat can cause gastric distress during activity. Athletes may also report feeling sluggish or "heavy" during exercise, which is likely due to the slow digestion of fat and inadequate consumption of carbohydrates. It is recommended that most athletes consume 20 to 30% calories from fat. Research has shown no benefits (and perhaps negative effects) of very low-fat diets (<15% of calories) (Position of the American Dietetic Association, 2000).

As described earlier in this chapter, fat is used as fuel during low- to moderate-intensity exercise. Because fat stores are abundant, athletes are much more likely to run out of carbohydrate stores than fat. Accordingly, researchers developed a theory that "fat loading"—eating a very high-fat diet for the days leading up to an endurance event—may enhance time to fatigue by promoting the use of fat rather than carbohydrates for energy production. However, research studies have not supported this theory. In addition, many athletes report that high-fat diets before exercise are unappetizing and cause gastrointestinal side effects.

Some types of fats are considered more healthful than others. Specifically, **unsaturated fats** (mono-unsaturated and polyunsaturated fats) typically have a favorable effect on blood cholesterol levels. Unsaturated fats are found in vegetable oils, olives and olive oil, nuts and seeds, fish, oil-based salad dressings, flax, and avocado. Some of these sources also contain omega-3 fatty acids, which can play an important role in immunity, recovery, and reducing inflammation. Athletes are encouraged to emphasize consumption of unsaturated fats while limiting the other two categories of dietary fats: saturated fats and trans fats. **Saturated fats** are solid at room temperature and are primarily found in animal products such as meats, poultry skin, full-fat dairy products, butter, and eggs. Saturated fats are linked to elevated blood cholesterol levels, and it is recommended that intake be limited to less than 10% calories/day. **Trans fats** are produced in the food industry by chemically manipulating oils. Examples include many fried foods, snack products such as cookies, crackers, and chips, pastries, and margarines. A public health effort is currently under way to reduce trans fats used in restaurants and in processed foods.

Athletes often have busy schedules and must frequently eat on the go, so strategies for selecting healthy meals at fast food restaurants, in vending machines, and at concession stands can be a valuable component of reducing dietary fat.

Micronutrients

Micronutrients are substances the body requires in small amounts, including a number of vitamins and minerals. Nutrition research has addressed the question of whether or not athletes have higher vitamin and mineral needs than inactive individuals. Although there are some exceptions, in most cases athletes should strive to attain the same amount recommended to the general population. In the United States, this guideline is expressed in the form of **dietary reference intakes** (DRI). For most micronutrients, athletes should aim to meet the RDA (a subgroup of the DRI that is considered sufficient to meet the needs of nearly all healthy individuals) without exceeding what is considered the tolerable upper intake level (UL). The UL is set at the maximum amount unlikely to pose adverse health risks. A complete set of DRI tables can be obtained by visiting the Institutes of Medicine Web site at **http://www.iom.edu**.

Even if micronutrient needs for athletes aren't specifically higher than those for the general population, the consequences of micronutrient deficiencies in athletes may appear earlier and have greater impact. For example, if a female college runner from a Division I cross country team has consumed inadequate levels of calcium during most of her teenage years, she is more likely to develop a stress fracture or other bone problem than a nonrunning peer with a similar dietary deficiency. This higher risk of injury occurs simply because she regularly puts her body through the stress and impact of training.

Reviewing exercise and sports-related issues for all vitamins and minerals is beyond the scope of this book. However, a few micronutrients with specific relevance to athletes are highlighted here.

CALCIUM In addition to supporting bone health, calcium also is directly involved in muscle contraction and nerve function—all three roles are critical for athletes. Nevertheless, many athletes struggle to meet their daily needs, which range, based on DRI values, from 1,000 mg/day to 1,300 mg/day. Because small amounts of calcium are lost through sweat, athletes with extremely high sweat rates may have greater calcium needs.

The most familiar dietary sources of calcium are milk and dairy products. One 8-ounce cup of milk or yogurt and 1 ounce of cheese have approximately 300 mg of calcium. Other dietary sources include salmon, spinach, and the wide variety of calcium-fortified products that are now available (juices, cereals, snacks). Lactose intolerant individuals or those with milk allergies or aversions may need specific dietary calcium counseling in addition to supplementation.

IRON Iron is a mineral involved in oxygen transport and energy production, thus playing an important role in exercise, particularly aerobic exercise. **Iron deficiency** (low levels of storage and transport iron in the blood) and **iron deficiency anemia** (a more progressed stage involving low levels of storage and transport iron in addition to decreased hemoglobin, the protein that carries oxygen throughout the body) can have a significant impact on performance and health. It has been reported that as many as 30 to 60% of competitive athletes have iron deficiency, and approximately 5% suffer from iron deficiency anemia (Volpe, 2006). Common deficiency symptoms include early fatigue during workouts, decreased cardiovascular stamina, decreased strength, decreased resistance to infection, easy bruising, inability to tolerate cold temperatures, and poor concentration.

Females are more likely to develop iron deficiency due to blood lost through menstruation (and thus iron loss) and lower calorie intake. Other contributors to iron deficiency include intense aerobic training (especially when the individual is not accustomed to it), vegetarian diets, low-calorie diets, infections, chronic bleeding problems, or menstrual dysfunction.

Dietary sources of iron include beef and other meats (especially dark meat), eggs, fortified cereals, beans, potatoes, dried fruits, and green vegetables. As a precautionary measure, athletes should strive to include several of these in their daily diet and perhaps consider a multivitamin that contains the RDA for iron (8 to 18 mg/day depending on age and sex). Athletes should not supplement with individual iron supplements unless specifically diagnosed with iron deficiency through blood analysis because excess levels of iron can be hazardous to the body. If symptoms consistent with iron deficiency exist, athletes should be seen by a physician.

ANTIOXIDANTS **Antioxidants** are a category of vitamins and minerals that can combat the effects of free radicals, which are compounds that can cause oxidative damage to the body's cells. Exercise has been shown to produce free radicals, so the issue of whether or not athletes require higher levels of antioxidant nutrients has been considered. Several nutrients have antioxidant properties, but the primary nutrients studied with respect to exercise are Vitamin C, Vitamin E, Vitamin A (carotene or beta-carotene), and selenium. Some research supports the theory that levels slightly higher than the RDA

may be required for athletes to protect muscles from damage and soreness associated with free radicals (Watson, 2006). There is also evidence that elevated intake of Vitamin C may help prevent respiratory infections in endurance-trained athletes. The best way for athletes to meet or exceed the RDA for the four antioxidants mentioned is to regularly consume brightly colored fruits and vegetables (e.g., oranges, cantaloupe, berries, spinach, broccoli, peppers), potatoes, whole grains, vegetable oils, nuts, and seeds.

Fluids and Electrolytes

Meeting fluid needs is a common challenge for athletes. Dehydration is much more likely than overhydration, but both can be detrimental to health and performance. Many individuals have been instructed to follow the guidelines of consuming 8 glasses of water each day. In 2004 the Institute of Medicine (IOM) issued recommendations that most women require the equivalent of about 90 ounces (more than 11 cups) of fluids per day and that men require about 125 ounces (more than 15 cups) per day. The IOM report went on to say that fluid needs can be met by most healthy individuals by consuming a variety of different beverages and high-fluid foods *when thirsty* (the entire report from the IOM can be accessed at **http://www.iom.edu**). Because athletes frequently do a poor job meeting their daily fluid requirements which may be higher than those of the sedentary individual, a common recommendation is that athletes monitor the color of their urine. Pale yellow or clear urine is an indicator of good hydration status; amber-colored urine (that looks like apple juice) or small volumes of urine indicate poor hydration status. Many athletes report to training sessions already dehydrated (Stover, 2006), and the likelihood that they will improve their fluid balance during activity is minimal, meaning that performance and safety may be at risk.

Most athletes do a poor job of matching their fluid loss (through sweat and urine) during activity (Murray, 2006). Inadequate fluid consumption during activity can result in decreased strength, stamina, and speed in addition to posing a risk for heat illness. Heat illness can range from muscle cramping to more severe conditions such as heat exhaustion and heat stroke (which can be deadly).

The American College of Sports Medicine recommends the following fluid guidelines for athletes:

Two hours before exercise: Drink 14 to 22 ounces of water or sports drink.

During exercise: Drink 6 to 12 ounces of water or sports drink every 15 to 20 minutes.

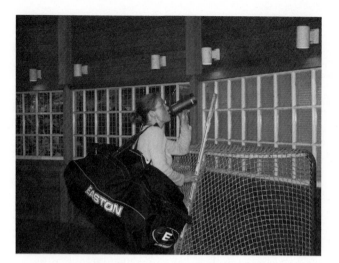

Proper hydration during intense activity is critical for performance and safety. It is recommended that athletes weigh themselves before and after exercise to monitor fluid loss. A fluid loss of >1–2% of body weight can impair performance and increase risk of heat illness. Athletes are encouraged to drink 16 to 24 ounces of fluids for every pound lost during an exercise session.

After exercise: Drink 16 to 24 ounces of water or sports drinks for every pound lost during activity (weighing athletes, especially in hot environments, can be critical for monitoring fluid intake).

Sports drinks have become a staple in many athletic environments. They have been shown repeatedly to better support athletes' hydration needs than plain water and also to enhance performance. Sweat contains not only water but also **electrolytes** such as sodium, potassium, chloride, calcium, and magnesium (with the most significant loss coming from sodium). Many sports drinks contain electrolytes in a formulation designed to mimic sweat loss. This can help the body maintain fluid balance, prevent muscle cramping and other heat-related problems, and promote further drinking. Many sports drinks also contain carbohydrates. Carbohydrates consumed during intense or long (more than 1 hour) exercise have been shown to enhance athletic performance by maintaining blood sugar levels and providing an energy "boost." Carbohydrates in sports drinks should be included at a level of less than 8% (about 15 grams/8 oz serving); higher levels can cause gastric distress and pull water into the digestive tract, promoting dehydration. Another advantage of consuming sports drinks over water during activity is that the appealing flavors make the beverage more palatable than plain water; therefore, athletes are likely to drink more of it. Sports drinks are most appropriately used before, during, and after exercise and not necessarily as all-day beverages, especially if the athlete is easily meeting his or her calorie

needs. Sports drinks should not be a frequently consumed beverage for sedentary people.

There are many different types of sports drinks available, and some companies have added ingredients to or instead of carbohydrates and electrolytes. The benefits of these ingredients (such as protein, caffeine, and various vitamins, minerals, and herbs) are still being investigated. Note that the highly popular energy drinks now widely available differ significantly from sports drinks. They are usually highly concentrated with sugars (although some are sugar-free) and some type of stimulant (such as caffeine) and rarely contain electrolytes. These drinks may have negative effects for athletes and should be used with caution, especially in youth athletes.

Sometimes using sports drinks isn't enough to replace the electrolytes lost through sweat. An old tradition was using salt tablets, which presented problems for some athletes, especially when they failed to consume enough fluids with the tablets. Current recommendations advise athletes training in intense heat or those who seem to sweat a lot or sweat out a high volume of salt to add salt to their food and make high-sodium food choices (soups, pretzels, popcorn, pickles, tomato juice, etc.). This recommendation can be confusing to athletes due to the broad public health message to decrease sodium intake as a means of controlling blood pressure. Athletes' sodium needs can be drastically greater than those of inactive individuals.

Weight Control and Body Composition

Achieving a healthy body weight without excessive dieting or exercising is becoming increasingly more difficult in today's food environment. The Centers for Disease Control and Prevention ([CDC], 2007) reports from the 1999–2002 National Health and Nutrition Examination Survey (NHANES) that an estimated 65% of U.S. adults were either overweight or obese. Further, in 2006 only four states had obesity prevalence rates less than 20%, and 22 states had prevalence rates equal to or greater than 25%. Athletes are not unaffected by the challenges of navigating daily food choices. Effectively controlling body weight often becomes a primary goal.

WEIGHT CONTROL An understanding of energy balance is the foundation of weight control. However, it is also important to consider genetic, physiological, lifestyle, and psychosocial factors when evaluating weight goals. Genes influence body size, shape, and fat distribution, as well as metabolic rate. These components can be managed but not necessarily changed. Lifestyle factors of eating

TABLE 3.5 Example 3,500 Calorie Meal Plan

Breakfast	Lunch	Dinner
1 ½ cups oatmeal, cooked with 2 tsp. brown sugar	Club sandwich: 4 oz turkey breast, 2 slices Swiss cheese, mixed lettuce greens, mustard, on 3 slices whole grain bread	4 oz skinless chicken breast
1 boiled egg	1 ½ cups sliced raw vegetables	2 ears corn on cob
1 cup calcium fortified orange juice	2 T ranch style dressing	2 tsp. butter or trans fat free margarine
	1 ½ cups fresh fruit salad	1 cup oriental style vegetables, with 1 tsp. olive oil
	1 oz pretzels	Tossed salad
		1 T Italian dressing
		1 whole grain roll
Snack	**Snack**	**Snack**
1 apple	1 cup skim milk	1 cup skim milk with one packet instant breakfast mix
1 oz almonds	2 crunchy granola bars	6 graham cracker squares
		1.5 T peanut butter

and physical activity greatly contribute to weight control measures. Nutrient density, portion size, and eating habits as well as amount and type of physical activity are all important considerations. The cultural and family meaning of food, economic status, and adopted emotional coping mechanisms are psychosocial factors that can also influence food choice and ultimately weight control.

An athlete's weight control interest may relate to goals for weight loss or weight gain. Recommendations that reduce body weight or body fat will only enhance performance if the guidelines and calorie intake are realistic and the diet is balanced. Similarly it is important to activate weight loss strategies during an appropriate time in an athlete's training, for example, during the off-season. It is recommended that weight loss occur at a rate not more than 1–2 pounds per week; weight loss greater than this amount could indicate loss of muscle tissue, and it is less likely that the weight loss will be maintained (Position of the American Dietetic Association, 2000). The use of extreme weight-control measures should be avoided because these practices can jeopardize the health of the athlete and possibly trigger behaviors associated with eating disorders.

Weight gain can be as challenging as weight loss for some athletes. Like the male soccer player (3,500-calorie/day) and female swimmer (5,500 calorie/day) discussed earlier in this chapter, avid exercisers with high

energy expenditures will consequently have very high calorie needs. Translating these needs into adequate food quantities with high nutrient density can be difficult without focused assessment and planning. Table 3.5 provides an example of a 3,500-calorie meal plan. With knowledge of nutrition and physical activity, sports nutrition professionals can help athletes achieve the body weight goal that best matches their exercise and performance goals.

BODY COMPOSITION Another component of an individual's weight that can be important to evaluate is **body composition**. The human body can be divided into fat-free mass (i.e., bone, water, muscle, tissue, etc.) and body fat. Nonessential, or storage fat is the component most athletes want to optimize. To set appropriate goals, an assessment is often needed. The body mass index (BMI) is a ratio of body weight to height; standards correlate with body fat but do not measure it directly. BMI may not always be an appropriate measurement for some athletes because it does not take into account the weight of muscle mass. Several other body composition assessment techniques exist to take a more accurate measurement of body fat. However, no technique is completely free from measurement error. For example, the Bod Pod generally reports a less than 2% measurement error. Table 3.6 summarizes five body composition analysis techniques.

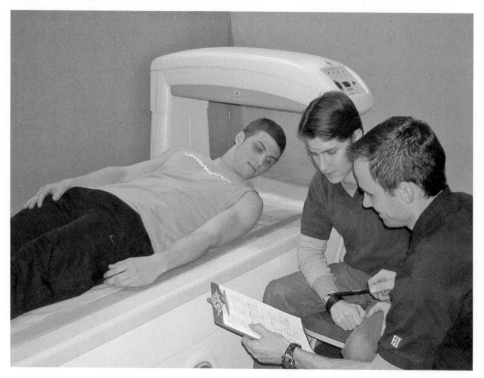

DEXA (Dual X-Ray Absorbpitometry) is a very accurate method of assessing body composition and bone density.

Each technique has its own advantages and disadvantages, and the limitations must be considered in order to achieve applicable results. For example, the Bod Pod has reliable accuracy but is expensive, the bioelectrical impedence analysis is practical but does not accurately assess short-term changes, and skinfold measurements are subject to a high degree of technician error if the technician is not properly trained and experienced. Training on body composition equipment, technique, measurement calcula-

TABLE 3.6 Body Composition Measurement Techniques

Technique	Equipment	Method
Underwater weighing (hydrostatic weighing)	UWW tank	Person is submerged and weighed under water with the assumption that the leaner persons have higher under water weight; whole-body density is calculated from mass and volume, which can then be applied to body fat calculations.
Air displacement (plethysmography)	Plethysmograph (Bod Pod)	Person is seated inside a chamber where the volume of air the person's body displaces is measured; whole-body density is calculated from mass and volume, which can then be applied to body fat calculations.
Dual X-ray absorbpitometry	DEXA machine	Person lies on a table while a low dose X-ray passes through a scanner as it moves across the body; estimates of fat mass, lean body mass, and bone mass are derived.
Bioelectrical impedance analysis (BIA)	BIA machine	Electrodes are attached to the body, which circulate a low-level electrical current; resistance (impedance) to this current is measured and can be applied to body fat calculations.
Skinfold measurements	Calipers	A technician measures folds of skin at specific locations on the body; data can then be used with formulas to predict body fat.

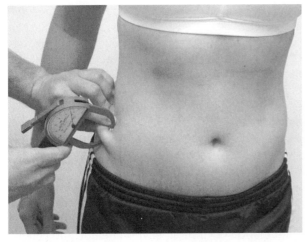

Skinfold calipers are one of the least expensive methods of assessing percent body fat. Amount of subcutaneous fat is typically measured at 3 or 7 sites and translated into a body fat percent estimate using established equations. It is critical that those administrating skinfold analyses are well-trained and practiced to ensure accuracy.

tion, and evaluation of results are important skills for sports nutrition professionals.

Eating Disorders and the Female Athlete Triad

EATING DISORDERS Adopting and maintaining sensible eating habits, regular and appropriate physical activity, along with mastering positive methods to handle emotions and stress are challenging goals for many. This can be especially so for athletes who participate in sports where appearance or body weight can be a factor in performance, such as track, gymnastics, crew, dancing, and wrestling, or for those who may be prone to eating disorders. Genetics and personality traits can play a role in the development of eating disorders. Athletes are encouraged to eat to provide the necessary fuel for performance, yet they often face self- or team-imposed weight restrictions or body image pressures that can put them at risk for developing an **eating disorder** or *disordered eating pattern* (displaying symptoms of abnormal eating behaviors without meeting all criteria for one of the defined eating disorder classes).

Eating disorders are psychological illnesses with medical complications resulting from nutrition-related behaviors. The incidence of eating disorders is on the rise, and such illnesses can be further characterized by severely disturbed food behaviors and eating patterns that are associated with negative body image and excessive concern for body weight or body fat. Three of the most common eating disorders are anorexia nervosa, bulimia nervosa, and binge eating disorder. Criteria for each condition have been outlined by the American Psychological Association in their *Diagnostic and Statistics Manual* (vol. 4), and general symptoms follow.

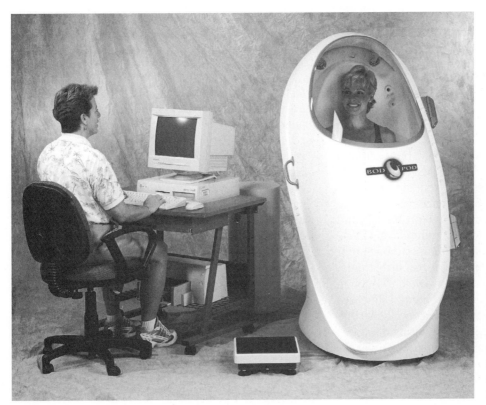

The Bod Pod is an instrument that utilizes air displacement (plethysmography) for body composition analysis. It works similar to principles involved in hydrostatic weighing. Cost is typically >$40,000.

ANOREXIA NERVOSA Anorexia nervosa is characterized by a person's refusal to maintain a minimally healthy body weight coupled with an intense fear of gaining weight or becoming fat. Body image is distorted to the degree of causing regular and often compulsive self-induced starvation. People suffering from anorexia are often extremely thin or emaciated.

Due to the extreme weight loss, anorexia is associated with many health complications and risks. For example, females with anorexia often lose the ability to regularly menstruate, develop low blood pressure and heart rate, and experience digestive problems, insomnia, and weakness. Anorexia also has been linked to more severe health problems including cardiovascular complications, endocrine disorders, increased susceptibility to infection, stress fractures, and chemical imbalances. Anorexia nervosa is often associated with other mental illnesses such as depression (Berkman, Lohr, & Bulik, 2007). Athletes with anorexia nervosa typically cannot complete their normal training regimen and perhaps should not be cleared medically to do so due to the serious nature of their condition. Exercise can cause further weight loss and further stresses organs that may already be affected by the eating disorder.

BULIMIA NERVOSA Bulimia nervosa is characterized by recurrent episodes of binge eating and purging. The binge often results in thousands of calories being rapidly consumed in an out-of-control fashion, followed by an attempt to rid the body of those calories with a purge. The purge can consist of compensatory behaviors such as vomiting, laxative or diuretic abuse, fasting, or excessive exercise. Bulimia is also associated with a loss of control and inability to stop or limit the amount of food being consumed. People suffering from bulimia deal with distorted body image and fear of gaining weight and are often ashamed of their behavior. In contrast to anorexia, a bulimic person is often of average or slightly above average weight for height. The binge-purge cycle poses a tremendous strain on the body. Health consequences can include dehydration, constipation, dental problems, and muscle weakness. If not treated, bulimia can cause chronic hoarseness, esophageal tears, stomach rupture, liver and kidney damage, cardiac arrhythmia, and difficulty maintaining a healthy weight. Bulimia nervosa often times coexists with mental illnesses such as anxiety disorder, obsessive compulsive disorder, or depression. Athletes with eating disorders should be specifically observed for risk of heat illness because hydration and electrolyte status may be impaired.

BINGE EATING DISORDER Binge eating disorder is characterized by binge eating and a lack of control over eating behaviors, followed by feelings of guilt and shame with weight gain. Hunger is rarely the cause for the excessive consumption; rather, food is used as a means of coping with stress or difficult emotions. Binge eaters are often overweight or obese and therefore face all the health risks associated with excessive weight gain and obesity. Rates of depression and anxiety are often higher in people suffering with binge eating disorder (Maughan, 2005).

Eating disorders are more prevalent in women; however, eating disorders also occur in men. There is no one specific cause for eating disorders. A combination of cultural, environmental, and genetic factors determine a person's risk and ultimately development of an eating disorder. This growing health problem requires everyone involved in the care of athletes to be watchful for those who may be prone to eating disorders or who participate in high-risk sports.

Treatment for disordered eating and eating disorders often involves the expertise of an interdisciplinary team that may include a sports dietitian, athletic trainer, physician, psychologist, psychiatrist, and perhaps even the athlete's coach or family.

FEMALE ATHLETE TRIAD Female athletes are at risk for three interrelated medical conditions collectively known as the **female athlete triad.** The triad consists of

- Disordered eating
- Amenorrhea (lack of menstrual periods)
- Low bone mineral density

Disordered eating is the first component of the triad and is marked by an inadequate energy balance. This energy imbalance can result from a diagnosed eating disorder or a failure to nutritionally compensate for increased energy demands due to training and activity. Over time, abnormal eating patterns can lead to malnutrition and poor intake of vitamins and minerals such as Vitamin D and calcium. Disordered eating can lead to *amenorrhea*, which is defined as the lack of menstrual cycles for 3 months or longer. Amenorrhea is a symptom of inadequate hormone function in a female. When monthly periods cease, estrogen production slows and becomes inadequate to continue normal physiologic function. Prolonged amenorrhea results in a weakening of the bones and, ultimately, osteoporosis as normal estrogen levels are needed for bone health. *Osteoporosis* develops due to the lack of estrogen and inadequate intake of the bone building nutrients, calcium, and Vitamin D.

TABLE 3.7 Medical Issues With Nutritional Considerations

Chronic Diseases	Diabetes High blood pressure (hypertension) High cholesterol (hypercholesterolemia)	Kidney disease Osteoporosis Eating disorders
Gastrointestinal Issues	Gastroesophageal reflux disease Gastroenteritis Irritable bowel syndrome	Celiac disease Chrohn's disease
Injury and Rehabilitation	Stress fractures Soft tissue injury	Wound healing Dental injury or surgery
Pharmacological Issues	Medication side effects	Drug nutrient interactions
Other	Sickle cell Iron deficiency anemia	Food allergies Menstrual irregularities

Left untreated, the triad can lead to poor physical and mental performance, an increased risk for fractures and broken bones, and metabolic disturbances. All active females can be at risk for the triad; however, endurance athletes and those who are highly competitive or elite are likely at highest risk.

Medical Issues Facing Athletes

A well-founded knowledge of exercise physiology positions a sports nutrition professional to best understand and manipulate nutritional recommendations for athletes faced with clinical health issues. The nutritional care process in the treatment of disease is termed **medical nutrition therapy** (MNT). The list of diseases amenable to MNT and nutritional intervention continues to grow. With continued research and understanding, in many cases it is possible to both treat and postpone disease progression by incorporating nutrition and exercise strategies. The prevention of degenerative diseases such as cancer, heart disease, hypertension, and osteoporosis is even more substantiated. Consequently, as society's population ages and people become more proactive health consumers, the sports nutrition professional will play a vital role in the care of athletes and active individuals. Table 3.7 presents examples of diseases and health issues with nutritional considerations. It should be recognized that providing MNT for athletes requires a high level of education and training on the systems of the body and the various disease states, as well as proper nutrition therapies and exercise response and adaptation. It is against the law in most states to practice MNT without the proper qualifications (i.e., Registered Dietitian).

Sports Nutrition for Special Populations

Nutrition recommendations are influenced by a number of factors. Age, health status, physiological condition, food preference, and personal beliefs all affect the individual energy needs, micro- and macronutrient requirements, fluid recommendations, and health and performance risk factors. The following populations having specific, specialized nutritional needs:

- Child and adolescent athletes
- Master's athletes
- Pregnant athletes
- Vegetarian/vegan athletes

It is important to have sports dietitians available to design appropriate nutrition recommendations for these populations. Children have many physiologic differences as compared to adults. For example, young athletes have a relative increase in energy expenditure due to decreased movement efficiency (Maughan, 2005). Since growth and physical activity are occurring simultaneously, it is important that nutrient needs are assessed properly. Similarly, older athletes require specific nutritional consideration due to their physiologic progressions. For example, attention to fluids becomes critical due to, among others, an age-related decrease in thirst sensation and a decrease in sweat production resulting from changes in sweat glands (Maughan, 2005). And since exercise and pregnancy are both sources of altered requirements, energy, carbohydrate, protein, fat, and fluid needs are all affected. This can present unique challenges for nutritional assessment. Vegetarian athletes also require special attention and may benefit from specific discussion and planning regarding protein, fat, calcium, iron, and vitamin B-12 intakes in order to optimize health and performance.

Dietary Supplements and Ergogenic Aids

In 1994 Congress amended the Federal Food, Drug, and Cosmetic Act and passed the **Dietary Supplement Health and Education Act** (DSHEA), which established dietary supplement standards. Congress defined dietary supplements as products (other than tobacco) that meet the following criteria:

- Is intended to supplement the diet
- Contains one or more dietary ingredient: including vitamins, minerals, herbs or other botanicals, amino acids, and other substances or their constituents
- Is intended to be taken by mouth as a pill, capsule, tablet, or liquid
- Is labeled on the front panel as being a dietary supplement

Whether a product is classified as a dietary supplement, conventional food, or drug is based on its *intended use*. The DSHEA can be accessed at **http://www.fda.gov/opacom/laws/dshea.html#sec3.** The DSHEA defines the dietary supplement but does not outline industry provisions for quality, accuracy, or purity of label ingredients. Dietary supplements often lack evidence supporting their claims or contain potentially hazardous ingredients or banned substances. Therefore, it is up to the consumer to make informed, educated decisions regarding nutritional supplement use. For the typical athlete, health and safety should be a primary concern when considering supplement use. Many ingredients can interact with prescription medication or cause harmful side effects. Competitive and elite athletes must be equally cautious because many governing sport bodies have banned substances lists and conduct routine drug testing. Many of the banned substances are also ingredients in dietary supplements, (e.g., ephedra and synephrine). Table 3.8. lists the NCAA's 2007–2008 banned substances list. If an athlete tests positive for any of these substances, he or she can be disqualified from competition and rendered ineligible for future events. The issue of supplement contamination with dangerous or banned substances is a concern. Some studies have shown that 15 to 25% of dietary supplements contain ingredients not listed on the label (Maughan, 2005). Sports nutrition professionals need to recognize and understand the lure of improved performance while maintaining a current knowledge and understanding of dietary supplement ingredients so as to make safe and effective recommendations to safeguard the athlete's health and performance.

In many cases, evaluating dietary supplements is challenging because there is little scientific research to back up manufacturers' claims. Creatine, which remains popular with athletes, can be considered an exception. Numerous research studies have linked creatine supplementation with enhanced creatine stores in some athletes, which has been shown to improve performance of repeated, high-intensity exercise (such as brief, exhaustive intervals on a cycle or sets of weight-lifting repetitions). It's important to consider, however, that these claims have not been tested in all ages and populations, and long-term safety is not known. Caffeine is another dietary supplement for which there is some research showing enhanced athletic performance with moderate doses consumed before exercise. Mechanisms for these improvements may be enhanced central nervous system stimulation or increased mobilization of fatty acids. Individuals have very different responses to caffeine, and some side effects are deleterious to performance. With the increased popularity of energy drinks and stimulant-containing dietary supplements, there is concern regarding side effects and possible positive drug tests (high levels of caffeine are banned by the NCAA and other groups).

The media has kept us up-to-date on the incidence of positive drug tests for anabolic steroids and human growth hormone (HGH) in professional athletes. In addition to being banned and illegal, both have numerous health and safety side effects, and athletes should be counseled against use of both steroids and HGH. As drug testing procedures continue to improve and sport governing bodies work to penalize substance abusers, it is likely that use will drop, creating a more level playing field for all.

Enhancing Competitive and Elite Athletic Performance Through Nutrition

Nutrition manipulations can play a direct role in performance enhancement, and some of these strategies have already been mentioned. The following techniques have been effective for some athletes:

- *Carbohydrate loading:* Increasing carbohydrate intake while decreasing physical activity during the 24 to 72 hours before an intense sporting event can increase muscle glycogen stores and improve performance.

TABLE 3.8   2006–2007 NCAA Banned Drug List

Stimulants

Amiphenazole	Doxapram	Pemoline
Amphetamine	Ephedrine (ephedra, ma huang)	Pentetrazol
Bemigride	Ethamivan	Phendimetrazine
Benzphetamine	Ethylamphetamine	Phenmetrazine
Bromantan	Fencamfamine	Phentermine
Caffeine (guarana)	Meclofenoxate	Phenylpropanolamine (ppa)
Chlorphentermine	Methamphetamine	Picrotoxine
Cocaine	Methylene-dioxymethamphetamine	Pipradol
Cropropamide	(MDMA) (Ecstasy)	Prolintane
Crothetamide	Methylphenidate	Strychnine
Diethylpropion	Nikethamide	Synephrine (citrus aurantium, zhi shi,
Dimethylamphetamine	Octopamine	bitter orange) and related compounds*

Anabolic Steroids

Androstenediol	Fluoxymesterone	Oxandrolone
Androstenedione	Gestrinone	Oxymesterone
Boldenone	Mesterolone	Oxymetholone
Clostebol	Methandienone	Stanozolol
Dehydrochlormethyl-testosterone	Methyltestosterone	Testosterone
Dehydroepiandrosterone (DHEA)	Nandrolone	Tetrahydrogestrinone (THG)
Dihydrotestosterone (DHT)	Norandrostenediol	Trenbolone and related compounds*
Dromostanolone	Norandrostenedione	
Epitrenbolone	Norethandrolone	

Other Anabolic Agents

Clenbuterol

Substances Banned for Specific Sport (Rifle)

Alcohol	Nadolol	Timolol and related compounds*
Atenolol	Pindolol	
Metoprolol	Propranolol	

Diuretics and Other Urine Manipulators

Acetazolamide	Finasteride	Polythiazide
Bendroflumethiazide	Flumethiazide	Probenecid
Benzthiazide	Furosemide	Spironolactone (canrenone)
Bumetanide	Hydrochlorothiazide	Triamterene
Chlorothiazide	Hydroflumethiazide	Trichlormethiazide and related
Chlorthalidone	Methyclothiazide	compounds*
Ethacrynic acid	Metolazone	

Street Drugs

Heroin	Marijuana	THC (tetrahydrocannabinol)3

Peptide Hormones and Analogues

Corticotrophin (ACTH)	Human chorionic gonadotrophin	Luteinizing hormone (LH)
Darbepoetin	(hCG)	Sermorelin
Erythropoietin (EPO)	Insulin like growth hormone	
Growth hormone (HGH	(IGF-1)	
somatotrophin)		

Anti-Estrogens

Anastrozole	Clomiphene	Tamoxifen and related compounds

*All the respective releasing factors of the above-mentioned substances also are banned.

Source: National Collegiate Athletic Association (NCAA), 2007.

TABLE 3.9 Sports Nutrition-Related Organizations and Web Sites

Scientific Organizations

American Dietetic Association (ADA)	**www.eatright.org**
Sports Cardiovascular and Wellness Nutritionists (SCAN)	**www.scandpg.org**
American College of Sports Medicine (ACSM)	**www.acsm.org**
International Society of Sports Nutrition (ISSN)	**www.theissn.org**
Academy for Eating Disorders (AED)	**www.aedweb.org**
National Strength and Conditioning Association (NSCA)	**www.nsca-lift.org**
National Athletic Trainer's Association (NATA)	**www.nata.org**

Associated Organizations

International Olympic Committee (IOC)	**www.olympic.org**
National Collegiate Athletic Association (NCAA)	**www.ncaa.org**
Center for Drug Free Sport	**www.drugfreesport.com**
Resource Exchange Center (REC)	**www.drugfreesport.com/REC**
Gatorade Sports Science Institute (GSSI)	**www.gssiweb.org**

■ *Carbohydrate feedings during exercise*: Consuming carbohydrates at a rate of 30 to 60 grams per hour during continuous or stop-and-go exercise lasting 45 minutes to one hour can enhance performance.

■ *Delaying central fatigue*: In addition to providing fuel to last throughout the exercise bout, some research has shown that consuming carbohydrates and maybe even specific amino acids during activity may delay fatigue of the central nervous system.

■ *Pregame meal*: Consuming a pregame meal 3 to 4 hours prior to activity containing about 200 to 300 grams of carbohydrates (low in fiber), with a little protein, and minimal fat can improve performance. Many athletes require guidance in selecting their precompetition meals.

■ *Recovery nutrition*: The immediate postexercise period seems to be an optimal time to restore energy lost during activity and promote muscle gains. Consuming carbohydrates, protein, and fluids during this period can enhance the process.

PROFESSIONAL ORGANIZATIONS

Many well-respected organizations exist to promote and further the field of nutrition for sports and exercise. Most are available to both interested students and practicing sports nutrition (dietetics) professionals offering membership, journal access, newsletters, informational listservs, and various learning opportunities. As with other exercise science-related organizations, membership in sports nutrition-related organizations often include discounted rates to annual meetings and workshops, scholarship opportunities, career mentoring, and networking opportunities. Membership in a professional nutrition organization is a great way to keep abreast of the dynamic field of sports nutrition. Table 3.9 provides a list of the organizations discussed below.

American Dietetic Association (ADA)

The ADA (2007) is the largest organization of nutrition and food professionals in the United States with approximately 65,000 members. The membership includes registered dietitians (RD), dietetic technicians registered (DTR), clinical and community dietetics professionals, food service managers, researchers, educators, and students representing a spectrum of interest and practice areas, one being nutrition for sports and exercise.

There are 29 areas of interest and practice officially represented within the ADA by divisions called Dietetic Practice Groups (DPGs). The field of sports nutrition is recognized within the Sports, Cardiovascular, and Wellness Nutritionists (SCAN) DPG. The SCAN DPG is one of the largest and most active DPGs of the ADA with membership totaling more than 5,300. SCAN's mission is to promote healthy, active lifestyles through dietetic practice (see Box 3.3). The SCAN practice group publishes the quarterly newsletter PULSE, which includes research updates, book reviews, conference offerings and more. They also published *Sports Nutrition: A Practice Manual for Professionals*, *4th edition* (2006) and collaborated with Dietitians of Canada and the American College of Sports Medicine (ACSM) in developing the nutrition and athletic performance position stand (see Box 3.4).

EXPLORE MORE **BOX 3.3**

Sports, Cardiovascular, and Wellness Nutritionists Mission Statement

"The SCAN Dietetic Practice Group is leading the future of dietetics by promoting healthy, active lifestyles through excellence in dietetics practice in sports, cardiovascular, and wellness nutrition, and the prevention and treatment of disordered eating" (SCAN, www.scandpg.org).

EXPLORE MORE **BOX 3.4**

Nutrition and Athletic Performance: Position of the American Dietetic Association, Dietitians of Canada, and the American College of Sports Medicine

"It is the position of the American Dietetic Association, Dietitians of Canada and the American College of Sports Medicine that physical activity, athletic performance and recovery from exercise are enhanced by optimal nutrition. These organizations recommend appropriate selection of food and fluids, timing of intake, and supplement choices for optimal health and exercise performance" (Position of the American Dietetic Association, 2000).

In addition to SCAN's publications, the ADA publishes the *Journal of the American Dietetic Association* (JADA), which often includes original research and articles regarding active individuals as well as competitive athletes. Subscription to the JADA is an example of an ADA membership benefit.

American College of Sports Medicine (ACSM)

The field of sports nutrition represents a blend of nutritional science and exercise science, and ACSM is a valuable organization for students and professionals interested or working with active individuals. ACSM is the largest exercise science and sports medicine organization in the world with more than 20,000 members worldwide. Members represent a variety of people working in various medical specialties, allied health professions, and scientific disciplines. ACSM's official journal, *Medicine and Science in Sports and Exercise*, is a monthly publication that includes original research, clinical studies, and reviews on sports medicine and exercise science topics. The ACSM mission statement can be found at their Web site (**www.ascsm.org**). ACSM also recognizes the role of nutrition in an active lifestyle through the establishment of the Nutrition Interest Group. The interest group allows for focused discussion and active debate within the field of sports nutrition. The nutrition group aims to promote the science of nutrition within ACSM, to be a reliable nutrition resource for the organization, and to critically evaluate nutrition and sport nutrition information in the marketplace.

Understanding the science of exercise is crucial to being able to apply appropriate nutrition concepts and principles to affect an individual's athletic performance or active lifestyle goal. For example, as discussed earlier in this chapter, nutrient requirements differ depending on the energy system being utilized by a person's activity or exercise. Therefore, as an organization that serves to promote the advancement of science relating to physical activity and exercise, ACSM is a well-positioned partner in the field of sports nutrition. Chapter 6 has more information on ACSM.

International Society of Sports Nutrition (ISSN)

The ISSN is a professional organization in the field of sports nutrition. The society promotes and supports the science and applied principles of sports nutrition (Box 3.5). Membership includes annual meeting opportunities, sport nutrition-related certificate eligibility, bimonthly newsletter subscription, access to the peer-reviewed *Journal of the International Society of Sports Nutrition* (JISSN), as well as the opportunity to view job postings in sports nutrition and related fields. The

---

EXPLORE MORE **BOX 3.5**

International Society of Sports Nutrition Mission Statement

"The International Society of Sports Nutrition is the leading professional organization in the field of sports nutrition. The ISSN is dedicated to promoting and supporting the science and application of sports nutrition" (ISSN, www.sportsnutritionsociety.org).

ISSN offers two sports nutrition certificates to qualified individuals: the Certified Sports Nutritionist from the International Society of Sports Nutrition (CISSN) certification and the Body Composition Certification by the International Society of Sports Nutrition (BCC-ISSN). The CISSN and BCC-ISSN certificates are discussed in further detail later in this chapter.

Academy for Eating Disorders (AED)

Nutrition-related behaviors are inherent in eating disorders and are a growing health problem, and the AED is a worldwide eating disorder organization. The AED was established in 1993 with a meeting convened to discuss effects and concerns of managed care and insurance practices on the provision of quality treatment for patients with eating disorders. It has grown and developed into an organization with international membership that promotes effective treatment, develops prevention initiatives, expands and supports research opportunities, and acts as an advocate of the field for those providing, receiving, and supporting eating disorder care (Box 3.6).

EXPLORE MORE **BOX 3.6**

The Academy for Eating Disorders Mission Statement

"The Academy for Eating Disorders is an international transdisciplinary professional organization that promotes excellence in research, treatment and prevention of eating disorders. The AED provides education, training and a forum for collaboration and professional dialogue" (AED, www.aedweb.org).

Membership in AED affords many professional and continuing education benefits as well as access to a worldwide network of eating disorder specialists. Subscription to the *International Journal of Eating Disorders*, the official journal of the AED, is a member benefit along with the quarterly newsletter featuring research, treatment information, job opportunities, and workshop and conference listings. The AED also holds an annual international conference and many seminars and workshops throughout the year.

The AED community offers several avenues for connection and support through the AED listserves, various committee and task force involvement, and Special Interest Group (SIG) participation. SIGs are designed as forums for individuals with a particular interest in a specific topic regarding eating disorders. Two SIGs of specific interest to those working with and interested in

sports nutrition are the Nutrition SIG and Athlete SIG (ASIG). The ASIG was formed in 2001 and is a multidisciplinary association of academic and health care professionals with expertise in the field of eating disorders. The ASIG is founded on the philosophy that athletes are a unique population best served through specialized approaches to identification, treatment, and prevention of eating disorders. They pursue the mission of promoting effective treatment and care of eating disordered athletes by information exchange on listserves, workshops, and conferences and developing and providing education materials to athletes and sport-related personnel.

National Strength and Conditioning Association (NSCA)

Professionals in the field of sports nutrition have ample opportunity and need to interact with related disciplines. One field with a particular interest and requirement for an effective interface is strength and conditioning. Often an athlete's health and performance goals can successfully be reached with dual attention from both the strength and conditioning and nutrition profession. Therefore, the NSCA is a valuable organization for anyone involved and interested in sports nutrition. Membership in the NSCA represents strength coaches, sports scientists, sports medicine and allied health professionals, and many others. This international nonprofit association supports three publications and two professional certifications. The NSCA exists for the common goal of utilizing proper strength training and conditioning to improve athletic performance and fitness (Box 3.7). Refer to Chapter 6 for a detailed discussion of the NSCA.

EXPLORE MORE **BOX 3.7**

National Strength and Conditioning Association Mission Statement

"As the worldwide authority on strength and conditioning, we support and disseminate research-based knowledge and its practical application to improve athletic performance and fitness" (NSCA, www.nsca.org).

National Association of Athletic Trainers (NATA)

Another organization from a related discipline that routinely works closely with sports nutrition professionals is the NATA. The NATA is the professional membership association for certified athletic trainers and those who support the athletic training profession

(Box 3.8). The organization was founded in 1950 and now registers almost 30,000 members worldwide. The NATA is involved with sports nutrition-related topics such as fluid and hydration status and the female athlete triad. The *Journal of Athletic Training* often publishes nutrition-related topics.

EXPLORE MORE **BOX 3.8**

National Athletic Trainer's Association Mission Statement

"The mission of the National Athletic Trainers' Association is to enhance the quality of health care provided by certified athletic trainers and to advance the athletic training profession" (NATA, www.nata.org).

Other Organizations

Several other organizations connect the practice of sports nutrition to the research and governing bodies associated with the field. For example, the International Olympic Committee (IOC) is the foremost authority for the Olympic Games. A Medical Commission was originally formed to oversee anti-doping issues but quickly expanded to incorporate three fundamental principles:

- Protection of the athlete's health
- Respect for both medical and sport ethics
- Equality for all competing athletes

The Medical Commission is now recognized as the main body addressing all medical issues in the Olympic Games. An example of the IOC's involvement in sports nutrition-related topics is the 2005 Consensus Statement and Position Stand on the Female Athlete Triad, which can be accessed at **http://www.olympic.org/uk/organisation/ commissions/medical/.** The commission also serves to advise athletes on the appropriateness of nutritional supplements.

In a similar manner, the National Collegiate Athletic Association (NCAA) is the governing body of its member institutions. The NCAA provides ruling and oversight of nutrition and food-related bylaws and has established permissible and nonpermissble substances that institutions may or may not provide to student athletes. In addition, the NCAA has adopted type and time limits on the provision of foods to athletes. The NCAA also maintains a banned substance list and provides nutrition education materials and guidelines for identification and treatment of nutrition related health issues.

Another valuable resource on the topic of nutritional supplements is the Center for Drug Free Sport. In 2001 the dietary supplement Resource Exchange Center (REC) was created as a part of the center. Its purpose is to offer subscribers a confidential hot line and Web site to answer athletes' questions about dietary supplements and banned substances. Current organizations utilizing the REC include NCAA, the National Football League, Major League Baseball, and the International All-Around Weightlifting Association.

In addition, the Gatorade Sport Science Institute (GSSI) can provide a wealth of knowledge on the latest sport nutrition research by respected scientists and nutrition professionals. The GSSI also dedicates efforts to translate the latest research-based findings into practical recommendations and useable educational tools.

These organizations and centers employ well-qualified researchers and practitioners to help promote their missions and advance the knowledge and application of sport nutrition-related principles. They can be valuable databases for respected information, despite the fact that they do not provide membership.

PROFESSIONAL CERTIFICATIONS

Many of the professional nutrition and nutrition-related organizations discussed offer credentials and certifications that designate special areas of skill and expertise. Obtaining a credential or certification beyond undergraduate education can help facilitate career development by expanding knowledge and skill, increasing marketability, creating employment opportunity options, and possibly justifying salary negotiations. Holding certifications and membership in professional organizations is a valuable attribute in a potential employee as it demonstrates interest in the field and active advancement of the learning process.

Commission on Dietetic Registration

The Commission on Dietetic Registration (CDR) is the major credentialing body of nutrition practitioners and the ADA. The CDR currently offers six distinct credentials. Two relevant credentials to the field of sports nutrition are Registered Dietitian (RD) and Certified Specialist in Sports Dietetics (CSSD). These credentials allow identification of knowledgeable and skilled practitioners in the field of sports nutrition. CDR also offers the Registered Dietetic Technician (DTR) degree as well as a Weight Management Certificate and state licensure.

REGISTERED DIETITIAN (RD) RDs are highly qualified allied health care professionals educated in nutrition and foods. An RD receives specific education and training to provide medical nutrition therapy and nutrition counseling to promote optimal nutrition, health, and well-being. There are several types of dietitians practicing in many different arenas, including hospital dietitians, private practice or consultant dietitians, public health or research dietitians, and, of course, sports dietitians.

RDs have successfully proven the following:

- Completion of a baccalaureate degree by an accredited college or university, or foreign equivalent
- Met current minimum academic requirements (Didactic Program in Dietetics) as approved by the Commission on Accreditation for Dietetics Education (CADE) of the ADA
- Completion of a minimum 900 supervised practice hours of preprofessional experience accredited by CADE
- Successful completion of the Registration Examination for Dietitians
- Remitted the annual registration maintenance fee
- Accrued 75 units of approved continuing professional education every 5 years

BOARD CERTIFIED SPECIALIST IN SPORTS DIETETICS (CSSD) The CSSD credential is designed for RDs who have specialized education, training, and experience in sports nutrition. Being Board Certified as a CSSD designates knowledge, skill, and expert ability in sports dietetics practice. CSSDs, or sports dietitians, apply evidence-based nutrition knowledge to exercise and sport to design, implement, and manage safe and effective nutrition strategies that optimize health, fitness, and performance. Sports dietitians work with athletes and active individuals by utilizing assessment, education, and counseling skills. CSSDs are RDs who have met the following criteria:

- Received current RD status by the Commission on Dietetic Registration
- Held RD status for a minimum of 3 years from original examination date
- Documentation of 1,500 sports specialty practice hours as an RD within the past 5 years

REGISTERED DIETETIC TECHNICIANS (DTRs) DTRs are also credentialed nutrition professionals, and they often work alongside RDs in many

settings. DTRs have completed a 2-year educational program, 450 hours supervised practice, and passed a national exam.

WEIGHT MANAGEMENT CERTIFICATE Successful management of weight and body composition is an important service provided by nutrition professionals, and CDRs weight management certificate can add to the foundation of knowledge and training. The program is open to ADA members, RDs, and DTRs and is designed to produce providers of comprehensive weight management care who also know when and how to refer patients to other specialists. The training program consists of three parts: a self-study module, a 2 ½ day workshop, and a posttest. After successful completion of the course requirements, the Certificate of Training in Adult Weight Management is awarded. Some of the topics covered in the certificate program include the following:

- Clinical management of overweight and obesity
- Medical complications of weight loss
- Behavior modification
- Role of exercise
- Over-the-counter dietary supplements
- Bariatric surgery as a treatment option

STATE LICENSURE In addition to RD credentialing, many states have regulatory licensure laws for dietitians and nutrition practitioners. State licensure helps to ensure that "only qualified, trained professionals provide nutrition services or advice to individuals requiring or seeking nutrition care or information." Licensing is defined by CDR as having statutes that include a defined scope of practice, therefore engaging in this practice without obtaining a license from the state is considered illegal. In 46 states, nutrition counseling is restricted to only those state licensed RDs; nonlicensed practitioners may be subject to prosecution for practicing without a license. In addition, states with certification laws limit the use of particular titles, such as dietitian or nutritionist. Often state licensure requirements are met through the same education and training required to become an RD. A summary of the laws by state of residence can be found at **http://www.eatright.org/ada/files/STATE_LICENSURE_SUMMARY_7_07_PDF.pdf.**

International Society of Sports Nutrition

As described earlier in this chapter, the ISSN offers two sports nutrition-related certifications.

Neither the CISSN nor the BCC-CISSN is restricted by prerequisite credentials or certifications, and RD status is not required. The society recognizes the need for any health or fitness professional working with athletes to possess a "fundamental understanding of the adaptive response to exercise and the role that nutrition plays in the acute and chronic response to exercise" (ISSN, 2007). The CISSN or the BCC-ISSN could be used by all of the following professionals:

- Exercise physiologists
- Health/medical professionals
- Nurse practitioners
- Certified personal trainers
- Strength and conditioning professionals
- Sports dietitians

CERTIFIED SPORTS NUTRITIONIST FROM THE INTERNATIONAL SOCIETY OF SPORTS NUTRITION (CISSN)
CISSNs must satisfy one of the two following criteria to qualify to take the CISSN examination:

- Hold a 4-year undergraduate degree in exercise science, kinesiology, physical education, nutrition, biology, or related biological science

or

- Have earned the CSCS (Certified Strength and Conditioning Specialist) from the National Strength and Conditioning Association

Criteria for those who do not meet the initial qualifications are available. It should be noted that only registered dietitians are legally allowed to provide medical nutrition therapy (MNT).

BODY COMPOSITION CERTIFICATION BY THE INTERNATIONAL SOCIETY OF SPORTS NUTRITION (BCC-ISSN)
One must pass a three-part practical exam to earn the BCC-ISSN. The exam includes skinfold measurements, girth measurements, and calculations of body composition variables. Either of the following requirements must be met for exam eligibility:

- Bachelor's degree in exercise science, nutrition, biology, or a related field

or

- Hold a valid CISSN, CSCS (Certified Strength and Conditioning Specialist), or NSCA-CPT (Certified Personal Trainer) certification

As with the CISSN, eligibility requirements are available if neither of the above criteria are met.

Advanced Degree Programs in Sports Nutrition

In addition to specialized sports nutrition credentials and certifications, there are many advanced degree programs with dedicated sports nutrition curriculums. The SCAN DPG Web site publishes a list of academic institutions offering courses and degree programs in sports nutrition and exercise. The December 2006 Internet update lists 47 institutions, their contact information, and available degree programs.

EMPLOYMENT OPPORTUNITIES

Strong recommendations for appropriate food choice and physical activity coupled with society's impending health status issues continues to create a marketplace with an increasing interest and demand for professionals who can consolidate the knowledge and practice of nutrition and physical activity. Sports nutrition professionals will be particularly well positioned in the job market for years to come and will be presented with a variety of employment options and career possibilities.

Sports nutrition professionals can be found working in a variety of settings, including positions within fitness clubs, corporate wellness facilities, sports organizations, food companies, university health centers, cardiac rehabilitation programs, sports medicine and family practice clinics, and more. Choosing to complete an advanced degree program can further opportunities in education, research, and management. Whichever career environment one pursues, being able to help people make healthful food choices and achieve their personal goals can be a gratifying career experience. Table 3.10 lists some of the available sports nutrition career settings; most require RD status.

SUMMARY

Consuming, absorbing, and utilizing foods and fluids are processes that outline the scope of human nutrition. The role the various nutrients and nutrient combinations, quantities, and ratios play in the health and performance of athletes defines the foundation of the sports nutrition field. The field arrived on the scientific scene in the mid-1900s and has grown into a well-respected and dynamic state of research and development. Findings of the past decades have left us with evidence-based guidelines and recommendations that help fuel, hydrate, and optimize the health of even the most elite of athletes. Topics

TABLE 3.10 Job Settings for Sports Nutrition Professionals

Setting	General Job Functions
Professional Sports Teams	Provide individual nutrition counseling, conduct seminars, design menus, implement game time nutrition strategies, evaluate supplements.
Collegiate Athletic Departments	Provide individual nutrition counseling, make team presentations, design menus, implement game time nutrition strategies, write policies and procedures, evaluate supplements.
Health Clubs/Fitness Centers	Work with clients, design health promotion programs, perform body composition assessments, present workshops.
Corporate Wellness Programs	Design health promotion programs, participate in health fairs and screenings, facilitate treatment groups, conduct classes, present seminars, work with clients.
Sports Medicine Clinics	Assess patient needs for rehabilitation, provide individual nutrition counseling, evaluate dietary supplements, present community seminars.
Family Practice Clinics	Assess patient needs for active population and clinical needs, provide individual nutrition counseling, evaluate dietary supplements, present community seminars.
Cardiac Rehabilitation Clinics	Prescribe individual nutrition plans for clinical needs, assess biochemical tests, provide nutrition counseling, conduct group workshops.
Private Practice	Provide individual nutrition counseling for clients, facilitate groups, present seminars.
Private Consulting	Assess client needs, provide recommendations, conduct seminars, serve as an external expert.
Academia	Teach courses, conduct research, write and publish print and other media, serve as a community resource.
Food Companies	Assist research and development, design marketing plans, evaluate new products, serve as a liason to consumers.

generally studied include energy balance, macro- and micronutrients, fluids and electrolytes, weight control strategies, body composition analysis, dietary supplements, and ergogenic aids. Sports nutrition courses also address the needs and concerns of those athletes with eating disorders or other medical issues and those populations that have special requirements and recommendations.

Many professional organizations exist to further the development and understanding of the field and to serve the continuing education needs of students, clinicians, and educators. The ADA, ACSM, ISSN, and AED are well established. Several other organizations form collaborative networks and allies for the field of sports nutrition (e.g., NSCA and NATA). Career and employment opportunities are in an exciting state of growth, and the field offers many different work environments to choose from. Today, sports dietitians work with professional and collegiate teams, in health clubs, wellness programs, and sports medicine clinics, with family practice and cardiac rehabilitation clinics, or establish private practice or consulting opportunities. Still others work in academia or with corporate food companies in various capacities.

■ Key Resources

Key Journals

Canadian Journal of Applied Physiology
European Journal of Applied Physiology
Exercise and Sport Sciences Reviews
International Journal of Eating Disorders
International Journal of Sport Nutrition and Exercise Metabolism

Journal of Applied Physiology
Journal of Strength and Conditioning Research
Journal of the American Dietetic Association
Journal of the International Society of Sports Nutrition
Medicine and Science in Sports and Exercise

Key Websites

General Nutrition

American Dietetic Association (http://www.eatright.org)

Sports Nutrition

Australian Institute of Sport Sports Nutrition (http://www.ais.org.au/nutrition/)

Gatorade Sports Science Institute (http://www.gssiweb.org)

International Society of Sports Nutrition (http://www.sportsnutritionsociety.org)

Iowa State University Extension, Eat to Compete, Sport Nutrition (http://www.extension.iastate.edu/nutrition/sport/)

SCAN: Sports, Cardiovascular and Wellness Nutritionists (ADA Practice Group) (http://www.scandpg.org)

University of Arizona Nutrition, Exercise, and Wellness (http://nutrition.arizona.edu/new/publications.phtml)

University of Illinois Extension, Sports Nutrition (http://www.urbanext.uiuc.edu/hsnut/)

Eating Disorders

Anorexia Nervosa and Related Eating Disorders, Inc. (ANRED), Athletes and Eating Disorders (http://www.anred.com/ath.html)

National Eating Disorders Association (http://www.edap.org)

National Institute of Mental Health (NIMH) Eating Disorder Information (http://www.nimh.nih.gov/publicat/eatingdisorders.cfm)

Dietary Supplements

American Botanical Council (http://abc.herbalgram.org)

Consumer Lab (http://www.consumerlab.com)

Herbmed (http://www.herbmed.org)

Natural Medicines Comprehensive Database (http://www.naturaldatabase.com)

National Center for Drug Free Sport, Inc. (http://www.drugfreesport.com)

NCAA Banned Drug List and Bylaw 16.5.2.2 (http://www.ncaa.org)

Office of Dietary Supplements (http://dietary-supplements.nih.gov/)

President's Council on Physical Fitness Anabolic Steroids and Athletes (http://www.fitness.gov/Digest-March2005.pdf)

■ Review Questions

1. Describe the distinction between general nutrition and sports nutrition.
2. What type of work requires Registered Dietitian (RD) status?
3. If a particular food item contains 100 kcals from protein, how many grams of protein does it have? Which nutrient provides the greatest kcals per gram?
4. Calculate the average daily energy expenditure for a 175-pound moderately active male.
5. What is the recommended macronutrient breakdown for exercising individuals (expressed in %)?
6. Describe some symptoms of protein deficiency? Of iron deficiency?
7. Give two examples of foods containing the following fats: saturated, trans, unsaturated.
8. Describe the general fluid needs before, during, and after activity.
9. Explain the benefits of evaluating body composition during a weight loss or weight gain program.
10. List the three components of the female athlete triad.
11. List several issues individuals should consider prior to taking dietary supplements.
12. What is the primary certification for individuals qualified to provide individualized nutrition counseling? What letters would these people list after their names?
13. What are two key concepts from the Nutrition and Athletic Performance Position Stand?
14. What does the ADA list as SCAN DPG member benefits?
15. There are currently 114 advanced degree nutrition programs. Does the ADA list an accredited advanced nutrition degree or dietetics program in your home state?
16. What do Part 1 and Part 2 measure on the BCC-ISSN certification practical exam?
17. What are three tips the SCAN DPG recommends for beginning a career in sports nutrition?
18. Which state currently offers the most sports nutrition degree programs?

■ References

American Dietetic Association. (2007). Eatright.org. Retrieved February 2007, from http://www.eatright.org/cps/rde/xchg/ada/hs.xsl/index.html

Berkman, N. D., Lohr, K. N., & Bulik, C. M. (2007, May). Outcomes of eating disorders: A systematic review of the literature. *International Journal of Eating Disorders*, 40(4), 293–309.

Berning, J. R., & Steen, S. N (1998). *Nutrition for sport & exercise* (2nd ed.). Gaithersburg, MD: Aspen.

Centers for Disease Control and Prevention. (2007, July 27). U.S. obesity trends 1985–2006. Retrieved February 10, 2007, from http://www.cdc.gov/nccdphp/dnpa/obesity/trend/maps/index.htm

Commission on Dietetic Registration. (2007). Laws that regulate dietitians/nutritionists. Retrieved February 10, 2007, from http://www.cdrnet.org/certifications/licensure/index.htm

Dunford, M. (2006). *Sports nutrition: A practice manual for professionals* (4th ed.). Chicago, IL: American Dietetic Association.

Ebine, N., Rafamantanantosa, H. H., Nayuki, Y., Yamanakak, K., Tashima, K., Ono, T., Sactoh, S., & Jones, P. J. (2002, May). Measurement of total energy expenditure by the doubly labeled water method in professional soccer players. *Journal of Sports Science*, 20(5), 391–397.

Foster-Powell, K., Holt, S. H., & Brand Miller, J. C. (2002). International tables of glycemic index and glycemic load values: 2002. *American Journal of Clinical Nutrition*, 76, 55–56.

International Society of Sports Nutrition. (2007). Sportsnutritionsociety.org. Retrieved February 2007, from http://www.sportsnutritionsociety.org/site/index.php

Knechtle, B., Enggist, A., & Jehle, T. (2005, July–August). Energy turnover at the Race Across AMerica (RAAM)—a case report. *International Journal of Sports Medicine, 26*(6), 499–503.

Koh-Banerjee, P., & Rimm, E. B. (2003, February). Whole grain consumption and weight gain: A review of the epidemiological evidence, potential mechanisms and opportunities for future research. *Proceedings of the Nutrition Society, 62*(1), 25–29.

Maughan, R. J. (2005). Contamination of dietary supplements and positive drug tests in sport. *Journal of Sports Science, 23*(9), 883–889.

Murray, B. (2006). Fluid, electrolytes, and exercise. In M. Dunford (Ed.), *Sports nutrition: A practice manual for professionals* (4th ed.). Chicago, IL: American Dietetic Association.

National Collegiate Athletic Association. (2007). NCAA banned drugs classes 2006–2007. Retrieved February 10, 2007, from http://www1.ncaa.org/membership/ed_outreach/health-safety/drug_testing/banned_drug_classes.pdf

Position of the American Dietetic Association, Dietitians of Canada, and the American College of Sports Medicine: Nutrition and athletic performance. (2000, December). *Journal of the American Dietetic Association, 100*(12), 1543–1556.

Ravussin, E., & Bogardus, C. (1989). Relationship of genetics, age and physical fitness to daily energy expenditure and fuel utilization. *American Journal of Clinical Nutrition, 49,* 968–975.

Stover, E. A. (2006). Consistently high urine specific gravity in adolescent American football players and the impact of an acute drinking strategy. *International Journal of Sports Medicine, 27,* 330–335.

Tarnopolsky, M. A., Atkinson, S. A., MacDougall, J. D., Chesley, A., Phillips, S., & Schwarez, H. P. (1992, November). Evaluation of protein requirements for trained strength athletes. *Journal of Applied Physiology, 73*(5), 1986–1995.

Thompson, J. L. & Manore, M. M. (1996). Predicted and measured resting metabolic rate of male and female endurance athletes. *Journal of the American Dietetic Association, 96,* 30–34.

Trappe, S., Trappe, T., & Costill, D. (1997, July). Energy expenditure of swimmers during high volume training. *Medicine and Science in Sports and Exercise, 29*(7), 950–954.

Volpe, S. L. (2006). Vitamins, minerals, and exercise. In M. Dunford (Ed.), *Sports nutrition: A practice manual for professionals* (4th ed.). Chicago, IL: American Dietetic Association.

Watson, T. (2006). Commentary B: The science of antioxidants and exercise performance. In L. Burke & V. Deakin (Eds.), *Clinical sports nutrition* (3rd ed.). Sydney: McGraw-Hill.

Williams, M. (2006). *Nutrition for health, fitness, and sport* (8th ed.). San Francisco: McGraw-Hill.

PART 3

Exploring the Behavioral

CHAPTER 4
Exercise and Sport Psychology
Gregory Wilson, PED, FACSM, University of Evansville

CHAPTER 5
Motor Learning and Motor Control
Kelly Cole, PhD, University of Iowa

Exercise and sport psychology and motor behavior comprise the behavioral knowledge base of exercise science. Exercise and sport psychology is a rapidly growing field of study that examines both the relationship of exercise participation to mental health and the various mental factors that influence athletic performance. Exercise and sport psychology originated from an area of psychology known as motor behavior, which studies various neural and behavioral factors associated with learning movement skills. The chapters in Part 2 describe the behavioral and neural aspects of exercise participation and how we learn to perform complex physical activities. Chapter 4 explores the relationship between regular exercise participation and mental well-being, as well as factors associated with positive adherence to an exercise program. The second half of this chapter discusses mental factors such as anxiety, motivation, confidence, mental imagery, and goal setting, which are associated with improvements in sport performance. Chapter 5 surveys the areas of motor learning, motor control, and motor development that make up the subdiscipline of motor behavior. Concepts such as sensory integration, brain plasticity, postural control, conditions for optimal learning, and the principles of skill learning are central to an understanding of motor behavior and are discussed in this chapter.

CHAPTER 4

Exercise and Sport Psychology

Gregory Wilson, PED, FACSM, University of Evansville

■ Chapter Objectives

After reading this chapter, you should be able to:

1. Define the terms *exercise psychology* and *sport psychology* and relate their significance to the exercise science curriculum.

2. Provide a brief overview of the history of exercise and sport psychology, including the "father of American sport psychology."

3. Describe the typical course content taught in most exercise and sport psychology classes, including personality characteristics associated with athletes and how they influence sport performance and performance enhancement techniques used in sport psychology.

4. Identify important peer-reviewed journals in the field of exercise and sport psychology.

5. List the important professional organizations in exercise and sport psychology.

6. Explain the various academic and career possibilities available for students interested in exercise and sport psychology.

■ Key Terms

acute exercise
adherence
catastrophe model
chronic exercise
distraction hypothesis
endorphins
extrinsic motivation
health belief model
Iceberg Profile

individualized zone of optimal
 functioning (IZOF) model
intrinsic motivation
inverted-U hypothesis
mental health model
monoamine hypothesis
outcome goals
performance goals
process goals

profile of mood states (POMS)
psychoneuromuscular theory
reversal theory
state anxiety
theory of planned behavior
thermogenic hypothesis
trait anxiety
transthoretical model

The study of human behavior is complex, and when the stresses of athletic competition are included, behavioral responses become important ingredients to success. Moreover, there is a growing recognition of the role exercise plays in a person's mental well-being. As is the case with the other subdisciplines of exercise science, the field of exercise and sport psychology encompasses a wide variety of clinical, research, educational, and applied activities, focusing on the relationship of physical activity to mental well-being and various mental factors related to performance enhancement.

Recently a great deal of interest has been given to the role of exercise on mental states and how exercise affects mood states and feelings of depression and levels of anxiety. Increasing evidence points to a positive association between mental health and exercise; however, causal explanations for this relationship have not yet been adequately determined. The first part of this chapter examines the role of exercise and mental health and explores several popular theories explaining this association. In addition, this section looks at the problem of exercise adherence and how behavioral issues affect exercise participation.

Enhancing individual levels of sport performance is often considered the primary focus of sport psychology, and the second half of this chapter examines how psychological variables may affect sport performance. For instance, it is believed that a wide variety of factors, ranging from personality differences to individual levels of precompetition anxiety, may directly affect how an athlete performs. Issues related to performance enhancement such as motivation, confidence, mental imagery, and goal setting are important contributors to athletic success, and this chapter examines the influence of each.

In the exercise science curriculum, it is difficult to separate physiological and mental aspects of human responses. Hence, knowledge of cognitive factors related to both exercise and sport performance is important to the understanding of both exercise participation and sport success. Often, exercise and sport psychology courses are taught as upper-level classes in the junior or senior year of study, and advanced classes are typically required of most exercise science graduate programs as well.

BRIEF HISTORY OF EXERCISE AND SPORT PSYCHOLOGY

The historical beginnings of sport psychology can be found in the writings of the ancient Greeks and Romans who referred to the mind–body relationship. However, the true empirical beginnings of this science can be identified with a reaction-time experiment conducted by Besell in 1796. He found individual differences in reaction time as astronomers attempted to record stellar events by determining when a star moved through the cross hairs of their telescopes (Boring, 1950). In fact, much of the early research in psychology was done in the area of *motor psychology*, which can be considered the forerunner to what we today call sport psychology.

American psychologist William James published an important textbook in 1890 called *Principles of Psychology*. James was influenced by work in motor psychology, and he felt that motor explanations for both emotions and cognitions provided the basis for understanding human behavior. In fact, James suggested that the physiological and muscular process that occurs simultaneously with emotions such as fear or sadness strongly influences our interpretations of these feelings (Kroll & Lewis, 1970).

However, the beginning of sport psychology in North America is often attributed to an experiment conducted by Norman Triplett in 1897 (Weinberg & Gould, 2003). Triplett was a psychologist at Indiana University who was interested in *social facilitation*, or how the presence of other people affects how an individual performs. To study the effects of an audience on participation, Triplett (1898) reviewed the racing records of cyclists and discovered that those races that were paced produced times 25% faster than times in unpaced races. Triplett next performed an experiment in which he required young children to reel in a fishing line as quickly as possible. Children did this both alone and in the presence of another child, and once again Triplett found that times were faster when another individual was present (Kroll & Lewis, 1970). This landmark study is often considered an important event in the history of sport-related research in the United States.

The founder of the modern Olympic movement, Baron de Coubertin, wrote *Essays in Sport Psychology* in 1913, in which he promoted sport as a means to better overall emotional well-being (Vanek & Cratty, 1970). A variety of other similar philosophical writings appeared throughout the early 20th century, that supported the association of physical activity and mental health, but little empirical work was done until the arrival of Coleman Roberts Griffith at the University of Illinois.

Griffith is often acclaimed as America's first sport psychologist and given the title of "father of American sport psychology" (Kroll & Lewis, 1970). In 1925 Griffith became the director for the Athletic Research Laboratory, funded by the University of Illinois Athletic Department. He wrote two classic books, *Psychology of Coaching* (1926) and *Psychology of Athletics* (1928), while teaching courses in sport psychology at the university and working with its athletic teams. Griffith also corresponded with legendary Notre Dame football coach Knute Rockne about psyching up and motivation techniques, both of which Rockne was renowned for using with his football teams. Perhaps his best remembered work was done with Red Grange, the famous Illinois and future NFL Hall of Fame running back. Griffith wanted to know what Grange thought about while playing in a game, and his observations lead to what is known as the *automatic skill response theory*, which purported that as performance increases, cognition decreases. Few sport psychologists picked up where Griffith left off, and most academic programs in the United States continued to rely primarily on studies conducted in work physiology and biomechanics as the foundation for their sport psychology curriculum (Kroll & Lewis, 1970).

The next major event took place during the 1963 Sports Medicine Congress in Barcelona when the first discussions concerning the formation of the International Congress of Sport Psychology (ICSP) were held (Kroll & Lewis, 1970). By 1965 this idea came to fruition with the initial meeting held in Rome, and Feruccio Antonelli was elected the first president of the ICSP. In 1966 the North American Society for Psychology in Sport and Physical Activity (NASPSPA) was formed in the United States, and a year later the first NASPSPA conference was convened. The Canadian Society for Psychomotor Learning and Sport was founded in 1969. During this time, Bryant Cratty, a highly respected professor at UCLA, published the *Psychology of Physical Activity* (1968), which became the leading textbook in the field.

There have been several other important professional milestones in terms of organizations related to exercise and sport psychology. The American Psychological Association (APA), representing the largest psychological organization in the world, formed the Exercise and Sport Psychology Interest Group (Division 47) in 1983. The Association for Applied Sport Psychology (AASP) was founded in 1986 and has since become the largest applied sport psychology organization worldwide. In 1991 the AASP established a "certified consultant" program, which specifically trains sport psychologists to work with athletes. In 1995 the American College of Sports Medicine (ACSM) established the Psychobiology and Behavior Interest Group to promote the advancement and knowledge of exercise and sport psychology.

Today, it is estimated that more than 2,700 exercise and sport psychologists are working in a variety of exercise and sport-related settings (Salmela, 1992). College and professional teams are increasingly utilizing the knowledge provided by sport psychologists, and since 1985 the U.S. Olympic organization has hired full-time sport psychologists (Weinberg & Gould, 2003). Moreover, the field of sport psychology has grown to include not only work in sport performance enhancement but also work in exercise psychology in which researchers examine the effects of physical activity on mental health. Influential exercise and sport psychologists have many areas of interest today, including exercise and mental health (William Morgan, University of Wisconsin; Jack Raglin, Indiana University; Patrick O'Connor, University of Georgia; Rod Dishman, University of Georgia; and Steven Pettuzzello, University of Illinois), goal setting with athletes (Robert Weinberg, Miami University), and anxiety and performance (Yuri Hanin, Finland; Daniel Gould, Michigan State University; and Daniel Landers, Arizona State University).

GENERAL COURSE CONTENT

Most courses in exercise and sport psychology are typically structured along two lines: how mental factors affect athletic performance and the relationship of exercise to mental health. Topics commonly include the following:

- Exercise and mental health
- Exercise adherence
- Personality characteristics and athletic performance
- Preperformance anxiety and sport performance
- Performance enhancement techniques

A variety of other topics may be covered in exercise and sport psychology classes, including the effects of positive and negative reinforcement on motivation, disordered eating behavior in athletes, career termination, focus, perceived exertion, and the psychology of sport injuries.

EXERCISE PSYCHOLOGY COURSE CONTENT

Exercise psychology examines such questions as the relationship between physical activity and mental health, behavioral factors related to exercise adherence, and perceived exertion. This section provides an overview of the relationship of exercise to mental health and discusses possible explanations for this relationship.

Exercise and Mental Health

In addition to having a positive impact on physical well-being, exercise has long been thought to have the potential to influence human moods and emotions. In recent years, research has sought to examine the relationship between exercise and mental health, particularly as it relates to anxiety and depression.

When examining the effects of physical activity on mental health, research has generally looked at either changes associated with **acute exercise** (a single exercise session) or **chronic exercise** (long-term participation in an exercise program) (Raglin, Wilson, & Galper, 2006). In exercise and mental health research, investigators measure psychological responses to both acute and chronic exercise through questionnaires given to the exercise participant. Typically, these questionnaires measure aspects of mental health such as anxiety or mood states. In the case of acute exercise, researchers use questionnaires that measure transitory emotions known as **states** that can quickly change in intensity in a few moments or seconds (Raglin, 1997). Acute exercise research has also examined different types of activity that have varied in duration from as long as 9 hours (e.g., triathlon) to as short as 5 minutes (Petruzzello, Landers, Hatfield, Kubitz, & Salazar, 1991).

On the other hand, research in chronic exercise involves the evaluation of stable psychological measures known as **traits.** Traits reveal how a person generally feels and are not changed through an acute exercise bout. Since traits are considered stable, exercise programs of long duration are used when measuring the health benefits of physical activity (Raglin, et al., 2006). Results from this research have demonstrated that chronic exercise programs often produce positive mental health benefits for participants who suffer from mild to moderate forms of anxiety of depression (Raglin, et al., 2006). Interestingly, for individuals suffering from mild to moderate levels of depression, both aerobic and anaerobic forms of exercise appear to be beneficial. However, for those suffering from mild to moderate anxiety, only aerobic exercise seems to lead to improved mental health (Raglin, et al., 2006).

The measurement of psychological outcomes of acute or chronic exercise has mostly been conducted using a standardized inventory of mood states known as the Profile of Mood States (McNair, Lorr, & Dropplemann, 1992), or anxiety such as the State-Trait Anxiety Inventory (Spielberger, Gursuch, Lushene, Vagg, & Jacobs, 1983).

While exercise is generally regarded as having a positive effect on mental health, there is data that suggests it may also negatively impact mental well-being (Raglin, et al., 2006). For instance, prolonged periods of intense training, known as overtraining, have been associated with negative mood changes in some athletes (Raglin & Wilson, 2000). Overtraining research indicates a dose-response relationship exists between training and mood and that increases in training can lead to negative mood alterations in athletes, which can lead to a condition known as staleness (Raglin & Wilson, 2000).

EXPLAINING THE MENTAL HEALTH BENEFITS OF EXERCISE Even though an increasing amount of research supporting the notion that exercise is associated with improvements in mental health has been done in recent years, the reasons for these positive effects have not been identified (Raglin, 1997; Raglin et al., 2006). This section presents a brief overview of the current physiological and cognitive mechanisms that have been proposed as explanations for the psychological benefits of exercise.

Several neuroscientific studies have provided possible explanations of why exercise may improve mood and reduce symptoms of depression and anxiety. A prominent neurochemical hypothesis is that certain endogenous opioids such as endorphins may play a significant role in the mental health benefits associated with exercise. **Endorphins** are chemical substances produced by the brain, pituitary glands, and other bodily tissues. Endorphins act as natural opiates in the body and have been linked to positive emotions. Any sort of physical stress, such as exercise, can stimulate the production of endorphins, and this has led many researchers to conclude that endorphins are responsible for the popular phenomenon known as the "runners' high." However, conflicting findings have been reported concerning the effects of endorphins following bouts of exercise. This remains a popular theory, and one often mentioned in the popular media, but it is difficult to prove its efficacy (Raglin et al., 2006).

A second chemical change that has been proposed is known as the **monoamine hypothesis.** Monoamines are neurotransmitters such as norepinephrine (NE), dopamine, and serotonin (5-HT) that are believed to play a role in depression. Similar to the endorphin hypothesis, it has been suggested that physical activity may increase production of these brain monoamines, causing positive changes in mood. However, as with the endorphin hypothesis, research in this area is inconclusive. Some animal studies have shown that increases in central and peripheral levels of monoamine hormones occur following exercise, but such findings cannot necessarily be generalized to humans (Raglin et al., 2006).

A third physiologic explanation is the **thermogenic hypothesis,** which suggests that the increase in body temperature associated with vigorous exercise can stimulate neurological changes that are associated with improved mood. Studies have shown reduction in muscular tension and anxiety following elevations in body temperature, and it is thought that exercise may provide the same therapeutic effect (Raglin, 1997). However, once again, studies examining this hypothesis have not shown a direct cause-effect relationship of temperature to the mood changes that occur following exercise (Raglin et al., 2006).

In addition to these physiological explanations, other cognitive or behavioral factors such as social interaction and support, feelings of achievement, self-mastery, and distraction have been suggested as being responsible for the mental health improvements associated with exercise. For instance, the **distraction hypothesis** suggests that exercise results in psychological benefits because it typically is performed in a setting that removes the individual from the cause of stress (e.g., workplace or other stressful environments), resulting in relaxation or a form of pleasant diversion (Raglin et al., 2006).

Researchers in exercise psychology currently have not agreed on a single explanation for the positive association of participation in physical activity and mental health. Because of the complexity of this relationship, it is possible that no single explanation can truly explain this phenomenon. In fact, multiple mechanisms may interact together to produce such positive effects (Raglin et al., 2006).

Exercise Adherence

In addition to the mental health benefits of participation in physical activity, the physical benefits of exercise are well known. However, it is estimated that only 25% of adults in the United States are active enough to maintain fitness levels (U.S. Department of Health and Human Services, 2000). Moreover, for those who do start an exercise program, roughly 50% will drop out within the first 6 months (Buckworth & Dishman, 2002). Discovering how to get people started on an exercise program, and keep them on a regular program once initiated, is another important area for exercise psychology.

Adherence refers to conforming to a standard of behavior that has been set as a part of a program. Research in exercise behavior generally defines adherence as regular participation in an exercise program that reaches 60 to 80% attendance (Buckworth & Dishman, 2002). The reasons some people are successful in adhering to an exercise program and others are not often revolve around behavioral issues.

Exercise psychology attempts to explain the process of exercise participation and adherence through theoretical models. The **health belief model** suggests the chances of a person participating in positive health behaviors (like physical activity) depends on individual beliefs about the importance of good health and the likelihood of developing a health-related problem (Weinberg & Gould, 2003). A second theoretical model states that intentions are the best predictor of future action. This model, called the **theory of planned behavior,** suggests that intentions are related to a person's attitude toward a specific behavior and the norms concerning this behavior. Hence, if people believe that exercise is good, and that others will look favorably upon their exercise participation, then they are more likely to adhere to an exercise program (Ajzen & Fishbein, 1980). The

transtheoretical model suggests that people go through stages of change (Prochaska, DiClemente, & Norcross, 1992). According to this model, a person passes through six stages in any lifestyle change: (1) precontemplation stage, (2) contemplation stage, (3) preparation stage, (4) action stage, (5) maintenance stage, and (6) termination stage.

Theories such as those discussed here assist in understanding the process in adopting an exercise program, but the exercise psychologist is still left with the question of who is most likely to start a regimen. To answer this question, we need to examine *behavioral determinants*, or factors that influence whether or not a person will exercise. In general, determinants can be divided into two categories: personal and environmental determinants. *Personal determinants* include things such as gender, self-efficacy, health knowledge, socioeconomic status, and lifestyle behaviors. *Environmental determinants* include concerns such as social support, access to facilities, weather, and the characteristics of the exercise program itself; that is, its intensity, duration, mode, and frequency (Willis & Campbell, 1992). Any number of personal and environmental determinants may act singly or together to influence the chances that a person will participate in physical activity.

Given the difficulty of exercise adherence, a number of behavioral strategies have been suggested to increase participation. For instance, positive reinforcement such as awarding incentives (such as T-shirts or discount tokens) and awards for attendance are often used to motivate individuals. Social support, such as group exercise or working out with a friend, also seems to foster higher adherence rates. Setting goals (such as weight loss or smoking cessation) have shown to be effective in maintaining regular exercise participation, as has the enthusiasm of the exercise leader in a group program (Weinberg & Gould, 2003).

Exercise adherence is an important issue in today's society. With an increasing number of Americans overweight and inactive, ways to involve and keep them exercising is important. Continued research in exercise psychology is needed to identify ways to make exercise more meaningful to those not engaged in an exercise routine.

SPORT PSYCHOLOGY COURSE CONTENT

Whereas exercise psychology focuses on how mental health can be improved through physical activity, sport psychology looks at those mental factors related to improving sport performance. This section examines how mental factors such as anxiety, confidence, motivation, goal setting, and mental imagery may affect athletic performance.

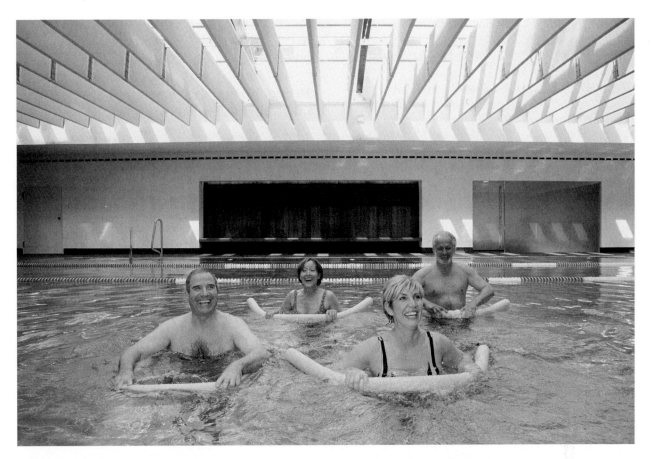

Exercise adherence rates are very low, but social support, such as group exercise or working out with a friend, seems to foster higher adherence rates.

Personality Characteristics and Athletic Performance

The association between personality traits and sport performance is one of the most discussed topics in sport psychology. Although most coaches and athletes believe an athlete's personality plays an important role in sporting success, the empirical evidence for this relationship has not always confirmed this (Raglin & Wilson, in press). The earliest studies that looked at this relationship found that athletes who were successful were generally more extroverted and emotionally stable (Cooper, 1969; Warburton & Kane, 1966). However, research conducted during the following decade offered very different conclusions. These studies suggested that personality had little or no impact on athletic performance (Martens, 1975; Rushall, 1970).

Fortunately, Morgan (1978, 1980) was able to reconcile these conflicting findings by demonstrating that much of the research that rejected the role of personality in sport had a variety of methodological problems. In fact, when such problems were carefully controlled, Morgan discovered that athletes did indeed exhibit unique personality traits when compared to nonathletes.

Morgan (1985) later extended these findings into what he called the **mental health model** of sport performance. The mental health model states that a negative relationship exists between psychopathology and performance. In other words, athletes who are depressed, anxious, or possess other forms of mental illness perform more poorly than athletes possessing average or above-average mental health (Raglin & Wilson, 2000). As measured by the **Profile of Mood States (POMS)** (McNair et al., 1992), the combination of low scores for undesirable (negative) mood factors (e.g., anger, fatigue, depression, confusion) and a high score for the desirable (positive) trait of vigor is commonly referred to as the **Iceberg Profile** (Morgan, 1980).

Further support for the mental health model was garnered through a review of a series of studies (Morgan, 1985), and these findings were later replicated by Mahoney (1989) and Newcombe and Boyle (1995). In these studies, measures of personality and mood state were measured in both college and elite athletes from a variety of sports. The psychological profiles of the successful and unsuccessful athletes were then compared, and it was found that the successful athletes had significant differences in mood state as demonstrated by their scores on the POMS.

Specifically, it was found that the successful athletes had higher levels of the positive trait vigor and displayed lower values for the negative states measured by the POMS.

Importantly, the mental health model also can be used to predict athletic performance. For instance, in a landmark study conducted by Morgan and Johnson (1978), psychological profiles were used to make predictions about the future success and failure of athletes attempting to earn a spot on the Olympic rowing team. These findings allowed Morgan and Johnson to successfully predict 70 to 85% of athletes that would eventually make the Olympic team. This level of success exceeded chance levels of prediction and supported the basis for the mental health model: successful athletes typically possessed lower scores for such personality factors as introversion, depression, neuroticism, and trait anxiety when compared with the unsuccessful athletes.

However, despite the high rate of accuracy, Morgan (1985) cautioned against using the mental health model in the selection of athletes for competition. In virtually all mental health model research, some mistakes have been made. For example, some athletes possess intermediate psychological scores, and these values prevent them from being categorized as either successful or unsuccessful. Furthermore, Morgan cautioned that the rate of prediction accuracy achieved through these studies is not sufficient to select athletes, and there is no evidence that psychological prediction models can be made more accurate than their current status (Eyseneck, Nias, & Cox, 1982; Morgan, 1997; Vanden Auweele, DeCuyper, VanMele, & Rzenicki, 1993).

Moreover, it is important to note that a dose-response relationship exists between the volume of training and an athlete's mood state. It is commonly accepted that athletes must undergo periods of intensive training, known as overtraining, to improve performance, but this can lead to unintended negative consequences for some athletes (Raglin & Wilson, 2000). Studies involving athletes from sports such as swimming and distance running have consistently found that intensive endurance training is associated with mood disturbances in both men and women athletes, even though these athletes possessed better than average mental health values prior to hard training (Raglin & Wilson, 2000). Results from these studies have found that increases in negative moods such as anxiety, anger, or depression are closely associated with increases in either the volume or intensity of training. At the peak of training, mood disturbances are also at their highest, with scores that typically exceed the population average (Raglin et al., 2006). On the other hand, reductions in training (called tapers) result in corresponding reductions in mood disturbances and increases in vigor. By the end of the training season when training volumes are low, the mood profiles of most athletes resemble their healthy preseason values.

Preperformance Anxiety and Sport Performance

Perhaps no area in sport psychology has received as much attention as the relationship of preperformance anxiety to sport performance. In fact, considerable debate continues over which theory provides the best explanation for this relationship, and there are more than 30 different anxiety measures designed specifically for athletes (Raglin et al., 2006).

The first and most widely recognized theory of anxiety and performance was the **inverted-U hypothesis,** which is sometimes referred to as the Yerkes-Dodson Law (Taylor & Wilson, 2002). Yerkes and Dodson (1908) originally conceptualized this idea as an explanation of the relationship between performance and stimulus intensity following an experiment involving maze discrimination in rats. By varying the degree of electrical stimulation while at the same time altering illumination, Yerkes and Dodson identified an optimal level of intensity at which the greatest learning occurred. However, as the degree of learning difficulty increased, the optimal level of stimulus intensity decreased (Raglin & Hanin, 2000). Specifically, Yerkes and Dodson suggested that increases in intensity produced associated improvements in performance, but only up to a specified point, after which greater intensity inhibited performance. Hence, when performance was plotted against intensity, a curvilinear portrayal in the shape of an inverted-U was shown.

This concept was further popularized and applied to sport performance by Oxendine (1970). Oxendine proposed that while moderate levels of anxiety were appropriate for most motor tasks, optimal levels of anxiety are dependent upon the specific type of sport task to be performed. In other words, for gross motor activities involving speed and strength (e.g., soccer, throwing the shot put), high levels of anxiety would be the most beneficial for sport performance. However, for those sports requiring fine muscle movements, steadiness, coordination, and general concentration (e.g., golf, throwing darts) low anxiety levels would prove beneficial.

Despite the intuitive commonsense appeal of the inverted-U hypothesis, extant empirical research supporting it is absent (Fazy & Hardy, 1988; Gould & Krane, 1992; Kleine, 1990; Neiss, 1988; Raglin & Turner, 1992). In addition, the inverted-U hypothesis has commonly been misinterpreted (Wilson, 1999), and Morgan and Ellickson (1989) have noted that the majority of these studies have examined the effect of intensity on learning a novel motor skill as opposed to athletic performance.

Despite such problems with the inverted-U hypothesis, the most important criticism of this view is that it implies that only moderate levels of anxiety are appropriate for all athletes and does not account for individual differences in the way athletes respond to the stress of competition (Fazey & Hardy, 1988; Kleine, 1990; Raglin & Hanin, 2000). Because of the inability of the inverted-U hypothesis to explain these individual differences, alternative models developed specifically from research with athletes have been used to explain differences in optimal anxiety.

INDIVIDUAL ZONE OF OPTIMAL FUNCTIONING (IZOF) MODEL

Because of the differences found in anxiety levels of successful athletes, the **individual zones of optimal function (IZOF) model** was conceptualized by Yuri Hanin (1986). Originally referred to as the individual optimum zone (IOZ) model (Cratty & Hanin, 1980), Hanin later redefined this paradigm as the zone of optimal function (ZOF) model (Hanin, 1986) before settling on the current individual zone of optimal function (IZOF) model (Hanin, 2000).

Based on data collected from a variety of Soviet athletes, Hanin found that regardless of the sport some athletes performed best at very low levels of anxiety (very relaxed), and others performed best while at very high levels of anxiety (extremely energized) (Raglin & Hanin, 2000). As a result, the IZOF model suggests that there is not one ideal level of anxiety for all athletes; rather, wide variation exists in the optimal level of anxiety between athletes.

Moreover, the optimal anxiety zone may range on a continuum anywhere from very high to very low depending on the unique characteristics of the individual athlete (Ebbeck & Weiss, 1988). For instance, in a study of college track and field athletes, Raglin and Turner (1992) found 51% of the men and 48% of the women reported best performances when anxiety levels were high, whereas in a study of 9- to 12-year-old track and field athletes, Wilson and Raglin (1997) found that 26% performed best with high anxiety levels.

Although the IZOF model has received considerable support, aspects of it have been questioned. For instance, the mechanism responsible for individual differences in optimal anxiety levels has not been fully explained. However, recent evidence suggests that experience is an important contributor to both an athlete's precompetition anxiety and optimal level of anxiety (Wilson, Raglin, & Pritchard, 2001; Wilson & Steinke, 2002). Findings from these studies suggest that those athletes labeled "optimistic" tended to have lower precompetition and optimal anxiety values than athletes who were more pessimistic in nature. Interestingly, however, no performance differences have been found between optimistic and pessimistic athletes. Hence, the study of personality differences in athletes is also important when evaluating the effects of precompetition anxiety upon performance.

The difficulty in conceptualizing and measuring the multifaceted psychobiological states of performance is complex, and this has led some sport psychologists (Fazey & Hardy, 1988; Gould, Tuffey, Hardt, & Lochbaum, 1993; Hardy, 1990; Martens, Vealy, & Burton, 1990) to question the unidimensional conceptualizations of the IZOF model and to propose theories that involve multiple components that may affect sport performance.

CATASTROPHE THEORY

In response to the emerging multidimensional views of the relationship of intensity to sport performance, more complex theories have been developed suggesting an interaction of cognitive, somatic, and self-confidence components within the individual athlete (Martens, Vealey, & Burton, 1990). Hardy (1990, 1996) has suggested that these components, when taken together, exert an interactive three-dimensional influence on sport performance that he has called catastrophe theory.

The **catastrophe model** purports that the impact of physiological arousal on performance depends on the level of cognitive anxiety possessed by the athlete (Wilson & Taylor, 2005). For example, in competitive situations in which physiological arousal is high, further increases in cognitive anxiety will have a debilitating effect upon performance. On the other hand, in cases where physiological arousal is low, increases in cognitive anxiety may act to enhance sport performance (Edwards & Hardy, 1996). Hence, poor levels of performance occur only under conditions of high physiological arousal and high intensity. When this happens, "catastrophe" occurs, resulting in a rapid and dramatic drop in performance (Cox, 1998).

Although limited support has been found for the catastrophe model, (Edwards & Hardy, 1996; Hardy, Parfitt & Pates, 1994; Woodman, Albinson & Hardy 1997), several investigators have criticized its basic tenants (Krane, 1993; Krane & Williams, 1994). Researchers have questioned whether the interaction effects upon performance are stable characteristics within the athlete (Gill, 1994). Moreover, Gould and Tuffey (1996) have suggested that more specific affective components of anxiety may exist, which has led some theorists (Hanin, 2000) to state that research may need to examine a wider range of emotions that influence sport performance. Finally, the catastrophe model has not been able to account for successful performances that occur under conditions of high cognitive anxiety in some athletes (Wilson & Taylor, 2005).

REVERSAL THEORY

Based on research conducted by Apter (1984), **reversal theory** has been applied to sport settings in an attempt to explain the effects of arousal on performance based on the athlete's appraisal of arousal (Kerr, 1997). Some sport psychologists believe that an individual athlete's interpretation of perceived anxiety is important to understanding its effects on performance (Jones, 1995). That is, high anxiety levels can be beneficial if an athlete perceives these levels as pleasant or positive. However, if anxiety is viewed as negative, it can have a negative effect on performance. Hence, for best performances to occur, athletes must view their anxiety as positive rather than negative (Kerr, 1997).

Reversal theory further suggests that there are shifts in perceptions of anxiety throughout the duration of a competition (Kerr, 1989). For example, an athlete may begin a competition in a positive mood state and interpret the accompanying anxiety as positive. However, as the competition progresses and the athlete starts to perform poorly, there is a shift in the mood state of the athlete, and the same level of anxiety is now seen as negative. Reversal theory suggests that perceptions of anxiety are not static but are dynamic, constantly changing throughout the course of a competition.

Since relatively little empirical work has been done in support of reversal theory, Weinberg and Gould (2003) have suggested that conclusions regarding its efficacy to sport performance cannot yet be made.

As can be seen, personality differences are considered important in understanding how athletes respond to the demands of competition. Although the ways in which responses occur are not yet fully understood, this is an important area of research in sport psychology.

Another aspect of sport psychology is how athletic performance can be enhanced through mental factors. The next section examines several common mental factors that are often considered important contributors to athletic performance.

Performance Enhancement Techniques

MENTAL IMAGERY Although many different psychological interventions have been promoted as a way to improve sport performance, mental imagery, or visualization, has received the greatest attention. However, despite the widespread popularity of mental imagery—both how it works and how beneficial it is to athletes—this technique remains unproven (Feltz & Lander, 1983; Raglin & Wilson, 2000).

Mental imagery can best be described as a process of internalized mental rehearsal that involves multisensory representations of an athlete's competitive experiences (Hale & Seiser, 2005). The goal of mental imagery is to reproduce the athletic experience as closely as possible so that the individual "feels" as if he or she is actually performing the sport.

A leading explanation for how mental imagery works is the **psychoneuromuscular theory,** which suggests that the imagery of motor performance results in increased neural activity in the motor cortex and causes associated physiological changes such as increases in electromyographic activity (EMG) and heart rate response. Other possible explanations have included symbolic learning, in which it is thought that imagery helps performers learn and focus on important elements of the skill while reducing distractions (Sackett, 1934), and that mental imagery leads to increased self-confidence and motivation (Callow & Hardy, 2001).

The greatest impact of mental imagery appears to be its positive effect on motor skill learning. For example, research has indicated that the positive effects of mental imagery are greater for tasks with a significant cognitive component as opposed to those relying on physical capacity or strength (Driskell, Cooper, & Moran, 1994; Feltz & Landers, 1983). The use of mental imagery may also assist the athlete in the identification and correction of technical errors by allowing the athlete to focus on the sequence and timing of movements (Hale & Seiser, 2005).

GOAL SETTING Another intervention often used to enhance athletic performance is goal setting. The term *goal* refers to the attainment of a specific level of proficiency on a task (Locke, Shaw, Saari, & Lathan, 1981). It is believed that goals influence performance by focusing an individual's attention on the relevant cues and tasks needed for success. In sport settings goals are often further categorized into outcome, performance, and process goals (Weinberg & Harmison, 2005). **Outcome goals** refer to the desired result of a specific competition; **performance goals** indicate the individual athlete's desired standard of performance. **Process goals** are concerned with how an athlete performs a specific skill or strategy.

Although the use of goal setting is an often popular method for improving sport performance, results from athletic studies are mixed. For example, Burton, Naylor, and Holliday (2001) reviewed 56 sport-related studies and found that 44 of these demonstrated moderate or strong effects, which represented a 78% effectiveness rate in enhancing sport performance through the setting of goals.

However, despite such equivocal findings, goal setting remains a popular means of increasing motivation in athletes (Weinberg, Burton, Yukelson, & Weigand, 2000), and Weinberg and Harmison (2005) have offered the following 10 basic principles to effective goal setting: (1) set specific goals, (2) set realistic yet challenging goals, (3) set long- and short-term goals, (4) set both competition and training goals, (5) write down goals, (6) develop goal-achievement strategies, (7) prioritize process, performance, and outcome goals, (8) set individual and team goals, (9) provide support for goals, and (10) provide feedback.

MOTIVATION Motivation is a topic of obvious interest to any coach or athlete interested in improving performance, and it can be broadly defined as the as degree of effort or intensity exhibited by a person toward achieving a goal (Sage, 1977; Ryan & Deci, 2000). Edward Thorndike (1935), a pioneer in motivational research, believed that humans are motivated to primarily seek pleasure and to avoid pain. David McClelland (1961) later expanded on this definition by suggesting that motivation consists of five different components—personality factors, situational factors, resultant tendencies, emotional factors and, achievement-related behaviors—all of which make up what McClelland called *need achievement theory*. McClelland believed that a person's motivational level is determined through the interaction on these five variables.

However, Bernard Weiner's (1986) *attribution theory* is perhaps the most commonly applied motivation theory in sport. According to this view, there are many different variables that work together to influence motivation, but these influences can be grouped into one of three separate domains he called stability, locus of causality, and locus of control. Something is stable when an individual attributes success to a permanent state such as talent, while unstable if attributed to a transitory state such as "good luck." Locus of causality can involve either external or internal motivational influences, and locus of control involves whether or not a person has control over the situation at hand (Raglin & Wilson, in press).

More recently, Joan Duda and Howard Hall (2001) have suggested a view called *achievement goal theory*. According to Duda and Hall, a person's goals and the perceived ability to attain these goals influence a person's level of motivation, and in turn, what success and failure mean to that individual. For instance, some athletes are **extrinsically** motivated, seeking awards or the approval of others for their accomplishments. However, Sandra Foster and Brent Walker (2005) suggest that such a motivational strategy may be negative for some athletes since their primary source of self-esteem comes from athletic success and its resultant rewards. Conversely, the athlete who performs for the pure enjoyment of the activity possesses **intrinsic motivation** (Foster & Walker, 2005). While both extrinsic and intrinsic motivation may be beneficial, it is generally believed that intrinsic motivation holds the greatest benefit for athletes (Raglin & Wilson, in press).

CONFIDENCE ENHANCEMENT Confidence is widely regarded as a prerequisite to successful sport performance. Confident athletes are typically believed to be more positive, motivated, and focused when compared to those with lesser degrees of confidence (Manzo & Mondin, 2005). For example, Mahoney and Avener (1977) found that U.S. Olympic qualifiers in men's gymnastics exhibited higher levels of self-confidence when compared to those who did not qualify. More recently, Jones and Hardy (1990) reported that 80% of elite athletes associated high levels of confidence with sport success.

Although self-confidence is typically viewed as the belief that one will be successful in a desired behavior, Vealey (2001) has suggested that sport self-confidence is a construct with both trait and state properties that are dependent on the time frame of reference that is used. In other words, confidence may vary from day to day (state) or may be a stable personality trait within the individual athlete. Furthermore, Vealey and Knight suggest that within sport there may be different types of self-confidence, such as confidence concerning one's ability to execute physical skills, confidence about one's psychological skills, confidence in perceptual skills, confidence in one's current level of physical fitness and training status, and finally confidence in one's potential to improve (as cited in Weinberg & Gould, 2003).

Bandura (1997) has further advocated that confidence is strongly influenced by the way in which people interpret their experiences. He has suggested that

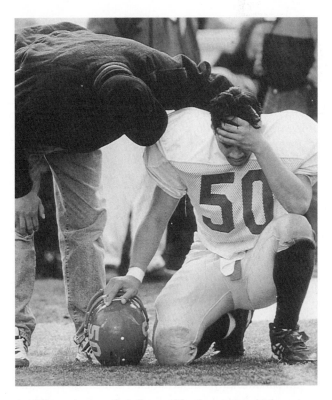

Confidence is strongly influenced by the way in which people interpret their experiences. Coaches must help athletes interpret their experiences in a constructive way to facilitate self-confidence.

TABLE 4.1 Current Textbooks in Exercise and Sport Psychology

Title	Authors	Edition/Year	Publisher	Web Site
Advances in Sport Psychology	Horn	2nd edition/2002	Human Kinetics	**www.humankinetics.com**
Applying Sport Psychology: Four Perspectives	Taylor & Wilson	1st edition/2005	Human Kinetics	**www.humankinetics.com**
Emotions in Sport	Hanin	1st edition/2000	Human Kinetics	**www.humankinetics.com**
Exercise Psychology	Buckworth & Dishman	1st edition/2002	Human Kinetics	**www.humankinetics.com**
Exploring Sport and Exercise Psychology	Van Raalte & Brewer	2nd edition/2002	American Psychological Association	**www.apa.com**
Foundations of Sport and Exercise Psychology	Weinberg & Gould	4th edition/2007	Human Kinetics	**www.humankinetics.com**
Sport Psychology	LeUnes & Nation	3rd edition/2002	Wadsworth	**www.wadsworth.com**
The Psychology of Exercise	Lox, Ginis, & Petruzzello	2nd edition/2006	Holcomb Hathaway	**www.hh-pub.com**
The Sport Psychology Handbook	Murphy	1st edition/2005	Human Kinetics	**www.humankinetics.com**
Sport Psychology: Concepts & Applications	Cox	5th edition/2002	McGraw-Hill	**www.mhhe.com**

there are four general ways people can facilitate self-confidence: through performance accomplishments (e.g., past successes), vicarious experiences (e.g., watching similar others succeed), verbal persuasion (encouragement, feedback from others), and physiological arousal. Other suggestions for enhancing confidence in athletes have included developing confidence through preparation/training (Taylor, 2001), the use of positive words or phrases that focus on the athletes' strengths (Taylor, 2001), or through social support and encouragement (Gould, Hodge, Peterson, & Giannini, 1989).

Other Topics

Additional topics in the area of sport psychology may include coach–athlete relationships, eating disorders in athletes, psychological factors of injury and rehabilitation, team cohesion, and attentional focus. The emphasis on these discussions is how mental factors can enhance physiological performance. On the other hand, other areas in exercise psychology may include theories of behavior change, programmatic factors associated with exercise adherence, and perceived exertion. Current textbooks on exercise and sport psychology are listed in Table 4.1.

PROFESSIONAL ORGANIZATIONS

The field of exercise and sport psychology has several different organizations open for membership at different levels. Typically, membership in these professional groups includes such benefits as subscriptions to publications, discounted fees to conferences and workshops, and access to various employment listings and notices. Although there has been debate in sport psychology concerning certification (e.g., who should certify and who should be certified), some prominent organizations have recently begun a rigorous certification process for their members. An overview of selected professional organizations in exercise and sport psychology is provided in this section (Table 4.2).

American College of Sports Medicine (ACSM)

ACSM was originally founded in 1954 in New York City during the annual meeting of the American Association for Health, Physical Education, Recreation and Dance (AAHPERD). In 1955 the name American College of

TABLE 4.2 Professional Organizations Related to Exercise and Sport Psychology

Organization	Address
American College of Sports Medicine (ACSM)	PO Box 1440 401 West Michigan Street Indianapolis, IN 46202 317-637-9200 **www.acsm.org**
American Psychological Association (APA)	750 1st Street NE Washington, DC 20002-4242 800-374-2717 **www.apa.com**
Association for Applied Sport Psychology (AASP)	2810 Crossroads Drive, Ste. 3800 Madison, WI 53718 608-443-2465 **appliedsportpsych.org**
North American Society for the Psychology of Sport and Physical Activity (NASPSPA)	Human Kinetics PO Box 5076 Champaign, IL 61825 800-747-4457 **www.naspspa.com**

Sports Medicine was formally adopted, and 1984 its National Center was moved to Indianapolis, Indiana. ACSM members are involved in a wide range of medical, allied health, and scientific disciplines. Due to the diversity and expertise of ACSM, it has become the largest and most respected exercise science organization in the world.

Because of the diversity of ACSM, interest groups were formed to promote research and communication among ACSM members with similar interests. In 1995 the Psychobiology and Behavior group was approved (Box 4.1).

EXPLORE MORE BOX 4.1

Psychobiology and Behavior Mission

"To promote research and the advancement of knowledge of sport psychology with a particular emphasis on psychobiology and health" (ACSM, 2007).

There are different levels of membership in ACSM, ranging from professional to student membership. The student membership category comes with a discounted membership fee. ACSM provides a variety of educational opportunities and publishes the respected journals *Medicine and Science in Sports and Exercise* and *Exercise and Sport Science Reviews*.

American Psychological Association (APA)

Based in Washington, D.C., the APA represents over 150,000 members and is the largest psychological organization in the world. The mission of the APA is to advance the science and profession of psychology, and 53 professional divisions within APA have been established that are devoted to specific areas of interest. The Exercise and Sport Psychology Interest Group (Division 47) was formed during the annual meeting of the APA in 1983 (Box 4.2).

EXPLORE MORE BOX 4.2

APA Division 47—Purpose and Goals

"Through the Division, scientists and practitioners with a common interest have the opportunity to interact and to further their personal and professional capabilities. Research interests of Division members include motivation to persist and achieve; psychological considerations in sport injury and rehabilitation; counseling techniques with athletes; assessing talent; exercise adherence and well-being; self-perceptions related to achieving; expertise in sport; youth sport; and performance enhancement and self-regulation techniques. The Division furthers scientific, education, and clinical foundations of exercise and sport psychology" (APA, 2007).

There are several different membership categories for the APA. Those who have received a doctoral degree in psychology or a related field can become an APA member, and thus belong to Division 47 through their membership. Both undergraduate and graduate students can join the APA by becoming student affiliates.

Association for Applied Sport Psychology (AASP)

The AASP was founded in 1986 and is now the largest applied sport psychology organization in the world. AASP was established to promote the science and practice of sport psychology and is made up of three focus areas: Health Psychology, Performance Enhancement/Interventions, and Social Psychology. Applied sport psychology extends research findings into real-life situations. The focus of the AASP is to work directly with coaches and athletes to facilitate sport performance (Box 4.3).

EXPLORE MORE BOX 4.3

AASP Purpose and Mission

"The purpose of the Association for Applied Sport Psychology (AASP) is to provide leadership for the development, research, and intervention strategies in sport psychology. Accordingly, the primary missions of AASP are:

A. To provide a professional forum for individuals who are committed to:

  1. research and theory development, and their applications in sport, exercise, and health psychology, and/or

  2. the delivery of psychological services to consumers in sport, exercise, and health contexts.

B. To support and disseminate new and relevant knowledge about research and practice in sport, exercise, and health psychology.

C. To establish and uphold professional standards for the competent and ethical practice of sport psychology.

D. To foster societal awareness of the relevance, and advocate the use, of sport psychology theory, research, and practice to enhance physical activity performance, health, and well-being" (AASP, 2007).

In 1989, the AASP initiated a Certified Consultant program that requires advanced training in both psychology and exercise science. This includes the attainment of a doctoral degree with coursework in psychology, health, exercise physiology, ethics, statistics, research design, cognitive behavior, health, psychopathology and biology. In addition, supervised counseling and practicum experiences are required.

The United States Olympic Committee (USOC) also maintains its own sport psychology registry. To work with U.S. Olympic athletes, a sport psychologist must be listed in this database. To be on the USOC registry, a sport psychologist must be a member in good standing of the American Psychological Association and a Certified Consultant of the AASP. The official journal of the AASP is the *Journal of Applied Sport Psychology*.

North American Society for the Psychology of Sport and Physical Activity (NASPSPA)

The North American Society for the Psychology of Sport and Physical Activity is a multidisciplinary association that is interested in a wide range of areas in the behavioral sciences. The purpose of NASPSPA is to advance the study of human behavior through the disciplines of sport psychology, motor development, and motor learning and control (Box 4.4).

EXPLORE MORE BOX 4.4

NASPSPA Mission Statement

"The North American Society for the Psychology of Sport and Physical Activity is a multidisciplinary association of scholars from the behavioral sciences and related professions. The Society functions to:

- Develop and advance the scientific study of human behavior when individuals are engaged in sport and physical activity.
- Facilitate the dissemination of information.
- Improve the quality of research and teaching in the psychology of sport, motor development, and motor learning and control" (NAPSPA, 2007).

CAREERS

Many students who pursue an interest in exercise and sport psychology typically are physically active or have experience as an athlete. These experiences have led them to an interest in learning "why" exercise is associated with feelings of improved mental outlook or with the mental aspects of sport performance. Typically, the subdiscipline of exercise and sport psychology is considered a graduate-level field, although undergraduate introductory classes are normally offered in most exercise science programs, and a growing number of schools are starting to offer academic minors in this area. To become fully credentialed as a "sport psychologist" an advanced degree in sport psychology is required (or a graduate degree in psychology, with specialized training working with athletes).

It is difficult to quantify professional opportunities in exercise and sport psychology because of the wide diversity in the field. The majority of employment opportunities are found at the college or university level and involve teaching, research, and working with a collegiate athletic program. However, there is a growing trend for professional sport teams and USOC national teams to employ sport psychologists as members of their overall support staff. Increasingly, sport psychologists are being utilized in the United States military, performing various motivational and behavioral functions. Other potential areas of employment may include working as a consulting sport psychologist for individual athletes or teams or as a clinical psychologist. However, it is once again important to remember that whether one seeks employment teaching at college or university level, with professional or USOC teams, or as a clinical psychologist, a doctorate degree is required.

SUMMARY

The history of exercise and sport psychology can be traced back to writings of the ancient Greeks and Romans, but the first true sport psychologist in the United States was Coleman Griffith Roberts in the early part of the 20th century. Today, researchers interested in the mental aspects of physical activity can be found working with athletes or studying the reasons for improvements in mental health through exercise. Exercise psychology examines the association between physical activity and mental health and seeks to establish a causal relationship between these two variables. Exercise psychology is also concerned with issues such as exercise adherence. Sport psychology, on the other hand, deals with issues important to sport performance enhancement such as motivation, the effects of anxiety on competition, confidence, mental imagery, or goal setting. A number of professional organizations serve the field of exercise and sport psychology, the most prominent of which include the ACSM, APA, AASP, and the NASPSPA. The AASP has instituted a certification program that specifically trains psychologists in working directly with athletes. Career options for the exercise and sport psychologist include working in educational or research settings or as an applied practitioner working directly with athletes.

■ Key Resources

Key Journals
International Journal of Sport Psychology
Journal of Applied Sport Psychology
Journal of Clinical Sport Psychology
Journal of Exercise and Sport Psychology
Journal of Health Psychology

Medicine and Science in Sports and Exercise
Perceptual and Motor Skills
Personality and Individual Differences
Research Quarterly for Exercise & Sport
The Sport Psychologist

■ Review Questions

1. Explain the difference in focus for those who work in exercise psychology and those practitioners who work in sport psychology.
2. Describe the role played by Coleman Griffith in the evolution of sport psychology in this country.
3. In what ways has exercise been associated with improvements in mental health?
4. Describe the four leading hypotheses used to explain the effects of exercise on mental health.

5. List the three theoretical models used to explain exercise participation and adherence, and give examples of each.
6. What is the mental health model of exercise and sport performance?
7. Compare and contrast the inverted-U hypothesis to the individual zones of optimal function (IZOF) model of anxiety and performance.
8. Explain the proposed benefits of both mental imagery and goal setting in terms of improving sport performance.

■ References

American College of Sports Medicine (2007). Mission statement. Retrieved from http://www.acsm.org
American Psychological Association. (2007) Mission statement. Retrieved from http://www.apa.org. division47

Association for Applied Sport Psychology. (2007). Mission statement. Retrieved from http://appliedsportpsych.org
Ajzen, I., & Fishbein, M. (1980). Understanding attitudes and predicting social behavior. Englewood Cliffs, NJ: Prentice-Hall.

Apter, M. J. (1984). Reversal theory and personality: A review. *Journal of Research in Personality*, 18, 265–288.

Bandura, A. (1997). *Self-efficacy: The exercise of personal control*. New York: W. H. Freeman.

Boring, E. G. (1950). *A history of experimental psychology* (2nd ed.). Englewood Cliffs, NJ. Prentice-Hall.

Buckworth, J., & Dishman, R. K. (2002). *Exercise psychology*. Champaign, IL: Human Kinetics.

Burton, D., Naylor, S., & Holliday, B. (2001). Goal setting in sport: Investigating the goal effectiveness paradigm. In R. Singer, H. Haubsenblaus, & C. Janelle (Eds.), *Handbook of sport psychology* (2nd ed.). New York: Wiley.

Callow, N., & Hardy, L. (2001). Types of imagery associated with sport confidence in netball players of varying skill levels. *Journal of Applied Sport Psychology*, 13, 1–17.

Cooper, L. (1969). Athletics, activity and personality: A review of the literature. *Research Quarterly* 40, 17–22.

Cox, R. H. (1998). *Sport psychology: Concepts and applications* (4th ed). Boston: McGraw-Hill.

Cratty, B. J. (1968). *Psychology of physical activity*. Englewood Cliffs, NJ: Prentice-Hall.

Cratty, B. J., & Hanin, Y. L. (1980). *The athlete in the sports team*. Denver, CO: Love.

Driskell, J. E., Cooper, C., & Moran, A. (1994). Does mental practice enhance elite performance? *Journal of Applied Psychology*, 79, 172–178.

Duda, J. L., & Hall, H. (2001) Achievement goal theory in sport: Recent extensions and future directions. In R. Singer, H. Hausenblas, & C. Janelle (Eds.), *Handbook of sport psychology* (2nd ed., pp. 417–443). New York: Wiley.

Ebbeck, V., & Weiss, M. R. (1988). The arousal-performance relationship: Task characteristics and performance measures in track and field athletics. *The Sport Psychologist*, 2, 13–27.

Edwards, T., & Hardy, L. (1996). The interactive effects of intensity and direction of cognition and somatic anxiety and self-confidence upon performance. *Journal of Sport and Exercise Psychology*, 18, 296–312.

Eysenck, H. J., Nias, K. B. D., & Cox, D. N. (1982) Personality and sport. *Advances in Behavioral Research and Therapy* 1, 1–56.

Fazey, J., & Hardy, L. (1988) The inverted-U hypothesis: A catastrophe for sport psychology? BASS *Monograph* 1. Leeds, UK: White Line Press.

Feltz, D. L., & Landers, D. M. (1983). The effects of mental practice on motor skill learning and performance: A meta-analysis. *Journal of Sport Psychology*, 5, 25–57.

Foster, S., & Walker, B. (2005). Motivation. In J. Taylor. & G. S. Wilson (Eds.), *Applying sport psychology; Four perspectives* (pp. 3–19). Champaign, IL: Human Kinetics.

Gill, D. L. (1994). A sport and exercise perspective on stress. *Quest*, 46, 20–27.

Gould, D., Hodge, K., Peterson, K., & Giannini, J. (1989). An exploratory examination of strategies used by elite coaches to enhance self-efficacy in athletes. *Journal of Sport and Exercise Psychology*, 11, 128–140.

Gould, D., & Krane, V. (1992). The arousal-athletic performance relationship: Current status and future directions. In T. S. Horn (Ed.), *Advances in sport psychology* (pp. 119–141). Champaign, IL: Human Kinetics.

Gould, D., & Tuffey, S. (1996). Zones of optimal functioning research. A review and critique. *Anxiety, Stress, and Coping*, 90(1), 53–68.

Gould, D., Tuffey, S., Hardt, L., & Lochbaum, M. (1993). Multidimensional state anxiety and middle distance running performance: An exploratory examination of Hanin's (1980) zones of optimal functioning hypothesis. *Journal of Applied Sport Psychology*, 5, 89–95.

Griffith, C. R. (1926). *Psychology of coaching*. New York: Scribner.

Griffith, C. R. (1928). *Psychology of athletics*. New York: Scribner.

Hale, B. D., & Seiser, L. (2005). Mental imagery. In J. Taylor & G. S. Wilson (Eds.), *Comprehensive perspectives on applied sport psychology: From researcher and consultant to coach and athlete*. Champaign, IL: Human Kinetics.

Hanin, Y. L. (1986). State-trait research in sports in the USSR. In C. D. Spielberger & R. Diaz Guerrero (Eds.), *Cross-cultural anxiety* (vol. 3, pp. 45–64). Washington, DC: Hemisphere.

Hanin, Y. L. (2000). *Emotions in sport*. Champaign, IL: Human Kinetics.

Hardy, L. (1990). A catastrophe model of performance in sport. In J. G. Jones & L. Hardy (Eds.), *Stress and performance in sport* (pp. 81–106). Chichester, UK: Wiley.

Hardy, L. (1996). Testing the prediction of the cusp catastrophe model of anxiety and performance. *The Sport Psychologist*, 10, 140–156.

Hardy, L., Parfitt, G., & Pates, J. (1994). Performance catastrophes in sport: A test of the hysteresis hypothesis. *Journal of Sport Sciences*, 12, 327–334.

Jones, G. (1995). Competitive anxiety in sport. In S. J. H. Biddle (Ed.), *European perspectives on exercise and sport psychology* (pp. 128–153). Leeds, UK: Human Kinetics.

Jones, G., & Hardy, L. (1990). Stress in sport: Experiences of some elite performers. In G. Jones.& L. Hardy (Eds.), *Stress and performance in sport* (pp. 247–277). Chichester: Wiley.

Kerr, J. M. (1989). Anxiety, arousal and sport performance: An application of reversal theory. In D. Hackfort & C. D. S pielberger (Eds.), *Anxiety in sports: An international perspective* (pp. 137–151). New York: Hemisphere.

Kerr, J. H. (1997). *Motivation and emotion in sport: Reversal theory*. East Sussex, UK: Psychology Press.

Klein, D. (1990). Anxiety and sports performance: A meta-analysis. *Anxiety Research*, 2, 113–131.

Krane, V. (1993). A practical application of the anxiety-athletic performance relationship: The zone of optimal function hypothesis. *The Sport Psychologist*, 7, 113–126.

Krane, V., & Williams, J. M. (1994). Cognitive anxiety, somatic anxiety and confidence in track and field athletes: The impact of gender, competitive level, and task characteristics. *International Journal of Sport Psychology*, 25, 203–217.

Kroll, W., & Lewis, G. (1970). American's fist sport psychologist. *Quest*, 13, 1–4.

Locke, E. A., Shaw, K. N., Sarri, L. M., & Smith, G. P. (1981). Goal setting and task performance. *Psychological Bulletin*, 90, 125–152.

Mahoney, M. J. (1989). Psychological predictors of elite and non-elite performance in olympic weight lifting. *International Journal of Sport Psychology*, 20, 1–12.

Mahoney, M. J., & Avener, M. (1977). Psychology of the elite athlete: An exploratory study. *Cognitive Therapy and Research*, 1, 135–142.

Manzo, L. G., & Mondin, G. W. (2005). Confidence. In J. Taylor.& G. S. Wilson (Eds.), *Applying sport psychology: Four perspectives* (pp. 21–32). Champaign, IL: Human Kinetics.

Martens, R. (1975). The paradigmatic crisis in American sport personology. *Sportwissenschaft*, 5, 9–24.

Martens, R., Vealey, R. S., & Burton, D. (1990). *Competitive anxiety in sport*. Champaign, IL: Human Kinetics.

McClelland, D. C. (1961). *The achieving society*. New York: Free Press.

McNair, D. M., Lorr, M., & Dropplemann, L. F. (1992). *Profile of mood states manual*. San Diego, CA: Educational and Testing Service.

Morgan, W. P. (1978). The credulous-skeptical argument in perspective. In W. F. Straub (Ed.), *An analysis of athlete behavior* (pp. 218–227) Ithaca, NY: Movement.

Morgan, W. P. (1980). The trait psychology controversy. *Research Quarterly for Exercise and Sport* 51, 50–76.

Morgan, W. P. (1985). Selected psychological factors limiting performance: A mental health model. In D. H. Clarke & H. M. Eckert (Eds.), *Limits of human performance* (pp. 70–80). Champaign, IL: Human Kinetics.

Morgan, W. P. (1997). Mind games: The psychology of sport. - In D. R. Lamb & R. Murray (Eds.), *Optimizing sport performance: Perspectives in exercise and sports medicine* (Vol. 10) pp 1–54. Cooper Publications, Carmel, IN.

Morgan, W. P., & Ellickson, K. A. (1989). Health, anxiety and physical exercise. In D. Hackfort & C. D. Spielberger (Eds.), *Anxiety in sports: An international perspective* (pp. 165–182). New York: Hemisphere.

Morgan, W. P., & Johnson, R. W. (1978). Personality characteristics of successful and unsuccessful oarsmen. *International Journal of Sport Psychology*, 9, 119–133.

Morgan, W. P., O'Connor, P. J., Sparling, P. B., & Pate, R. R. (1987). Psychological characterization of the elite female distance runner. *International Journal of Sports Medicine*, 8, 124–131.

Neiss, R. (1988). Reconceptualizing arousal: Psychobiological states in motor performance. *Psychological Bulletin*, 103(3), 345–366.

Newcombe, P. A., & Boyle, G. A. (1995) High school students' sports personalities: Variations across participation level, gender, type of sport, and success. *International Journal of Sport Psychology*, 26, 277–294.

North American Society of the Psychology of Sport and Physical Activity. (2007). Mission statement. Retrieved from http://www.naspspa.org

Oxendine, J. B. (1970). Emotional arousal and motor performance. *Quest* 13, 23–30.

Petruzzello, S. J., Landers, D. M., Hatfield, B. D., Kubitz, K. A., & Salazar, W. (1991). A meta-analysis on the anxiety reducing effects of acute and chronic exercise: Outcomes and mechanisms. *Sports Medicine*, 11(3), 143–182.

Prochaska, J. O., DiClemente, C. C., & Norcross, J. C. (1992). In search of how people change. *American Psychologist*, 47, 1102–1114.

Raglin, J. S. (1997). Anxiolytic effects of physical activity. In W. P. Morgan (Ed.), *Physical activity and mental health* (pp. 107–126). Washington, DC: Taylor & Francis.

Raglin, J. S., & Hanin, Y. L. (2000) Competitive anxiety. In Y. L. Hanin (Ed.), *Emotions in Sport* (pp. 93–111). Champaign, IL: Human Kinetics.

Raglin, J. S., & Turner, P. E. (1992). Predicted, actual and optimal precompetition anxiety in adolescent track and field athletes. *Scandinavian Journal of Medicine and Science in Sports*, 2, 148–152.

Raglin, J. S., & Wilson, G. S. (2000) Overtraining and staleness in athletes. In Y. L. Hanin (Ed.), *Emotions and Sport* (pp. 191–207). Champaign, IL: Human Kinetics.

Raglin, J. S., & Wilson, G. S. (in press). Psychological characteristics of athletes and their responses to sport-related stressors. In. R. J. Maughan (Ed.), *Olympic textbook of science in sport*. Oxford, UK: Wiley & Sons.

Raglin, J. S., Wilson, G. S., & Galper, D. (2006). Exercise and its effects on mental health. In C. Bouchard, S. Blair, & W. Haskell (Eds.), *Physical activity and health* (pp. 247–257). Champaign, IL: Human Kinetics.

Rushall, B. S. (1970). An evaluation of the relationship between personality and physical performance categories. In G. S. Kenyon (Ed.), *Contemporary psychology of sport* (pp. 157–165). Chicago: Athletic Institute.

Ryan, R. M., & Deci, E. L. (2000). Self-determination theory and the facilitation of intrinsic motivation, social development, and subjective well being. *American Psychologist* 55, 68–78.

Sackett, R. S. (1934). The influences of symbolic rehearsal upon the retention of a maze habit. *Journal of General Psychology*, 13, 113–128.

Sage, G. (1977). *Introduction to motor behavior: A neuropsychological approach* (2nd ed.). Reading, MA: Addison-Wesley.

Salmela, J. H. (1992). *The world of sport psychology source book* (2nd ed.). Champaign, IL: Human Kinetics.

Spielberger, C. D., Gursuch, R. L., Lushene, R. E., Vagg, P. R., & Jacobs, G. A. (1983). *Manual for the State-Trait Anxiety Inventory: STAI (form Y)*. Palo Alto, CA: Consulting Psychologists Press.

Taylor, J. (2001). *Prime sport: Triumph of the athlete mind*. New York: Universe.

Taylor, J., & Wilson, G. S. (2002). Intensity regulation and athletic performance. In J. L. Van.Raalte & B. W. Brewer (Eds.), *Exploring sport and exercise psychology* (pp. 99–130). Washington, DC: American Psychologist Association.

Thorndike, E. L. (1935). *The psychology of wants, interest, and attitudes*. New York: Appleton-Century-Crofts.

Triplett, N. (1898). The dynamogenic factors in pacemaking and competition. *American Journal of Psychology*, 9, 507–533.

U.S. Department of Health and Human Services. (2000). *Healthy people 2010: Understanding and improving health* (2nd ed.). Washington DC: Government Printing Office.

Vanden Auweele, Y., DeCuyper, B., VanMele, V., & Rzenicki, R. (1993). Elite performance and personality: From description and prediction to diagnosis and intervention. In R. N. Singer, M. Murphey, & L. K. Tennant (Eds.), *Handbook of research on sport psychology* (pp. 257–289). New York: Macmillan.

Vanek, M., & Cratty, B. J. (1970). *Psychology and the superior athlete*. New York: Macmillan.

Vealey, R. S. (2001). Understanding and enhancing self-confidence in athletes. In R. Singer, H. Hausenblas, & C. Janelle (Eds.), *Handbook of sport psychology* (pp. 540–565). New York: John Wiley and Sons.

Warburton, R. W., & Kane, J. E. (1966). Personality related to sport and physical activity. In J. E. Kane (Ed.), *Readings in physical education* (pp. 61–89). London: P. E. Association.

Weinberg, R. S., Burton, D., Yukelson, D., & . Weigand, D. (2000). Perceived goal setting practices of Olympic athletes: An exploratory investigation. *The Sport Psychologist*, 14, 280–296.

Weinberg, R. S., & Gould, D. (2003). *Foundations of sport and exercise psychology* (3rd ed.). Champaign, IL: Human Kinetics.

Weinberg, R., & Harmison, R. (2005). Goal setting. In J. Taylor & G. S. Wilson (Eds.), *Comprehensive perspectives on applied sport psychology: From researcher and consultant to coach and athlete*. Champaign, IL: Human Kinetics.

Weiner, B. (1986). *An attribution theory of achievement motivation and emotion*. New York: Springer-Verlag.

Willis, J. D., & Campbell, L. F. (1992). *Exercise psychology*. Champaign, IL: Human Kinetics.

Wilson, G. S. (1999). Personality variables in levels of predicted and actual test anxiety among college students. *Education Research Quarterly*, 22, 3–15.

Wilson, G. S., & Raglin, J. S. (1997). Sport anxiety variability in 9–12 year old track and field athletes. *Scandinavian Journal of Medicine and Science in Sports*, 7, 253–258.

Wilson, G. S., Raglin, J. S., & Pritchard, M. E. (2001). Optimism, pessimism, and precompetition anxiety in college athletes. *Personality & Individual Differences*, 32(5), 893–902.

Wilson, G. S., & Steinke, J. S. (2002). Cognitive orientation, precompetition and actual competition anxiety in collegiate softball players. *Research Quarterly for Exercise and Sport*, 73(3), 335–339.

Wilson, G. S., & Taylor, J. (2005). Intensity and athletic performance. In J. Taylor.& G. S. Wilson.(Eds.), *Applying sport psychology: Four perspectives* (pp. 33–49). Champaign, IL: Human Kinetics.

Woodman, T., Albinson, J. G., & Hardy, L. (1997). An investigation of the zones of optimal functioning hypothesis within a multidimensional framework. *Journal of Sport and Exercise Psychology*, 19, 131–141.

Yerkes, R. M., & Dodson, J. D. (1908). The relation of strength of stimulus to rapidity of habit-formation. *Journal of Comparative Neurology and Psychology*, 18, 459–482.

CHAPTER 5

Motor Learning and Motor Control

Kelly Cole, PhD, University of Iowa

■ Chapter Objectives

After reading this chapter, you should be able to:

1. Define the terms *motor control* and *motor learning* and explain their significance to understanding motor behavior.

2. Provide a brief overview of the history of the science of motor control and motor learning.

3. Describe conditions that are optimal for learning and refining skilled movements.

4. Describe key concepts of the current understanding of how skilled movement is produced.

5. Explain the career options for students with training in motor control and motor learning.

6. Identify the various professional scientific and clinical organizations that are relevant to the broad field of motor behavior and their associated certification programs.

■ Key Terms

anticipatory postural control
applied motor control
  physiologists
blocked practice
brain plasticity
central pattern generator
central representation

constant practice
deafferented
distributed practice
initial conditions
Law of Practice
massed practice
motor behavior

motor control
motor learning
posture
random practice
retention test
sensory information
variable practice

Consider the words of Sir Charles S. Sherrington (winner of the Nobel Prize in Physiology or Medicine, 1932):

> [E]ven in man the crown of life is an action, not a thought . . . to move things is all that mankind can do, and that for such the sole executant is muscle, whether in whispering a syllable or in felling a forest. (Linacre Lecture, Cambridge, England, 1924)

Sherrington was telling us that motor behavior is a fundamental human function that is essential to virtually all of our aspirations in life. This is why courses in motor behavior are found universally in exercise science curricula.

Motor behavior can be defined as the study of human movement[1] or action. Motor behavior involves two overlapping themes: motor control and motor learning. **Motor control** focuses on the processes that underlie the production of movement in health and disease; **motor learning** focuses on how skilled movements are acquired, including the optimal conditions for learning new motor skills.

Courses in motor control and motor learning often appear as intermediate- or upper-level components of an exercise science curriculum and follow courses in anatomy, physiology, and physics. An understanding of basic physics is essential because movements result from the interaction of our body with our environment. For example, gravity acts on the masses of our body segments, body segments affect each other as they move, and objects exert forces on our bodies (and vice versa) as we manipulate them. The process of producing coordinated, functional movements must account for these physical properties at some level, and so the study of motor behavior should be intertwined with the study of biomechanics. A course in general psychology is helpful because our everyday movements also depend on attention, perception, memory, motivation, and even decision making.

A BRIEF HISTORY OF MOTOR CONTROL AND MOTOR LEARNING

The origins of contemporary motor behavior are found in medicine, physiology, psychology, and engineering. Our understanding of how the nervous system participates in the production of movement began within the related disciplines of medicine and physiology. Several key events occurred during the late 1800s and early 1900s that propelled motor neuroscience into a modern discipline. Let's place the level of under-

standing (or lack of understanding) of basic neuroscience during the late 1800s in perspective. This was a time when anatomists and physiologists debated the existence of the synapse, the junction between neurons that is fundamental to information processing in the nervous system.

The Rise of Electrophysiology

In 1870 Gustav Theodor Fritsch (1838–1927) and Julius Eduard Hitzig (1838–1907) began the study of the brain's *electro*physiology. They applied localized, low-level electrical stimulation to the brains of dogs and demonstrated that brain areas previously thought to be involved exclusively in thought and emotion participated directly in producing movement. John Hughlings Jackson (1835–1911), "the father of British neurology," wrote extensively on the neural control of movement. He often gained insights from his observations of patients. For example, Jackson observed grand mal epileptic seizures and noticed that there was a progressive involvement of different body parts that followed a similar pattern across his patients, including his wife. This led him to deduce that seizures resulted from excessive electrical activity that began in one area of the brain and then spread. The regularity of the movement patterns allowed him to conclude, before the work of Fritsch and Hitzig, that the highest level of the brain—the cerebral cortex—participated in the generation of movement. He also deduced that the muscles of the body are represented in the cerebral cortex by a systematic body map (Figure 5.1).

These key observations were followed by those of Sir David Ferrier (1843–1924), who confirmed and elaborated the concept of cerebral cortical maps.

The modern era of motor neurophysiology began with the systematic research of Sir Charles S. Sherrington (1857–1952) who shared the Nobel Prize in 1932 for his study of *reflexes* (automatic motor responses in reaction to an external stimulus) and their role in the brain's control of movement and posture. Sherrington ushered in a highly productive era of increasingly sophisticated study of how the nervous system participates in the production of simple and skilled movements. This motor neuroscience tradition developed at an increasingly fast pace and was directed mostly at discovering the neural causes of movement with little regard to the properties of the movements themselves.

Early Contributions From Psychology

At the same time a completely separate tradition of research in the discipline of psychology developed. Beginning in the late 1880s, scientists focused on the study of highly skilled movements by observing and describing the properties of movements under a variety

---

[1]In this chapter *movement* is often used generically to refer to actions involving the production of force or motion.

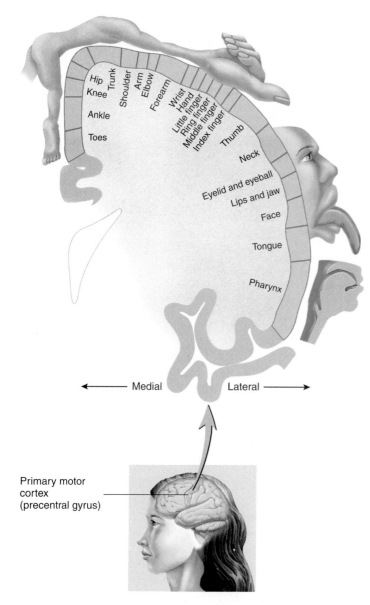

Primary motor
cortex
(precentral gyrus)

Figure 5.1   The somatotopic map of the primary motor cortex.

period of research concerning motor learning, optimal training methods, and the optimal design of equipment to minimize human-user errors (now known as ergonomics or human factors engineering). Seminal work during this time included research by K. J. W. Craik (1914–1945) and his theory that information processing in the brain occurs in bursts rather than continuously. A. T. Welford (1914–1995) built on Craik's work with his influential theory that information processing in the nervous system encounters delays because the information is processed in single channels. Paul M. Fitts (1912–1965) continued along this theme of the brain as an information processor by describing fundamental relations between movement duration, movement size, and movement accuracy in rapid, aimed movements. Finally, Franklin Henry (1904–1993) studied motor behavior in a physical education setting. He trained a generation of prominent scientists who began their careers in the 1960s and 1970s.

The 1920s, 30s, and 40s also saw the emergence of the field of motor development. This field began with seminal publications of observational research by Arnold Gesell (1928), Mary Shirley (1931), Myrtle McGraw (1935), and Nancy Bayley (1936).

Merging of Physiological and Psychological Approaches

Beginning in the 1970s there was a rapid merger of the traditions of psychology and motor neurophysiology. The work of the Russian neurophysiologist Nikolai Bernstein (1897–1966) was particularly influential in this merging of disciplines. Bernstein worked in obscurity in Russia during the 1930s and 1940s on the fundamental issue of how a system as complex as the neuromuscular system is coordinated. He used approaches to the study of motor control that merged the behavioral and neural levels of inquiry. In particular he observed how the body, as both a neural and mechanical system, interacted with the environment. He theorized that functional movement is the result of control that is distributed across many levels of the nervous system, and also among the neuromuscular and mechanical systems of the body. Bernstein's work was not widely known until an English translation appeared in 1967, one year after his death. This and other translations accelerated the combined neural and behavioral approach to the study of motor control, which continues today.

MOTOR LEARNING

The acquisition and refinement of new motor skills have a major impact on our lives as we take up new hobbies or jobs, participate in sports, or begin to

of conditions. R. S. Woodworth (1869–1962), who went on to serve briefly as an assistant to Sherrington, began by studying the principles of rapid hand movements, including the interaction of speed, accuracy, and vision. E. L. Thorndike (1874–1949), a colleague of Woodworth on the Columbia University faculty, studied the processes that underlie skill learning. His *Law of Effect* was influential in formulating early 20th century learning theory. This law states that rewarded responses tend to be repeated, whereas responses that are not rewarded tend not to be repeated.

World War II saw scientists in the United States and Great Britain study critical questions for the war effort, such as how to select and rapidly train pilots, bombardiers, and gunners. This research developed momentum that carried on into a productive postwar

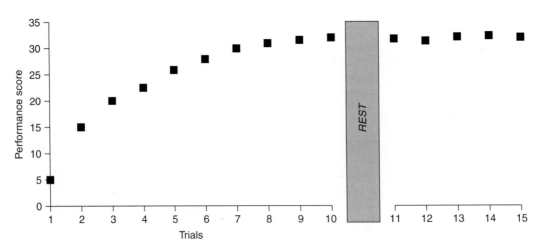

Figure 5.2 Hypothetical data demonstrating a typical performance curve in which performance increases more rapidly during the early phases of practice and less rapidly as the learner gains more experience with the task. Learning can be inferred from the retention of performance following a rest period.

engage in important activities of modern life like driving a car or typing on a keyboard. It is not surprising that considerable research effort has been expended over the past 70 years to understand how we learn and refine new motor skills. The results of this research have influenced how instructors, coaches, therapists, and others approach teaching and rehabilitation to optimize motor learning. Recently the study of motor learning has been reenergized by remarkable discoveries of rapid structural changes that occur in our brains as we learn new motor skills. These discoveries have fueled intense study of the neural mechanisms underlying learning and how this new knowledge can enhance the recovery of motor function following brain injuries. This part of the chapter considers the results of several decades of research on motor skill acquisition by examining the conditions that facilitate motor learning so that one can maximize the efficiency of training and practice sessions. Next recent exciting discoveries in the area of brain plasticity and its implications for motor learning and the recovery of motor function following brain injury are examined.

Schmidt and Lee (2005) defined motor learning succintly: "Motor learning is a set of processes associated with practice or experience leading to relatively permanent changes in the capability for movement" (p. 302). In other words, when we learn a motor skill, we permanently change our capability for producing a skilled action, and these changes occur through neural processes that are associated with practice or experience. Because motor learning is defined as a change in the *capability* for movement, rather than in movement itself, we must *infer* that motor learning has occurred from a change in motor performance. It is a common experience to improve

performance on a new task during the initial practice session. If we plot measures of performance over the course of practice, we may see a curve like that in Figure 5.2.

The curve shown in Figure 5.2 certainly reflects improving performance with practice, but does the increased performance from the 1st to the 10th trial reflect motor learning? Our definition specifies that only relatively permanent changes qualify as evidence for motor learning. One way to determine whether the increased performance is relatively permanent would be to test our performance on another day or after a suitable delay or rest, which would allow temporary effects (such as being warmed up or in a state of heightened attention) to dissipate. In this way we can estimate what we *retained* from the previous session. Examining the results of **retention tests** is one approach to inferring motor learning from measures of performance. In Figure 5.2, trials 11 through 15 represent the results of a retention test and show that the increased performance was maintained after a rest period. The opposite also can occur; that is, performance can improve after rest from dissipation of conditions such as fatigue that impair performance.

Schmidt and Lee's definition of motor learning also states that the processes that underlie learning are *associated with* practice or experience. Why not say instead that the learning *occurs during* practice or experience? One reason is that neural processes that help to make the changed motor performance permanent are active for many hours after practice and some may even require a night of sleep (Brashers-Krug, Shadmehr, & Bizzi, 1996; Cohen, Pascual-Leone, Press, & Robertson, 2005; Robertson, Pascual-Leone, & Miall, 2004). Consolidating motor memory into a relatively permanent state appears to occur gradually and may consist of several stages that involve different brain areas (Luft & Buitrago, 2005). This may be another reason performance on retention tests can exceed performance at the end of the previous training period.

Motor learning does not always require physical practice or experience. One can improve motor performance in a permanent way by imitating someone else's performance (observational learning) or by attempting a task following a verbal description of the task. Perhaps more surprising, there is a rich literature indicating that vividly imagining that you are performing a task yields increased performance on retention tests (Feltz & Landers, 1983; Jeannerod, 1995). Although these performance gains are not as great as those obtained by physical practice, they are substantial (Hird, Landers, Thomas, & Horan, 1991). One theory is that the motor learning comes about by the brain practicing the task internally, using the same brain regions and mechanisms as it would for performing the task, and then inhibiting the final commands that would produce muscle force (Jeannerod, 2001). The fact that increased strength has been demonstrated following mental practice indirectly support this mechanism (Yue & Cole, 1992). Another view is that the performance gains following physical versus mental training result from activity in different brain areas (Nyberg, Eriksson, Larsson, & Marklund, 2006), depending on the complexity of the task. Although we don't completely understand the mechanisms that underlie motor learning following mental practice, there is no doubt that we can learn new tasks, to a point, without physical practice.

Conditions for Optimal Learning

THE LAW OF PRACTICE Coaches, instructors, therapists, and students all seek, or should seek, to understand how one should practice in order to learn most *efficiently* (to achieve the most learning with the least practice). Maximizing the number of practice trials is the first principle of practice and has come to be known as the **Law of Practice.** It should come as no surprise that more practice leads to more learning. The change in performance typically is rapid early in practice and slows as performance improves (see Figure 5.2). After extensive practice, the performance gains may slow so much that it may be tempting to conclude that learning no longer occurs. However, there are reports of performance gains that continue even after millions of repetitions of a task over many years (Crossman, 1959).

An important application of this Law of Practice is the recent change in the treatment of individuals following a stroke affecting the motor areas of the cerebral cortex. It had been believed that little motor recovery could occur after 6 to 12 months following the stroke. Research over the past decade has now demonstrated that intense, repetitive practice of the impaired upper limb, practice lasting several hours per day over a few weeks, can substantially improve motor function even years after a stroke. This was true when the therapeutic technique included forced use of the impaired limb in functional tasks (Wolf et al., 2006) or when the impaired upper limb was assisted or resisted robotically during reaching movements (Fasoli et al., 2004). These findings have powered an exciting revolution in the approaches to therapy following stroke. What is more remarkable is that stroke recovery following these intense, repetitive practice therapies and motor learning in healthy individuals from repetitive practice appear to share common mechanisms involving brain plasticity (discussed later in this chapter).

MASSED VERSUS DISTRIBUTED PRACTICE

How should one schedule practice to maximize learning? Studies of practice distribution have focused on determining how much time should be spent in practice versus rest during a practice session, as well as the distribution of practice sessions during the day. A considerable amount of research has focused on whether you retain more with relatively short rest intervals during a practice session, termed **massed practice,** or if better retention occurs with relatively long rest intervals during a session, termed **distributed practice.** Practice sessions organized around distributed practice schedules will require more time if an equal number of repetitions are to occur compared to practice based on a massed practice schedule. The general finding is that massed practice tends to result in poorer performance during the practice session compared to distributed practice (Lee & Genovese, 1988). Participants who practiced under a distributed practice schedule also showed better retention when tested either a short time after the practice session (minutes) or a long time after practice (weeks, months).

This suggests that a practice session with adequate rest periods yields better motor learning. However, much of this research concerning practice distribution schedules has focused on motor tasks that are best described as continuous, such as attempting to follow, or track, the motions of something moving continuously, or climbing up and down a small ladder that you must balance while climbing. Do the findings from these studies on practice schedules for continuous tasks generalize to so-called discrete tasks that last less than a second, such as kicking or throwing? The answer, based on much less research, seems to be that massed practice yields better performance on discrete tasks compared to continuous tasks both during practice and on retention tests performed later. It seems fair to conclude that while a massed practice schedule may be best for learning a discrete task, continuous tasks that introduce the possibility of fatigue should be practiced under a distributed schedule. Clearly, instructors, coaches, and therapists teaching discrete skills will favor the efficiency of a massed practice schedule, but they should be prepared to alter their practice scheduling for continuous tasks. Consider how this statement would impact a physical therapist working with a client attempting to regain upper limb reaching skills versus walking, or the practice schedules that may favor the skills needed in baseball versus those of the musician.

Another issue of considerable practical importance is whether one should schedule multiple short practices during the day or week, or if fewer, longer practices yield better performance and retention. Results from an experiment in which postal workers were taught a typing task used for a mail sorting machine (Baddeley & Longman, 1978) indicated that massed practice schedules (e.g., two 1-hour sessions, twice per day for 15 days) yielded worse performance while practicing and poorer retention 1 to 9 months later than did more distributed practice schedules (e.g., 1-hour sessions once per day for 60 days).

At this point the astute reader may begin to wonder how the Law of Practice affects conclusions about practice schedules. Studies on practice distribution schedules are designed to hold constant the number of task repetitions or the actual time spent practicing. Thus, under distributed practice schedules it will take longer to achieve the same amount of time or number of task repetitions compared to a massed practice schedule. The Law of Practice states that performance and retention increase with increasing practice time or number of repetitions. Putting these concepts together one can ask if, during practice sessions of equal duration for massed versus distributed practice, the negative effects of massed practice (in the case of continuous tasks) can be offset by the increased practice that can be realized during the massed practice sessions compared to distributed practice sessions. While these issues require additional study, research confirms the benefits of massed practice in stroke recovery for upper limb skills, as noted previously (although many of the skills were discrete in nature).

VARIABLE VERSUS CONSTANT PRACTICE

Other issues come into play when designing practice sessions; one of these involves the repetitiveness of practice. When learning a brand new skill like throwing a curve ball in baseball, one tends to repeat the same movements again and again without interrupting this practice by throwing a different pitch, such as a fastball or change-up. This approach helps you to achieve the "feel" of the essential motions for throwing a curve ball. Once this first phase of learning is complete, your goal probably is to learn to throw the pitch accurately to different locations in the strike zone (e.g., close to the batter's body versus away from the batter) and also to throw the curve accurately after just having thrown a different type of pitch. How should you plan your practice sessions with these latter goals in mind? Should you practice throwing accurately to a single target and assume that this accuracy will generalize when you want to throw the ball to a different part of the strike zone? Or should you practice pitching to a variety of targets? Similarly, if you want to practice curve balls, fastballs, and change-ups during a single practice session, will you learn them more efficiently by practicing first one pitch to a desired level of performance before moving on to another? These examples raise the issue of two important factors in designing a practice session: variable versus constant practice and blocked versus random practice scheduling.

Variable practice refers to practicing the same skill under varying conditions or at different levels or targets. Our baseball pitcher could employ a **constant practice** scheme by repetitively pitching to one location, such as the middle of the strike zone. Variable practice would involve attempting to pitch to a variety of locations (e.g., high, low, left corner, right corner). Studies comparing constant versus variable practice schemes generally indicate that individuals who train under variable practice conditions perform *worse* during the training session but perform *better* during the later retention test, from which we infer better learning for the variable practice group. You can imagine as a coach it could be difficult to convince the athlete that he or she will learn more with variable practice when the athlete is experiencing worse performance while practicing compared to constant practice schemes.

The effects of variable practice also have been studied when individuals practice a variety of different target locations and then are tested later on a target upon which they never practiced. The performance of these individuals is compared against individuals who practiced only one target location before their test on the novel target location. Studies like this reveal that those who experienced variable practice performed worse during the training session than those who practiced a single target, but they performed better when tested on the novel target. Thus, it seems that variable practice also helps us learn how to adjust our motor commands to new circumstances. It has been suggested that variable practice is particularly beneficial to those who generally are less experienced in movement, such as children (Schmidt & Lee, 2005). In any case, variable practice has not been demonstrated to impede learning compared to constant practice.

BLOCKED VERSUS RANDOM PRACTICE

How should one schedule practice? In the case of throwing darts accurately to a variety of targets on the board, should you practice first at one target until you become proficient, then another target, and so on? This would be an example of a **blocked practice** schedule. Under a **random practice** schedule, you would attempt to hit a different target on each throw. Intuitively you might think that practicing different targets randomly would slow your learning. Perhaps constantly changing targets will interfere with your ability to concentrate and get into a groove. The results of experiments comparing blocked versus random practice schedules shows that blocked practice yields better performance than random practice *during the training sessions*, but practice under a random schedule yields better performance *on retention tests* compared to practice under a blocked schedule. One explanation for this often-reported finding is that we learn better when we don't "get into a groove," because we must engage in more elaborate and complete preparation for each movement rather than carrying over the preparation from repetition to repetition. This line of reasoning was derived from the theory of contextual interference (Battig, 1979). This supports the approach some basketball coaches take in which they intersperse free throw shooting practice in small blocks throughout a practice session rather than requiring players to repetitively shoot free throws in large blocks at the beginning or end of practice.

Before we leave this topic, it is important to note that scientists also have studied intermediate forms of random practice, in which small blocks of the same task are mixed randomly among small blocks of different tasks. Under these conditions, we find that one can achieve the same level of learning without resorting to a completely randomized practice schedule. For example, the softball pitcher may throw four rising pitches, followed by four change-ups, and then four curves or drop balls. In any case, the results of research lead us to conclude that once an individual can perform the task in a basic way, one should avoid drilling on the task by repeating it over and over and over again without performing an intervening skill. This conclusion should hold for efficiently learning just about any motor skill one can imagine, across sports, music, hobbies, and occupational skills.

PHYSICAL GUIDANCE After considering the earlier discussion of motor learning by mental imagery, and the reasoning behind the positive effects of random practice schedules, it may come as no surprise that we learn better when we perform movements as much as possible under our own power rather than with physical assistance or guidance. This is an important issue because physical assistance via a therapist or robotic device is frequently used in rehabilitation following nervous system injury or disease. There is no doubt that guidance, either physical or verbal (talking someone through the task), is useful at first. Likewise, physical guidance or feedback during a task will improve the performance during a training session. At this point in the chapter, you probably are skeptical about accepting the conditions that lead to a performance gain as representing conditions for learning, unless these gains are retained in later sessions. Your skepticism would be justified, as once again we find a condition of practice guidance, which is not as effective in producing sustainable gains in performance as other techniques. Techniques that force the performer to generate the actions on his or her own as much as possible provide greater performance gains during subsequent tests than when the actions are guided. In particular, feedback about performance at the end of the task, or at the end of a block of repetitions, is more effective in producing motor learning than are physical guidance or continuous feedback during each trial.

Current techniques in motor rehabilitation following brain injury attempt to wean the patient from physical guidance as quickly as possible. In stroke rehabilitation, when weakness is a problem, early stages of therapy may involve some assistance in producing reaching movements. Later stages of this therapy involve the patient working without assistance and even against resistance (to increase strength) as he or she progresses.

Brain Plasticity

Brain plasticity refers to the ability of the brain to show modification in response to experience (learning and memory) or injury. Research in motor learning has been reenergized during the past 20 years by exciting discoveries that revealed more rapid and extensive brain plasticity than was previously believed.

One of the remarkable findings emerging recently is that the motor areas that are active during movement of a particular joint, or the sensory areas that respond to stimulation of a particular body part, can reorganize within hours while acquiring new tactile perceptual skills or motor skills (Xerri, Coq, Merzenich, & Jenkins, 1996; for a review see Sanes & Donoghue, 2000). In experiments such as these, the brain areas that responded to the stimulation or movement of a particular part of the body expand as the skill is practiced, while nearby areas representing noninvolved body parts shrink. These findings reveal that the basic cortical areas involved in sensing stimuli and generating movement are not static but reorganize dynamically in response to experience. Quite simply, the demands placed upon us by our environment cause the brain to adapt.

We now know that this adaptation includes increases and decreases in the number and complexity of dendrites (the portions of neurons important for receiving information from other neurons) and their connections with other neurons, along with changes in the strength or effectiveness of these synaptic contacts. The role of these fundamental changes during the early phases of skill acquisition is under increased study. For example, drugs that affect the electrical excitability of cells in the brain can affect motor learning. Drugs that decrease excitability in the motor cortex (and act as central nervous system depressants), such as lorazepam (used to relieve anxiety) and dextromethorphan (used in cough suppressants), impair motor learning (Donchin, Sawaki, Ghangadar, & Cohen, 2002).

Although rapid changes in brain plasticity may be adaptive (helpful) to the organism, they may also be *maladaptive*. It is believed that plastic changes are partly to blame for a rare disorder known as focal dystonia, which is manifest as a crampinglike behavior that impairs the ability to produce highly practiced movements, such as those of master-level musicians (Byl, 2004).

Paralleling our expanding knowledge of brain plasticity during motor learning is a research effort aimed at discovering the mechanisms that underlie recovery of motor function following brain injury. It had long been believed that the primate brain was capable only of limited structural change following injury. The brilliant anatomist and Nobel Laureate Ramon y Cajal (considered by many as a father of modern neuroscience) believed that the axons and dendrites of mammalian neurons in adults were incapable of further growth and regeneration (Ramon y Cajal, 1928). We now know that this is not true and that after injury there is brain plasticity at molecular, synaptic, cellular, network, and systems levels (Nudo, 2006). Our rapidly expanding knowledge about what drives new growth and regeneration after brain injury holds promise for better recovery of function through behavioral and pharmacological therapies.

A key question is the extent to which these adaptive processes can be enhanced. Therapeutic interventions have been explored using drugs, electrical stimulation, and behavioral therapy. Scientists also are investigating issues like the timing of interventions to determine how best to take advantage of the adaptive mechanisms that are spurred into action following injury. An important finding is that postinjury behavioral experience facilitates the adaptive rewiring. It is thought that the activation of the intact areas through our attempts to move serves as some sort of signal that, in effect, calls out to the sprouting axons so that the area can be recognized as a target.

It is easy to see why there is so much interest now in studies focused on determining which therapeutic practices are most effective, how the therapy sessions should be scheduled and structured (timing, intensity, type of movements), and how the intervention should be modified, if at all, according to the site of lesion and size of lesion. In addition to the effectiveness of therapy, the *efficiency* of therapy is of great concern because therapy time is expensive. The role of robotic devices in stroke therapy is garnering considerable interest for this reason. Collectively these issues are rapidly reshaping the face of poststroke therapeutic practices.

MOTOR CONTROL

The movements that we produce require vast networks of neurons in our central nervous system that ultimately converge on the neurons that directly activate our muscles. These neuronal networks that plan and execute our movements also interact with networks concerned with motivation (it's time for me to go to school), attention (ignore the television program you've been watching and look for your backpack), sensory information about the state of the environment (my backpack is 1 foot in front of me and 6 inches to the right of my right shoulder, and it weighs 10 pounds) and the state of your body (I'm already standing up, my left hand is holding my jacket, and my right hand is at my side), and emotional or strategic factors (I'm running late, so I'd better move quickly).

Scientists don't completely understand how we produce even simple coordinated movements like reaching, so there is no single theory of motor control. This part of the chapter introduces some of the most fundamental observations that have been made about movement production. These observations begin to help us understand how skilled movements are produced from the interactions of the nervous system, musculoskeletal system, and the environment.

Central Motor Representations and the Role of Sensory Information

The central nervous system is continuously bombarded by sensory signals carrying information important for planning and executing our movements. Besides vision, sensory signals from receptors in our muscles, tendons, skin, vestibular system, joints, and ligaments can inform our motor system about the state of our body (particularly the musculoskeletal system) and the state of our surroundings. It is not surprising, therefore, that there is a long history of research focused on the problem of discovering exactly how sensory information contributes to motor control. An important finding of this research was that individuals who were deprived of sensory information through disease or injury still could produce voluntary movements. This means that the brain must store, or represent, motor actions in some way. In this section we'll focus on the movement capabilities of individuals deprived of sensory information, and in the process we'll learn a little about how action is stored or represented in the central nervous system.

An influential study by Mott and Sherrington (1895) reported that a monkey failed to use its forelimb after the sensory nerve roots to that limb alone were severed where they enter the spinal cord. They concluded, incorrectly, that sensory signals were absolutely essential to produce movement. This was vigorously disputed a few years later (Hering, 1897). Thus began a period of about 150 years of controversy regarding this topic. (We now know that monkeys *will* use their sensation-deprived forelimb when forced to; for example, when the normal forelimb is restrained [Taub, 1976]). These controversies were resolved in the 1980s when two reports were published concerning individuals who lost all sensory signals from their arms and legs from an unknown disease that affected sensory neurons of the arms and legs while leaving motor neurons unaffected (Rothwell et al., 1982; Sanes, Mauritz, Dalakas, & Evarts, 1985). These insensate (or **deafferented**) individuals were relatively unimpaired in muscle strength, but they could not feel when their skin was touched or when their joints moved. Also missing were the reflexive contractions of their muscles that normally occur when muscles are rapidly stretched (e.g., when the physician taps the tendon just below your knee with a reflex hammer).

The most revealing results were obtained when the patients closed their eyes, for it was then that the scientists could observe the capacity of the central nervous system to produce movement without sensory information. In the laboratory these patients were able to initiate and perform simple and complex movements, though poorly. Clearly, Mott and Sherrington (1895) were wrong! Learned, voluntary movements could be performed without sensory information. This means that movements are represented centrally in some form and, at our desire, can be reproduced or assembled from their essential elements by processes that continue to be the subject of considerable research (see Shumway-Cook & Woollacott, 2007, for a succinct review of contemporary theories of movement control).

One important clue to the nature of these **central representations** of skilled movements can be found in the observations of Sanes and his colleagues (1985). They observed that the movements that their insensate patients produced typically contained errors. When vision was removed, not only did profound errors of movement size occur in these patients but frequently even the direction of movement was incorrect. We must conclude that the brain does not store complete, well-formed actions that are simply replayed from memory. Instead, additional information from our sensory systems is needed, such as the current state of the body and the state of our immediate surroundings, to assemble the detailed movement commands so that accurate movements can be produced. (This topic is addressed in the next section.) Such observations support the widely held belief today that movements are elaborated in their details by a progression of neural processes, beginning with an abstract representation of the movement, and that sensory information is required at several steps in this process to generate accurate and efficient movements. How we acquire, maintain, and adapt these central representations are topics of intense study today.

Sensory Signals and Motor Control

We now come to the obvious issue: Exactly what is the role of **sensory information** in producing accurate actions? In 1941 the eminent neuroembryologist Paul Weiss wrote, "Nobody in his senses would think of questioning the importance of sensory control of movement. But just what is the precise scope of that control?" (p. 23). Scientists continue to address Weiss's question today.

POSTURAL CONTROL We can gain insight to this issue by further examining how insensate individuals behave while they attempt to produce various motor actions. First, sensory information is crucial in correcting for small errors that occur during slow movements and while attempting to hold a steady **posture.** One of the most profound behaviors of these insensate patients is their lack of postural stability. When attempting to hold a steady hand position, they do so reasonably well with vision of the hand, but without vision their hand position drifts substantially (Figure 5.3b). Thus, one critical role of sensory information from the limbs is to signal the nervous system to correct the small imbalances that occur in the forces around a joint as we contract our muscles and attempt to maintain a steady posture. Without sensory information (from our limbs or from vision of our limbs), these small errors in force and position accumulate, causing the limb to drift slowly out of the desired position.

ERROR CORRECTION DURING MOVEMENT
The gradual accumulation of error when sensory information is absent also may explain the behaviors we observe when an insensate individual attempts to touch the thumb to each of his or her fingers in rapid succession (Rothwell et al., 1982). The patient performs the task reasonably well with eyes closed at the start of the task (Figure 5.4a). However, after 30 seconds had

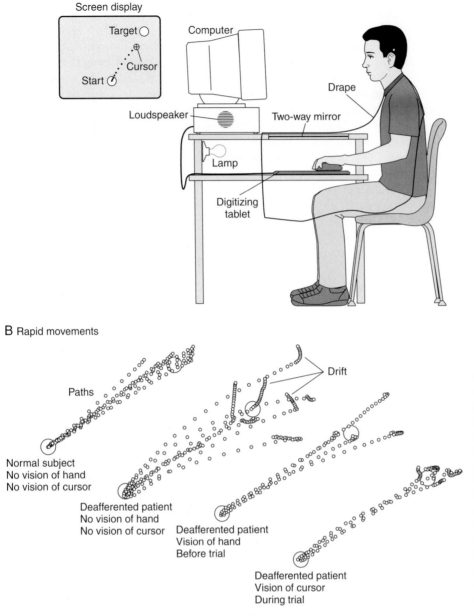

A Experimental setup

Screen display

Target ○

Cursor ⊕

Start ⊙

Computer

Loudspeaker

Two-way mirror

Drape

Lamp

Digitizing tablet

B Rapid movements

Paths

Drift

Normal subject
No vision of hand
No vision of cursor

Deafferented patient
No vision of hand
No vision of cursor

Deafferented patient
Vision of hand
Before trial

Deafferented patient
Vision of cursor
During trial

Figure 5.3 (a) The experimental setup for a study that examined the effect of removing vision of one's limb on sliding the hand to a target. (b) The paths that the hand followed when moving from the start position (left circles) to the target position (right circles), for normal subjects and for subjects who had an insensate limb due to disease ("deafferented").

Source: Kandel et al. (1991). Principles of neural science (3rd ed.). New York: Elsevier.

elapsed (Figure 5.4b), the fingers and thumb become increasingly misaligned until they miss each other completely. The conclusion that sensory information is used to correct small errors in movements as they evolve also is supported by many other lines of evidence and depends on movement characteristics such as speed, size, and the needed accuracy.

INITIAL CONDITION INFORMATION It may be tempting at this point to conclude that the main roles of sensory information for motor control are (1) to help correct or compensate for errors that develop in our forces and movements, during both movement and posture, and (2) to specify the locations of objects in space that we intend to contact or avoid (a role that we haven't discussed yet, but

which should seem obvious). Sensory information plays another, crucially important role that reveals to us a little more about the nature of our central representations of motor actions. Bernstein (1967) recognized that the same motor command will produce different results depending on the starting position of the limb. Perhaps sensory signals also provide information about the beginning state of our muscles, joints, and limbs.

Indeed, it is clear that central representations require this **initial condition** sensory information to generate the appropriate motor commands. Claude Ghez and his colleagues (1995) observed insensate (deafferented) individuals with this question in mind. They asked participants to slide a small object, similar to a computer mouse, to different

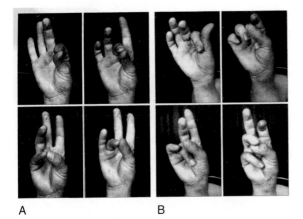

A   B

Figure 5.4 Photographs of the hand of a patient with no sensation in the upper limb who was instructed to tap each finger to the thumb. (a) Accurate performance in the seconds following the patient closing his eyes. (b) Inaccurate performance after the patient had been performing the task for 30 seconds.

Source: Rothwell, J. C., Traub, M. M., Day B. L., Obeso, J. A., Thomas, P. K., & Marsden, C. D. (1982). Manual motor performance in a deafferented man. *Brain, 10 5*, 515–542.

positions on a table using horizontal arm movements (see Figure 5.3a). A cursor on a computer monitor continuously indicated the position of the object so that participants could see the object's movement progress. A two-way mirror blocked participants' view of their arm, and they could only see their arm when the investigators illuminated a light under the mirror. Without vision of the cursor or their arm, the deafferented participants were significantly less accurate in movement direction and extent when compared to the healthy participants, and their movements tended to curve more than the healthy adults (Figure 5.3b). This finding reinforces the importance of sensory information from the upper extremity in producing targeted reaching movements. Once the deafferented participants stopped moving at the location that they believed to be the target, their arm began to drift, again demonstrating the role of sensory information in controlling posture.

The surprising new finding in this study was that compared to the no-vision condition, the deafferented participants improved their movement performance substantially simply by viewing their arm just *prior* to the start of their arm movement (but not *during* arm movement). In fact, viewing the arm prior to the movement (but not during the movement) yielded movements nearly as accurate as the movements that were produced when the patients could see their arm (or the cursor representing the position of their hand) continuously during the movement (Figure 5.3b; compare the rightmost two groups of data). Another surprising finding was that the improvements from

viewing the arm prior to the movement disappeared if the deafferented participants delayed their movement for any more than a minute. Ghez and his colleagues concluded that healthy individuals use sensory information from their upper limb to provide the nervous system with the starting position and configuration of the limb, and this information was essential to the process of generating accurate and well-planned movements. In the absence of this sensory information from the limb, the deafferented patients substituted *visual* information about the starting limb configuration (when they were allowed to see their arm before movement).

These findings indicate that our central motor processes require sensory information about initial body conditions to generate accurate motor commands. Also, these initial conditions are likely to change from moment-to-moment as we move our body and limbs slightly, so the sensory information about initial conditions is not stored for very long. Presumably, the streams of incoming information concerning the state of our body continuously replace our rapidly decaying memories about initial conditions. This means that the central motor processes *predictively* generate the needed commands as long as accurate information about the starting configuration of the limb and the location of the target are available. This type of predictive control has been call *feedforward*. Sensory information from the limb during movement can then correct for the typically small errors that remain, using *feedback* control.

Our central motor processes also require initial condition information about the ever-changing conditions of our surroundings. Consider what happens to your arm movement when you lift a pitcher of lemonade that is nearly empty if you expected that pitcher to be full, or how you walk across a frozen pond compared to unexpectedly encountering a patch of ice on the sidewalk. Clearly, our movement planning processes use sensory signals and memory to estimate the mechanical conditions of the surroundings with which we interact.

Thus far we have focused on the importance of sensory information in motor control for (1) correcting or compensating errors that develop during the movement, (2) providing initial condition information about our body and the external world, and (3) locating something that we wish to contact (or avoid).

The control of walking provides good examples of two additional roles for sensory information: (4) setting the springiness of our muscles and (5) signaling when our movement has reached a point so the next phase of the movement can be started. A continuous flow of sensory signals from receptors in our muscles and tendons back to neurons in our spinal cord influence the activation of our muscles.

These sensory signals to the spinal cord (along with commands converging on the spinal cord from other parts of the brain) appear to set properties like the "springiness" of our muscles (resistance to lengthening). While we walk, many of the muscles in our lower limbs rhythmically change from a relatively stiff condition, when supporting the load of our body, to much less stiff, when the limb is swinging forward in the air. Extensive experiments in animal locomotion indicate that the basic patterns of these rhythmic changes in muscle activation result from networks of neurons within the spinal cord that function as a **central pattern generator.** Once switched on, normally via higher brain centers, the central pattern generator issues the basic alternating rhythmic patterns of muscle activation within and across limbs, even in the absence of sensory information. This is akin to the ability of deafferented individuals to rhythmically tap their fingers to their thumb. However, just like the deafferented individuals' attempts at tapping the thumb and fingers together, without sensory information the muscle activations that are issued from the central pattern generator contain small errors that quickly accumulate until walking fails. The central pattern generator appears to issue motor commands under the assumption that sensory information from the limbs is returning to the spinal cord and that these signals will increase muscle springiness via reflexes. As a result, some features of a movement, like the lower part of our leg accelerating briefly during one part of its forward swing, occur not because the movement program explicitly commanded this feature but because it emerged out of the complex interactions of the nervous system and musculoskeletal system.

Finally, sensory information also signals the progress of our actions and can trigger the next phase of an action, which is a fifth role for sensory information. The leg bearing our body load (while the opposite leg swings forward) eventually must swing forward (while the other leg supports our body load) if we are to continue our forward progression. This can occur only when the opposite leg has contacted the ground and the extensor muscles, such as those in the front of the thigh, stiffen adequately to bear your entire weight. Sherrington suggested that receptors in the hip muscles of the leg that is waiting to become the swing leg may signal the appropriate time for the leg to begin its forward swing. Elegant studies of cat locomotion confirmed Sherrington's suggestion and also confirmed a similar role for receptors in the tendons that signal when the leg is no longer bearing a substantial portion of body load, so the leg can be lifted for swing. The rhythmic output of the central pattern generator shifting between standing on the leg and swinging it forward is prevented if the proper sensory signals are not received.

Putting It All Together: Postural Control

Let's consider a task that we've only briefly touched upon to this point, postural control. It is essential that we stabilize our body, or parts of our body, against external forces and against forces from our own movement. Maintaining our balance in the face of gravity is an example of postural control in relation to external forces. Maintaining a stable shoulder position while moving the forearm at the elbow is an example of how postural control is required whenever we move a body segment. Because forces come in pairs (equal and oppositely directed), the simple task of moving one segment of your limb requires that you stabilize the other segments, or suffer unintended movements of those segments. Sherrington recognized the fundamental importance of postural control when he eloquently stated that "posture follows movement like its shadow" (Creed, Denny-Brown, Eccles, Liddell, & Sherrington, 1932, pp. 147–148).

Maintaining our balance while standing upright solves the mechanical problem of keeping the vertical projection of our center of mass (the point at the center of our total body mass) within our base of support (the area of our body that contacts a support surface). While standing upright and supported only at our feet, our base of support is the area from the lateral edge of one foot to the lateral edge of the opposite foot.[2] The first requirement in this task of maintaining balance is the need to fight gravity and support our body load without sagging or collapsing toward the ground. To do this, we automatically activate the appropriate muscles from our neck to our ankles, reinforced by sensory signals from those muscles. This basic activation of our antigravity muscles has been termed *postural tone*. But this task is not so easily achieved. With nearly frictionless joints, very small imbalances in the forces on each side of a joint will result in the slow positional drift of the joint. We've already discussed studies of insensate individuals who find it impossible to hold an outstretched limb still unless they view that limb. It should come as no surprise that standing upright involves rapid processing of sensory information by the brain to select appropriate muscles and change their level of activation so as to minimize *sway*, motion around the vertical axis of the body.

The process of controlling sway usually does not require our attention, so we say that it is automatic. We have discovered that this control requires that we rapidly predict the direction and amount of

[2]In fact, the problem is a bit more complex because the speed at which the center of mass is moving also determines how close your center of mass can get to the edges of your base of support without losing your balance.

sway from sensory information and then select the actions that will minimize the sway. How we control forward and backward sway has been studied extensively using a platform that the person stands on that can unexpectedly move forward or backward. These studies have shown that a backward sway, from forward translation of the platform, triggers a coordinated activation of muscles that efficiently pull the body segments forward. The contractions begin first with muscles acting around the ankle, followed by activation of muscles acting around the knee, hips, and finally at the trunk and neck. The opposing muscles are activated if the platform moves backward.

These patterns work because the person can effectively exert forces against the support surface with his or her feet. What happens when you are standing on a narrow support surface such that your toes and heels have nothing to push against? In this case the initial conditions have changed compared to the flat support surface, and the brain, having processed sensory information about the new support conditions, selects a different pattern of muscle activation that focuses on muscles that will produce large movements around the hips (think about balancing on a tightrope).

The essentially *predictive* nature of these processes was demonstrated when investigators mixed in trials with a pure platform rotation, which caused the ankles to rotate without causing sway (Figure 5.5). No sway occurs in this case because the rotation didn't move the base of support in relation to the vertical projection of the center of mass. On these trials people reacted to the imposed ankle motion by generating the same sequence of muscle activations as if the platform had moved forward (when the platform rotated the toes up) or backward (when the platform rotated the toes down). As a result, the rotation triggered muscle responses that *caused* sway. Individuals quickly suppressed these responses within a few trials, demonstrating the ease with which these sensory-to-motor transformations can be adapted to new circumstances that arise in the environment.

As previously noted, postural control means more than controlling the orientation of the body in the face of gravity and other external forces. For example, the movements that we intentionally generate, like reaching out to grasp and lift an object, cause our center of mass to move, which can cause sway. We've seen how the nervous system can react to sway quite effectively by rapidly processing sensory signals about sway to generate actions to minimize sway in accordance with support conditions. Does the nervous system use the same strategy when the disturbance to our stability is of our own making? The answer is no.

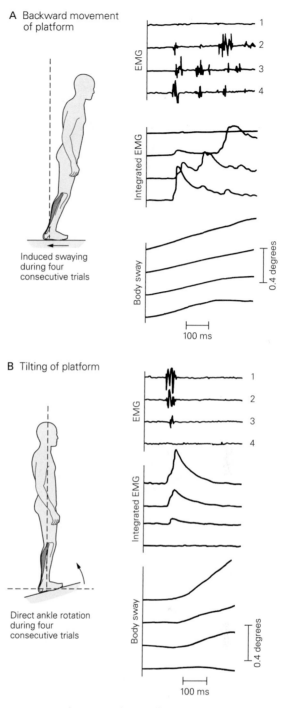

A Backward movement of platform

Induced swaying during four consecutive trials

B Tilting of platform

Direct ankle rotation during four consecutive trials

Figure 5.5 The postural control system responds to sway of the body around the vertical axis that is caused by the backward translation of a moveable platform upon which the person stands. The motor system learns to trigger the appropriate responses based on ankle rotation, and before much sway actually occurs. This prediction is wrong when the platform rotates because, while the ankles still rotate, no sway occurs.

Consider the simple act of lifting one leg to the side (Figure 5.6). As your leg rises, your center of mass will move to the side, which would lead to a sideways sway if your postural control system did nothing. Rather than reacting to this sway (as was the case for

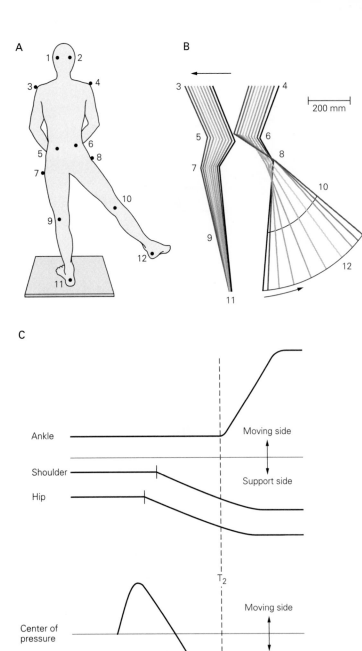

A

B

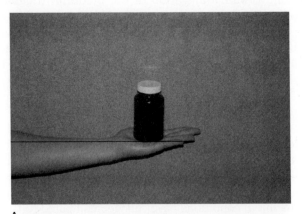

A

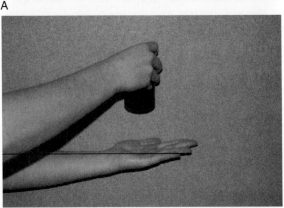

B

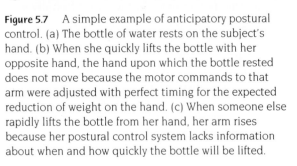

C

C

Figure 5.6 The act of lifting one's leg sideways while standing involves shifts in the body's center of mass away from midline *before* the leg begins to rise, illustrating an anticipatory postural action.

the experiments using platform translations discussed previously), the brain activates muscles just slightly in advance of the leg motion so that you lean slightly to the side away from the leg that you are about to lift. This type of postural control has been termed **anticipatory,** to distinguish it from the reactive adjustments that occur when our balance is disturbed unexpectedly. Apparently, while the nervous system builds the central commands for the intended arm movements, it also is determining the postural

adjustments needed to prevent sway in the face of those arm movements.

Here's a simple demonstration of anticipatory postural control that requires another person and an object like a bottle of water (Figure 5.7). Have your colleague balance the bottle of water in front of him or

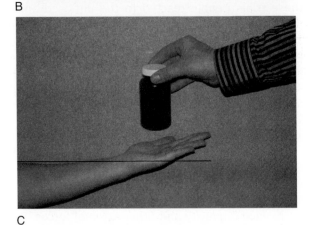

Figure 5.7 A simple example of anticipatory postural control. (a) The bottle of water rests on the subject's hand. (b) When she quickly lifts the bottle with her opposite hand, the hand upon which the bottle rested does not move because the motor commands to that arm were adjusted with perfect timing for the expected reduction of weight on the hand. (c) When someone else rapidly lifts the bottle from her hand, her arm rises because her postural control system lacks information about when and how quickly the bottle will be lifted.

her on an open palm with eyes closed. Ask the person to use the other hand to quickly lift the bottle off of the open hand. Observe the motion of the open hand. Replace the bottle on the open hand (your colleague's eyes should remain closed), and don't tell the person what is to come next. Without warning, quickly lift the bottle from his or her hand. You should observe a fairly large upward motion of the hand in the second case. The relatively small hand movement that should have occurred when your colleague lifted the bottle from his or her own hand was the result of a reduction in the drive to the arm muscles that were supporting the bottle. This reduction in muscle drive was precisely coordinated with the removal of the bottle from the hand. Your colleague couldn't produce this adjustment when *you* lifted the bottle because the central processes for producing anticipatory postural adjustments didn't have access to information concerning when and how quickly the load was to be removed. This demonstrates the predictive, rather than reactive, nature of the reduction in arm muscle commands to the support arm.

PROFESSIONAL ORGANIZATIONS AND CERTIFICATIONS

A wide variety of organizations and societies are dedicated to promoting the many professions that focus on the study and application of motor control and motor learning. Several of the more prominent organizations that also oversee professional certification are discussed here, along with professional societies that do not oversee professional certification but exist to organize and disseminate information about a discipline or field.

Many professional organizations and scientific societies foster a profession without necessarily overseeing the accreditation of educational programs or the certification of clinicians or practitioners. They aim to advance the scientific understanding of the discipline, provide professional development activities and resources, promote public information about the discipline, and many inform or lobby legislators about scientific information regarding the discipline that may affect public policy. The Society for Neuroscience is a long-standing society in this model that developed out of the American Physiological Society. It is dedicated to advancing the understanding of the nervous system by serving scientists and scientists-in-training, and the public, through the general activities noted previously. The annual meeting of the organization, based in the United States, draws approximately 25,000 to 30,000 attendees, most of whom are scientists and graduate students. The

International Brain Research Organization, based in Canada, also promotes the development and dissemination of scientific information about the brain but focuses in addition on international collaboration and interchange of scientific information.

Some scientific societies and organizations focus more directly on the fields of motor control and motor learning. The International Society for Motor Control is a relatively new society aimed at promoting basic and applied research in the area of the control of movements of biological systems. A much older society, the North American Society for Psychology of Sport and Physical Activity, describes itself as "a multidisciplinary association of scholars from the behavioral sciences and related professions." The society aims to advance the scientific study of human behavior related to sport and physical activity, disseminate information, and improve the quality of research and teaching in the psychology of sport, motor development, and motor learning and control. The American Alliance for Health, Physical Education, Recreation and Dance (AAPHERD) has been important in the development of scientists and the science of motor behavior and for professionals who apply this knowledge, especially in physical education, coaching, and dance instruction. As its name suggests, it is an alliance of several national organizations and research consortia. (The name of this organization may soon change.) The American College of Sports Medicine (ACSM) likewise is a professional organization for scientists and practitioners some of whom touch upon motor control and motor learning in their research and practices.

The Biomedical Engineering Society exists to "to promote the increase of biomedical engineering knowledge and its utilization." It also participates in the accreditation of educational programs. The definition of biomedical engineering is quite broad, reflecting the historical interplay between medicine and technology. According to the National Institutes of Health,

> Biomedical engineering integrates physical, chemical, mathematical, and computational sciences and engineering principles to study biology, medicine, behavior, and health. It advances fundamental concepts; creates knowledge from the molecular to the organ systems level; and develops innovative biologics, materials, processes, implants, devices and informatics approaches for the prevention, diagnosis, and treatment of disease, for patient rehabilitation, and for improving health." (**www.becon.nih. gov/bioengineering_definition.htm**)

It is easy to see how motor control and motor learning can interact with such a broadly defined engineering discipline.

A common feature of professionals that deliver health care is the requirement to obtain a license to practice their profession. Just like physicians and dentists must obtain the appropriate license to practice medicine and dentistry in their state, so too must physical and occupational therapists, speech-language pathologists, athletic trainers, teachers, and so on. Before applying for a license, most states require certification by an approved professional organization. This certification requires minimum standards of education including graduating from an accredited educational program. These issues are discussed further in the next section.

CAREERS

Knowledge about motor control can be applied to a wide variety of clinical, instructional, and engineering fields. Physical therapists, occupational therapists, speech-language pathologists, and athletic trainers apply their knowledge of motor control and motor learning on a daily basis as they determine how best to help their clients establish, modify, or regain motor function. Indeed, Vernon Brooks (1986) referred to physical therapists and occupational therapists as **applied motor control physiologists,** a phrase that can be applied as well to speech-language therapists and athletic trainers.

Physicians practicing in the fields of neurology, orthopedic surgery, physical medicine and rehabilitation, and other specialties also are concerned with how best to improve impaired motor performance. In instructional settings, physical educators, coaches, music instructors, and dance instructors can, and should, directly apply principles of motor learning to their teaching techniques. In industry, those who design devices and environments that humans engage also apply knowledge of motor control, from the design of user interfaces for machine control to the design of roadways. The fields of ergonomics and human factors engineering emerged partly out of the realization that injury or suboptimal performance and learning often occur unless we apply our knowledge of movement physiology and information processing to engineering design. Indeed, accident investigations (and subsequent court litigation) routinely make use of knowledge about motor control in determining who was at fault, how accidents occur, and how best to avoid future accidents. Likewise, biomedical engineers and those who design and fit orthotic and prosthetic devices routinely apply knowledge of motor physiology.

As should be clear from this chapter, the discipline of motor behavior has been driven strongly by research in psychology, medicine, physiology, and engineering. Careers focused on research in motor behavior are pursued in academic and industrial settings by persons who obtain doctoral degrees or their equivalent in the various disciplines discussed. For more information about these occupations, consult the *Occupational Outlook Handbook* (U.S. Department of Labor, 2006–2007). This excellent resource describes the nature of the work, the work environment, required education and certification, and the employment and salary outlook in the United States. It is updated regularly.

Physical Therapy

According to the U.S. Department of Labor, "Physical therapists provide services that help restore function, improve mobility, relieve pain, and prevent or limit permanent physical disabilities of patients suffering from injuries or disease. They restore, maintain, and promote overall fitness and health. Their patients include accident victims and individuals with disabling conditions such as low-back pain, arthritis, heart disease, fractures, head injuries, and cerebral palsy" (U.S. Department of Labor, 2006–2007). The American Physical Therapy Association (APTA) is a professional organization designed to foster advancements in physical therapy practice, research, and education. The vision statement for this organization states that by the year 2020 physical therapy services will be provided by physical therapists who are doctors of physical therapy. Currently individuals who obtain a master's degree from a school of physical therapy can seek certification from the APTA, which will allow them to apply for a license to practice in their state. The trend toward schools of physical therapy offering only the doctor of physical therapy degree is strong in the United States, and it appears that the vision of the APTA may well be realized. Mirroring the medical profession, this association also oversees board certification in specialty fields within the discipline of physical therapy (e.g., pediatric, gerentologic, orthopaedic specialties). Physical therapists often are assisted by physical therapist assistants who are educated and licensed within the discipline.

Occupational Therapy

The American Occupational Therapy Association, Inc. (AOTA) is a professional organization that serves a similar function to that of the APTA. The U.S. Department of Labor notes that occupational therapists help people improve their ability to perform tasks in their daily living and working environments. Occupational therapists serve individuals who have conditions that are mentally, physically, developmentally, or emotionally disabling. They help their clients to develop, recover, or maintain daily living and work skills, often by helping them to compensate for permanent loss of function. Beginning in 2007, a master's degree or higher will be the minimum educational requirement for entry into the field. To obtain a license to practice occupational therapy in the United States, one must graduate from an accredited educational program and pass a national certification examination. Upon passing the exam, you are awarded the title Occupational Therapist Registered (OTR). Some states also require therapists who work in schools or early intervention programs to have taken additional education-related classes, obtained an education practice certificate, or met early intervention certification requirements.

Speech-Language Pathologist

The American Speech-Language-Hearing Association (ASHA) is the professional, scientific, and credentialing association for speech-language pathologists in the United States. In nearly all states, speech-language pathologists must be licensed to work in a health care setting, and all states require a master's degree or equivalent and a passing score on the national examination on speech-language pathology. Additional requirements typically include 300 to 375 hours of supervised clinical experience and 9 months of professional clinical experience after graduation. Speech-language pathologists can acquire the Certificate of Clinical Competence in Speech-Language Pathology (CCC-SLP) offered by AHSA, which requires a graduate degree and 400 hours of supervised clinical experience, and a postgraduate clinical fellowship, in addition to passing the national examination. With this certificate, a speech-language pathologist can seek employment in hospital, clinic, and educational settings although in some states a teaching license in speech-language pathology can be obtained with lesser education. Many speech-language pathology programs are moving toward the clinical doctorate as an additional level of training.

Athletic Training

The National Athletic Training Association (NATA) oversees the professional certification of individuals who seek employment as athletic trainers. Athletic trainers are health care professionals who specialize in preventing, recognizing, managing, and rehabilitating injuries that result from physical activity (see chapter 7). They work under the direction of a licensed physician and cooperate with other health care professionals, athletics administrators, coaches, and parents. A bachelor's degree from an accredited college or university with a major in athletic training

is required for certification and for almost all jobs as an athletic trainer. Many trainers further their training with advanced degrees.

Orthotists and Prosthetists

Orthotists and prosthetists assist patients with disabling conditions of the limbs and spine, or with partial or total absence of limb, by fitting and preparing orthopedic braces and prostheses (devices that replace our own tissues, such as an artificial limb). The American Academy of Orthotists and Prosthetists was founded to foster the development of practitioners in orthotics and prosthetics. This organization has been spearheading the accreditation of schools of orthotics and prosthetics and is actively promoting the establishment of doctoral programs in the discipline. Currently the typical educational requirement is a bachelor's degree from an accredited program. Compared to the other disciplines that have been discussed, orthotics and prosthetics is a young field that is rapidly advancing as materials technology thrives and as technology contributes to the development and refinement of powered prostheses.

SUMMARY

As our knowledge of brain function has advanced in the past 30 years, it can be argued that motor control and motor learning are so intimately related in their physiology that the distinction between these fields today exists only as a historical legacy. Today many prominent scientists working on issues of motor control also work on questions concerning motor learning, and vice versa.

Because so much of our daily activity depends on moving, adapting skills to new conditions, and learning new movement skills, we are motivated to understand how all of this comes about for its own intrinsic value, to perform better, and to better recover function after injury. It is easy to see why the science of motor control and motor learning has been applied more and more to issues of health care, recreation, engineering, and design, and why professional organizations and scientific societies that relate in some way to motor behavior continue to grow. Career opportunities abound, particularly in the application of this knowledge to health care and recreation. In any case, the practitioner or scientist requires a broad knowledge base in physiology, physics, and psychology. This broad knowledge base is becoming increasingly important to understand the basis of motor behavior and to keep pace with the rapid advance of knowledge during this golden age of the brain.

■ Key Resources

Key Journals

Behavioral and Brain Sciences
Ergonomics
Experimental Brain Research
Human Movement Science
Journal of Applied Physiology
Journal of Experimental Psychology: Human Perception and Performance

Journal of Motor Behavior
Journal of Neuroscience
Journal of Neurophysiology
Nature Neuroscience
Perceptual and Motor Skills
Research Quarterly for Exercise and Sport

Key WebSites

American Academy of Orthotists and Prosthetists (www.oandp.org)
American Alliance for Health, Physical Education, Recreation and Dance (www.aapherd.org)
American College of Sports Medicine (www.asm.org)
American Occupational Therapy Association, Inc. (www.aota.org)
American Physical Therapy Association (www.apta.org)
American Speech-Language-Hearing Association (www.asha.org)

Biomedical Engineering Society (www.bmes.org)
International Brain Research Organization (www.ibro.org)
International Society for Motor Control (www.i-s-m-c.org)
National Athletic Training Association (www.nata.org)
North American Society for Psychology of Sport and Physical Activity (www.naspspa.org)
Society for Neuroscience (www.sfn.org)
U.S. Department of Labor's Bureau of Labor Statistics' Occupational Outlook Handbook (www.bls.gov/oco/home.htm)

■ Review Questions

1. In what key way did motor behavior research conducted before 1950 differ between neurophysiologists and psychologists? What was Bernstein's role in reducing this difference?
2. What evidence leads us to believe that the central nervous system internally stores or represents skilled movements?
3. What evidence leads us to believe that stored representations of movements interact with sensory information?
4. Give an example of how initial condition information contributes to programming a movement.
5. List three different ways in which sensory information can contribute to executing a movement accurately.
6. Describe what is meant by the term *anticipatory postural control*. Give an example of an anticipatory postural adjustment.
7. In motor learning experiments, what is meant by a retention test? Why are such tests important to discovering the practice conditions that are optimal for motor learning?
8. What is the Law of Practice?
9. List three conditions of practice known to affect motor learning.
10. Describe how you might structure a practice session for the optimal learning of three motor skills.
11. What is brain plasticity, and why is it important for motor learning and for recovery of motor function after a stroke?

■ References

Baddeley, A. D., & Longman, D. J. A. (1978). The influence of length and frequency of training session on the rate of learning to type. *Ergonomics*, 21, 627–635.

Battig, W. F. (1979). The flexibility of human memory. In L. S. Cermak .& F. I. M. Craik (Eds.), *Levels of processing in human memory* (pp. 23–44). Hillsdale, NJ: Erlbaum.

Bayley, N. (1936). The development of motor abilities during the first three years: A study of sixty-one infants tested repeatedly. *Monographs of the Society for Research in Child Development*, 1, 26–61.

Bernstein, N. (1967). *The co-ordination and regulation of movements*. Oxford: Pergamon Press.

Brashers-Krug, T., Shadmehr, R., & Bizzi, E. (1996). Consolidation in human motor memory. *Nature*, 382, 252–255.

Brooks, V. B. (1986). *The neural basis of motor control*. Oxford: Oxford University Press.

Byl, N. N. (2004). Focal hand dystonia may result from aberrant neuroplasticity. *Advances in Neurology*, 94, 19–28.

Cohen, D. A., Pascual-Leone, A., Press, D. Z., & Robertson, E. M. (2005). Off-line learning of motor skill memory: A double dissociation of goal and movement. PNAS, 102(50), 18237–18241.

Creed, R. S., Denny-Brown, D., Eccles, J. C., Liddell, E. G. T., & Sherrington, C. S. (1932). *Reflex activity of the spinal cord*. Oxford, UK: Clarendon Press.

Crossman, E. R. F. W. (1959). A theory of the acquisition of speed skill. *Ergonomics*, 2, 153–166.

Donchin, O., Sawaki, L., Ghangadar, M., & Cohen, L. G. (2002). Mechanisms influencing acquisition and recall of motor memories. *Journal of Neurophysiology*, 88, 2114–2123.

Fasoli, S. E., Krebs, H. I., Stein, J., Frontera, W. R., Hughes, R., & Hogan, N. (2004). Robotic therapy for chronic motor impairments after stroke: Follow-up results. *Archives Physical Medicine Rehabilitation* (85), 1106–1111.

Feltz, D. L., & Landers, D. M. (1983). The effects of mental practice on motor-skill learning and performance: A meta-analysis. *Journal of Sport Psychology*, 5, 25–57.

Gesell, A. (1928). *Infancy and human growth*. New York: Macmillan.

Ghez, C., Gordon, J., & Ghilardi, M. F. (1995). Impairments of reaching movements in patients without proprioception. 2. Effects of visual information on accuracy. *Journal of Neurophysiology*, 73(1), 361–372.

Hering, H. E. (1897). Uber centripetale Ataxie beim Menschen and beim Affen. *Neurol Centralblatt*, 16, 1077–1094.

Hird, J. S., Landers, D. M., Thomas, J. R., & Horan, J. J. (1991). Physical practice is superior to mental practice in enhancing cognitive and motor task performance. *Journal of Sport & Exercise Psychology*, 13, 281–293.

Jeannerod, M. (1995). Mental imagery in the motor context. *Neuropsychologia*, 33(11), 1419–1432.

Jeannerod, M. (2001). Neural simulation of action: A unifying mechanism for motor cognition. *Neuroimage*, 14, 103–109.

Lee, T. D., & Genovese, E. D. (1988). Distribution of practice in motor skill acquisition: Learning and performance effects reconsidered. *Research Quarterly for Exercise and Sport*, 59, 277–287.

Luft, A. R., & Buitrago, M. M. (2005). Stages of motor skill learning. *Molecular Neurobiology*, 32(3), 205–216.

McGraw, M. (1935). *Growth: A study of Johnny and Jimmy*. New York: Appleton-Century-Crofts.

Mott, F. W., & Sherrington, C. S. (1895). Experiments upon the influence of sensory nerves upon movement and nutrition of the limbs. Preliminary.communication. *Proceedings of the Royal Society of London, Series B* 57, 481–488.

Nudo, R. (2006). Mechanisms for recovery of motor function following cortical damage. *Current Opinion in Neurobiology*, 16, 638–644.

Nyberg, L., Eriksson, J., Larsson, A., & Marklund, P. (2006). Learning b y doing versus learning by thinking: An fMRI study of motor and mental training. *Neuropsychologia*, 44, 711–717.

Ramon y Cajal, S. (1928). *Degeneration and regeneration of the nervous system*. May RM, trans. London. Oxford University.

Robertson, E. M., Pascual-Leone, A., & Miall, R. C. (2004). Current concepts in procedural consolidation. *Nature Review Neuroscience*, 5(7), 576–582.

Rothwell, J. C., Traub, M. M., Day, B. L., Obeso, J. A., Thomas, P. K., & Marsden, C. D. (1982). Manual motor performance in a deafferented man. *Brain*, 105, 515–542.

Sanes, J. N., & Donoghue, J. P. (2000). Plasticity and primary motor cortex. *Annual Review of Neuroscience*, 23, 393–415.

Sanes, J. N., Mauritz, K. H., Dalakas, M. C., & Evarts, E. V. (1985). Motor control in humans with large-fiber sensory neuropathy. *Human Neurobiology*, 4(2), 101–114.

Schmidt, R. A., & Lee, T. D. (2005). *Motor control and learning: A behavioral emphasis* (4th ed.). Campaign, IL: Human Kinetics.

Sherrington, C. (1910). Flexion reflex on the limb, cross extension-reflex and reflex stepping and standing. *Journal of Physiology*, 40, 28–121.

Shirley, M. M. (1931). *The first two years, a study of twenty-five babies: Postural and locomotor development*. Minneapolis, MN: University of Minnesota Press.

Shumway-Cook, A., & Woollacott, M. H. (2007). *Motor control: Translating research into clinical practice* (3rd ed.). Philadelphia: Lippincott Williams & Wilkins.

Taub, E. (1976). Movement in nonhuman primates deprived of somatosensory feedback. *Exercise and Sports Science Reviews*, 4, 335–374.

U.S. Department of Labor. Bureau of Labor Statistics. (2006–2007). *Occupational outlook handbook*. Retrieved from www.bls.gov/oco/home.htm

Weiss, P. A. (1941). Self-differentiation of the basic patterns of coordination. *Comparative Psychology Monographs*, 17, 1–96.

Wolf, S. L., Winstein, C. J., Miller, J. P., Taub, E., Uswatte, G., Morris, D., et al. (2006). Effect of contraint-induced movement therapy on upper extremity function 3 to 9 months after stroke: The EXCITE randomized clinical trial. *JAMA*, 296(17), 2095–2104.

Xerri, C., Coq, J. O., Merzenich, M. M., & Jenkins, W. M. (1996). Experience-induced plasticity of cutaneous maps in the primary somatosensory cortex of adult monkeys and rats. *Journal of Physiology* (Paris), 90(3–4), 277–287.

Yue, G., & Cole, K. J. (1992). Strength increases from the motor program: Comparison of training with maximal voluntary and imagined muscle contractions. *Journal of Neurophysiology*, 67(5), 1114–1123.

Exploring the Biomechanical

CHAPTER 6
Biomechanics
Susan Hall, PhD, University of Delaware

Biomechanics investigates human movement through the application of mechanical principles such as linear and angular kinematics and kinetics qualities. Biomechanic principles are used in understanding the forces produced by the body for actions as simple as picking up a glass to the complicated movements performed in athletic competitions. Part 4 explores how biomechanics incorporates information from such areas as anatomy and physiology, physics, mathematics, and engineering to understand the complicated processes involved in human movement.

Biomechanics

Susan Hall, PhD, University of Delaware

■ Chapter Objectives

After reading this chapter, you should be able to:

1. Define the term *biomechanics* and discuss the range of topics studied by biomechanists.
2. Explain the historical development of biomechanics, including the key contributing scientists and discoveries.
3. Describe some of the essential elements of content taught in most undergraduate biomechanics classes.
4. List career options and related professional organizations available to students interested in biomechanics.
5. Understand how to find information related to biomechanics through Web sites, data bases, and journals.

■ Key Terms

acceleration
angle of projection
angular
angular acceleration
angular displacement
angular impulse
angular momentum
angular velocity
Archimedes' principle
center of gravity
center of volume
coefficient of friction
drag

fluid
force
form drag
free body diagram
friction
impulse
kinematics
kinetics
linear acceleration
linear displacement
linear momentum
linear velocity
mass

moment of inertia
net force
normal reaction force
qualitative
quantitative
radius of gyration
Sir Isaac Newton
skin friction
theoretical square law
torque
vector
wave drag

The term *biomechanics* combines the prefix *bio*, meaning "life," with the word *mechanics*, which is the study of the actions of forces. In the early 1970s the international community of scientists adopted biomechanics as the name of the science involving the study of the mechanical aspects of living organisms (Nelson, 1980). Within the field of exercise science, the living organism most commonly of interest is the human body. The forces studied include both the internal forces produced by muscles and the external forces that act on the body. An introductory course in biomechanics provides foundational understanding of mechanical principles and their applications in analyzing the human body.

The biomechanics of human movement is one of the subdisciplines of exercise science. It is important to recognize, however, that biomechanists may also have an academic background in a field such as zoology, medicine, engineering, or physical therapy, with the commonality being an interest in the biomechanical aspects of the structure and function of living things.

Biomechanics is a key course in undergraduate exercise science programs. The forces acting on the human body exert powerful influences over the body's physiological and neurological as well as mechanical functions. An understanding of biomechanics promotes a comprehensive understanding of human body function. Biomechanics is typically an upper-level course (junior or senior year of study), with prerequisite courses in anatomy and mathematics. Although the actions of forces can be discussed from a conceptual perspective, at more advanced levels biomechanics is strictly a quantitative field of study. Students likely to pursue advanced study of biomechanics are those who enjoy mathematics, computer applications, and problem solving in general.

After taking a course in biomechanics, students should be able to answer questions such as these: Why does jumping help increase bone density? How does the angle at a joint influence the amount of force the muscles at the joint can produce? Is it easier to push or pull a heavy object? Why must an athlete throw a ball and a discus at different angles to maximize the distance of the throw? Why is it easier to float in salt water than in fresh water?

BRIEF HISTORY OF BIOMECHANICS

Although modern day biomechanics coalesced as a recognized scientific discipline during the 1970s, the work of scientists from many previous centuries laid the foundation for this development. One of the earliest giants in the development of foundational knowledge for biomechanics was Aristotle (384–322 BC), who wrote *Parts of Animals*, *Movement of Animals*, and *Progression of Animals*. These papers characterized animals as mechanical systems, analyzed muscle actions, and described walking in terms of translating rotary motion at joints into the linear motion of the body. Another of the early Greeks, Archimedes (287–212 BC) explained the principle of floatation, which equates the size of the buoyant force to the weight of the volume of displaced fluid. The Roman physician Galen (131–201 AD), who treated injured gladiators, produced the equivalent of a medical textbook titled *On the Function of the Parts*. This volume elucidated the differences between sensory and motor nerves and between agonist and antagonist muscles, among other things.

With the Renaissance came the multifaceted genius of Leonardo da Vinci (1452–1519), who described the mechanics of the human body during standing, walking, going up and down hill, and rising from a seated position. He studied muscle origins and insertions and was able to analyze muscle forces in terms of vector components. His work also demonstrated understanding of friction, gravitational acceleration, and the concept of the center of gravity.

Known for his strong personality and wit, Galileo (1564–1642) was one of the central figures of the scientific revolution. He may have been the original proponent of what we now call the scientific method: the use of objective experiments to derive cause-effect relationships. Among his numerous contributions were the observations that projectiles follow parabolic paths and that bone strength increases with a hollow, rather than a solid, interior and with increasing diameter. Galileo is known as the father of mechanics, the father of modern physics, and the father of modern astronomy.

The title "father of biomechanics" goes to another Italian, Giovanni Alfonso Borelli (1608–1679), who was a physiologist and physicist. His book, *On the Movement of Animals*, described the location of the human center of gravity, explained the principles of leverage within the musculoskeletal system, and proposed that inspiration requires muscle activity but that expiration occurs due to tissue elasticity, among other observations.

Significant contributions to the developing study of biomechanics also came from **Sir Isaac Newton** (1643–1727), described by many as the single greatest figure in the history of science. Newton's groundbreaking *Philosophiae Naturalis Principia Mathematica* set forth the law of gravitation and the three laws of motion. He also proposed the concepts of conservation of linear and angular momentum, along with many other major contributions to physics, mathematics, and astronomy.

Advances in the study of animal and human locomotion occurred again during the 19th century when French astronomer Janssen, who had used sequential photographs to study planetary motion, suggested that investigators also use serial pictures to study locomotion. British landscape photographer Eadweard Muybridge (1831–1904) capitalized on this concept with 12 volumes of sequential photographs of men, women, children, and numerous species of animals walking and running. Muybridge was a colorful character who was not averse to writing press releases praising his own work. Much notoriety followed Muybridge's motion picture study of galloping horses, which demonstrated that, indeed, there is a point in the gait cycle during which all four hooves are simultaneously off the ground, thus resolving a well-publicized debate of the day.

During this same period, a German, Julius Wolff (1836–1902), was formulating his famous Wolff's Law: "Every change in the form and function of a bone or of their function alone is followed by certain definite changes in their internal architecture, and equally definite secondary alteration in their external conformation, in accordance with mathematical laws." In modern-day terms, bone material accrues in regions of increased stress and diminishes in regions of decreased stress.

On another front, Germans Christian Wilhelm Braune (1831–1892) and Otto Fischer (1861–1917) completed detailed dissection studies of cadavers to determine locations of body segment centers of gravity. The often-cited cadaver work of Wilfrid Taylor Dempster (1955) during the 1950s and 1960s extended our quantitative knowledge of the relative lengths, weights, and center of gravity locations of the individual body segments.

The next real breakthrough in the development of modern biomechanics came about with the availability of personal computers (PCs) in the mid-1970s.

The Scelbi, Mark-8 Altair, IBM 5100, Apple I, Apple II, TRS-80, and Commodore Pet were among the first personal computers widely available to consumers. These personal computers provided a quantum leap of improvement in data storage capability and computational power compared to the handheld calculators of the day. This first generation of PCs also set the stage for the subsequent development of motion analysis via automated tracking of body segments using digital cameras and reflective markers.

COURSE CONTENT

Several factors can influence the specific content of undergraduate biomechanics courses in an exercise science curriculum, including the philosophy of the instructor, the entrance criteria for the major, and the courses identified as prerequisites for biomechanics. Most first courses in biomechanics address the topical areas generally regarded as core content, which are described in this section: kinematics, kinetics, and fluid mechanics.

Kinematics

What we are able to observe visually when watching a body in motion is termed the **kinematics** of the movement. Kinematics involves the study of the size, sequencing, and timing of movement, without reference to the forces that cause or result from the motion. We refer to the kinematics of an exercise or a sport skill execution as *form* or *technique*.

Kinematic analysis can be both qualitative and quantitative (Figure 6.1). For example, **qualitatively**

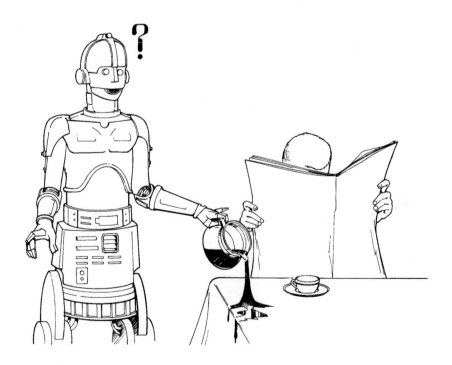

Figure 6.1 Quantitatively, the robot missed the coffee cup by 15 cm. Qualitatively, he malfunctioned.

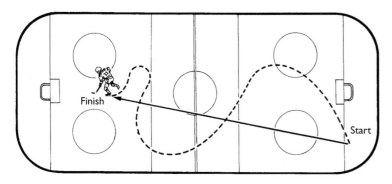

Figure 6.2 The distance a skater travels may be measured from the track on the ice. The skater's displacement is measured in a straight line from initial position to final position.

describing the kinematics of performing a squat exercise involves identifying the major joint actions, which are flexion at the hip and knee followed by extension at the hip and knee. A more detailed qualitative kinematic analysis might also include mention of maintaining erect trunk and head positions and balancing the barbell with no dipping or twisting of the weight during the descent and ascent phases. Although most assessments of human movement are visual and qualitative, **quantitative** analysis is also often necessary. Physical therapists, for example, typically measure the range of motion of a joint requiring postsurgery rehabilitation to help determine which range of motion exercises may be appropriate.

The kinematic quantities of interest in biomechanics are distance, displacement, speed, velocity, and acceleration. Displacement, velocity, and acceleration are **vector** quantities, which means that they have both size and direction. **Linear displacement** is a length or distance in a given direction along a straight line (Figure 6.2). **Angular displacement** is the change in the angular position or orientation of a line or a body segment (Figure 6.3). Analyzing human movement involves **angular** quantities because it is primarily rotational motion that occurs at the joints of the body. **Linear velocity** is speed in a given direction, or displacement divided by the time interval

over which the displacement occurs. Similarly, **angular velocity** is angular displacement divided by the time interval over which the angular displacement occurs. **Acceleration** is the rate of change in velocity, or the change in velocity divided by the time interval. **Angular acceleration** is the rate of change of angular velocity, or the change in angular velocity divided by the time interval.

Biomechanists often quantitatively study the kinematic features associated with skilled performances of exercises and other human movements to try to gain insight into what distinguishes successful performance from less skilled performance. Maximizing average speed is the objective of most racing events, and sport biomechanists have studied the kinematics of fast performances in running, skiing, skating, cycling, swimming, and rowing events. For human gait, both running and walking, speed is the product of stride length and stride frequency. The fastest male and female sprinters are distinguished from less-skilled competitors by extremely high stride frequencies and short ground contact times, although their stride lengths are usually only average or slightly greater than average (Dillman, 1985). In contrast, the fastest cross-country skiers have longer-than-average cycle lengths, with cycle rates that are only average (Nilsson, Tveit, & Eikrehagen, 2004). Research

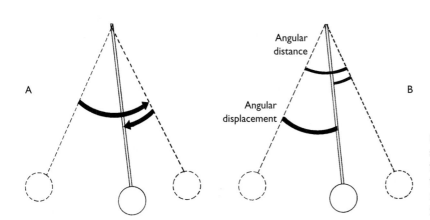

Figure 6.3 (a) The path of motion of a swinging pendulum. (b) The angular distance is the sum of all angular changes that have occurred; the angular displacement is the angle between the initial and final positions.

on skating kinematics has shown that better ice skaters appear to excel because of higher stride rates (McCaw & Hoshizaki, 1987), whereas elite roller skaters are distinguished by longer strides (Wilson, McDonald, & Neal, 1987). Interestingly, for elite swimmers in the 100-m and 200-m breaststroke events, the optimum stroke rate to stroke length ratio has been found to be unique to each individual swimmer (Thompson, Haljand, & MacLaren, 2000).

During running, stride length is not simply a function of the runner's body height, but can also be influenced by muscle fiber composition, footwear, state of fatigue, injury history, and the inclination (grade) of the running surface (Hardin, vanden Bogert, & Hamill, 2004). Runners traveling at a slow pace tend to increase running speed primarily by increasing stride length. At faster running speeds, recreational runners rely more on increasing stride frequency to increase velocity. Runners should avoid overstriding, or using an overly long stride length, because that is a risk factor for hamstring strains.

Those who run regularly for exercise tend to prefer a constant stride frequency during workouts. One reason for this may relate to running economy—the oxygen consumption required for performing a given task (Cavanagh & Kram, 1985). Most runners tend to choose a combination of stride length and stride frequency that minimizes the physiological cost of running (Cavanagh & Williams, 1982). Many species of animals do the same thing. Running on downhill and uphill surfaces tends to increase and decrease running speed, respectively, with these differences primarily a function of increased and decreased stride length (Paradisis & Cooke, 2001). The presence of fatigue, as would be expected near the end of a marathon event, tends to result in increased stride frequency and decreased stride length (Kyrolainen el al., 2000). Older runners also tend to prefer shorter strides as compared to younger ones (Conoboy & Dyson, 2006).

In the long jump, high jump, and pole vault, the primary factor influencing success is the athlete's ability to maximize velocity going into takeoff (Chow & Hay, 2005; Dapena & Chung, 1988). The other important kinematic variable influencing jump performance is takeoff angle. The takeoff angles measured among elite long jumpers range from approximately 18° to 27° (Hay, 1986). In the ski jump, however, where athletes have the advantage of a large elevation difference between takeoff and landing, takeoff angles are as small as 4.6° to 6.2° (Watanabe, 1989). In an event such as the high jump, in which the goal is to maximize vertical displacement, takeoff angles among skilled Fosbury Flop–style jumpers range from 40° to 48° (Dapena, 1980).

The **angle of projection** is also an important influence on shots in basketball because a more vertical approach to the basket provides a larger

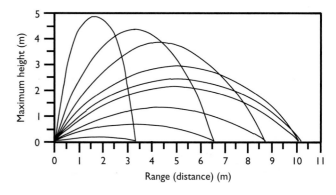

Figure 6.4 The influence of projection angle on the flight path of a projected ball can be seen in this scaled diagram of trajectories for a ball projected at 10 m/s.

margin of error than a shallow approach angle (Figure 6.4). Within 4.57 m of the basket experienced players tend to release shots at angles of about 52° to 55°, providing a relatively steep angle of entry. Alternatively, shots taken from outside the three-point line tend to be released at 48° to 50°, allowing for a minimum release speed, but a less steep angle of entry (Miller & Bartlett, 1996). When shooting in close proximity to a defender, players tend to release the ball at a larger release angle and from a greater height than is the case when a player is open (Rojas, Cepero, Ona, & Guitierrez, 2000). Although the strategy behind this is typically to keep the shot from being blocked, it may also result in more accurate shooting.

In the throwing events, the aerodynamic characteristics of the projected implements also influence the flight path and optimum angle of projection. In these events (shot, discus, javelin, and hammer), only the trajectory of the shot is not appreciably affected by aerodynamic forces. If projected by a cannon, the optimum angle for maximizing the distance traveled in the air by a shot is 45°. When the human musculoskeletal system is projecting a shot, however, the optimum projection angle must be one that does not restrict projection speed. The release angles reported among elite shot putters are approximately 36° to 37° (Hubbard, de Mestre, & Scott, 2001). As is often the case with athletic performance, however, optimum release angle for the shot put varies from athlete to athlete because of individual differences in the decrease of release speed with increasing release angle (Linthorne, 2001).

Sports involving a swinging implement, such as a bat or a racquet, involve the added complication of optimal timing of the swing to impart the desired projection speed and angle to the struck ball. The batter in baseball must time the swing precisely to make contact with the ball and direct it into fair territory. A 40 m/s pitch reaches the batter 0.41 seconds after leaving the pitcher's hand. Researchers estimate that a difference of 0.001 seconds in the time of initiation of the swing can determine whether the ball is directed to center field or down the foul line, and that a swing initiated 0.003 seconds too early or too late will result in no contact with the ball (Gutman, 1988). The racquet swings of male professional tennis players are also extremely fast, having been measured at 1900 to 2200 degrees per second (deg/s) just prior to ball impact (Elliott, 1989).

Moving the body segments themselves at a high rate of angular velocity is a characteristic of skilled performance in many sports. Angular velocities at the joints of the throwing arm in major league baseball pitchers range around 2320 deg/s in elbow extension and 7240 deg/s in internal rotation (Fleisig, Barrentine, Zheng, Escamilla, & Andrews, 1999). Surprisingly, these values are also very high in the throwing arms of youth pitchers, with 2230 deg/s in elbow extension and 6900 deg/s in internal rotation documented (Fleisig et al., 1999). Comparison of different types of pitches thrown by collegiate baseball pitchers showed internal rotation values of 7550 deg/s for fastball pitches, 6680 deg/s for change-up pitches, 7120 deg/s for curveball pitches, and 7920 deg/s for slider pitches (Escamilla, Fleisig, Barrentine, Zheng, & Andrews, 1998).

It is important to recognize, however, that most biomechanical studies of human kinematics involve nonathletes. For example, research has shown that infants begin to use stable patterns of coordination in reaching for objects at 12 to 15 months of age, with adultlike reaching movements occurring by about 2 years (Konczak & Dichgans, 1997). Scientists have also studied the kinematics of the developmental progressions in gait development and throwing ability in young children (Haywood & Getchell, 2001). Working with adapted physical education specialists, biomechanists have documented the characteristic kinematic patterns associated with relatively common disabling conditions such as cerebral palsy, Down syndrome, and stroke. Quantitative kinematic screening tests are used to evaluate treatment and progression of a wide variety of motor disorders (Ramos, Latash, Hurvitz, & Brown, 1997). For example, kinematic analysis indicates that walking on a treadmill with a grade of approximately 13 to 15% appears to be optimal for minimizing patellofemoral discomfort and potential strain on the anterior cruciate ligament (ACL) in post–ACL reconstruction patients (Lange, Hintermeister, Schlegel, Dillman, & Steadman, 1996).

Biomechanists typically use high-speed cinematography or videography to perform quantitative kinematic analyses. The process involves taking a carefully planned film or video of a performance, with subsequent computerized or computer-assisted analysis of the performance on a picture-by-picture basis. Reflective markers are typically placed over subject

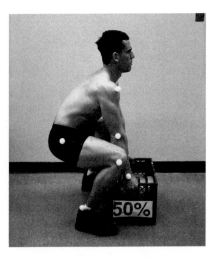

Reflective markers on this individual are automatically tracked by infrared cameras. The three-dimensional coordinates of each marker are stored in a computer file every 1/100th second for subsequent use in calculations of kinematic quantities of interest.

joint centers and other points of interest. Through a process called *digitizing*, the three-dimensional coordinates of these markers are stored in data files. Digitizing was originally a tedious and time-consuming process that involved activating a handheld pen or cursor over the image of the individual's joint centers. Today, however, systems that automatically track and digitize reflective markers are common.

Kinetics

Kinetics is the analysis of the actions of forces. **Force** can be thought of as a push or pull acting on a body. Being a vector quantity, force is characterized by magnitude, direction, and point of application to a body. Because most situations involve the actions of more than one force, the first step when analyzing forces is constructing a **free body diagram.** A free body is any body, body segment, or other object that is of interest for the analysis. A free body diagram consists of a drawing of the system being analyzed with vector representations of the acting forces (Figure 6.5). Even though a hand must be applying force to a tennis racket for the racket to be in motion, if the racket is the free body of interest, the hand is represented in the free body diagram of the racket only as a force vector.

A force rarely acts in isolation; the overall effect of many forces acting on a body is a function of the **net force,** which is the vector sum of all the acting forces. If all of the acting forces are balanced in both magnitude and direction, they cancel each other out and the net force is zero. If a net force is present, however, the body moves in the direction of the net force with an acceleration that is a product of the magnitude of the net force and the body's **mass.**

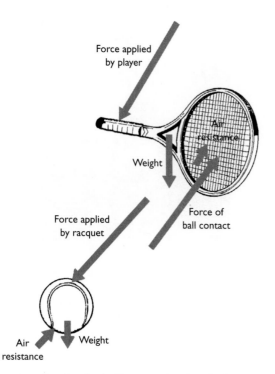

Force applied by player

Air resistance

Weight

Force applied by racquet

Force of ball contact

Air resistance

Weight

Figure 6.5 Two free body diagrams showing the forces acting on the racquet and ball.

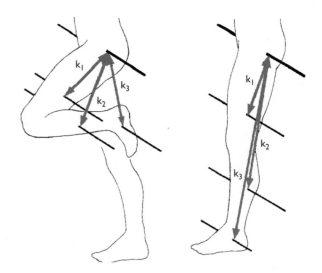

Figure 6.7 Knee angle affects the moment of inertia of the swinging leg with respect to the hip because of changes in the radius of gyration for the lower leg (k_2) and foot (k_3).

When a force causes an object to rotate, the rotary effect of the force is called **torque**. Torque is quantified as the product of the magnitude of the force (F) and the force's moment arm, or the perpendicular distance ($d_\perp$) from the force's line of action

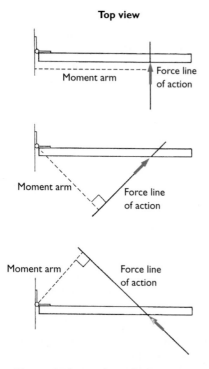

Top view

Moment arm

Force line of action

Moment arm

Force line of action

Moment arm

Force line of action

Figure 6.6 Torque is the product of a force's magnitude and the perpendicular distance from the force's line of action to the axis of rotation.

to the axis of rotation (Figure 6.6). Torque is a vector quantity with a magnitude and direction. The convention for the direction of rotational motion is that counterclockwise is positive and clockwise is negative.

As mentioned in the history section, Sir Isaac Newton discovered many of the fundamental relationships that form the foundation for the field of modern mechanics. Newton's first law of motion is the law of inertia, which states that a body will maintain a state of rest or constant velocity until acted upon by an external force that changes that state. Inertia is a body's tendency to resist acceleration. The more mass a body has, the greater its tendency to resist **linear acceleration.** The inertial property for angular motion is **moment of inertia,** which represents a body's resistance to angular acceleration. Moment of inertia (I) is influenced both by mass (m) and by the distribution of mass in the body with respect to the axis of rotation. Mass distribution is characterized by the **radius of gyration** (k), which is the distance from the axis of rotation to a point at which the mass of the body can theoretically be concentrated without altering the inertial characteristics of the rotating body (Figure 6.7). It is easier to swing a baseball bat when holding it by the barrel than by the grip, because when holding the bat by the grip there is more mass distributed farther away from the axis of rotation. Although the mass of the bat remains constant, when the axis of rotation is the barrel instead of the grip, the radius of gyration is dramatically reduced.

Newton's second law, known as the law of acceleration, may be stated as follows:

When a force acts on a body, the resulting acceleration of the body is in the direction of the force and of a magnitude inversely proportional to its mass.

The law is equally true for angular motion:

> When a torque acts on a body, the resulting angular acceleration is in the direction of the torque and of a magnitude inversely proportional to its moment of inertia.

The third law of motion is the law of reaction, which can be stated simply as follows:

> For every action, there is an equal and opposite reaction.

Or, as stated in terms of forces,

> When one body exerts a force on a second, the second body exerts a reaction force that is equal in magnitude and opposite in direction on the first body.

For angular motion, the law becomes:

> When one body exerts a torque on a second, the second body exerts an equal and opposite torque on the first.

During gait, every contact of a foot with the floor or ground generates an upward reaction force. These ground reaction forces (GRFs) can be measured with force platforms, which are typically built rigidly into a floor flush with the surface and interfaced to a computer. Force platforms transduce GRFs in vertical, lateral, and anteroposterior directions. Researchers have studied the GRFs generated during running to investigate factors related to both performance and running-related injuries. The magnitude of the vertical component of the GRF during running is generally 2 to 3 times the runner's body weight, with the pattern of force sustained during ground contact differing with running style. Runners are classified as rearfoot, midfoot, or forefoot strikers, according to the portion of the shoe first making contact with the ground (Figure 6.8).

Other factors influencing GRF patterns include running speed, running duration, knee flexion angle at contact, stride length, fatigue, footwear, surface stiffness, surface smoothness, light intensity, and grade (Derrick & Mercer, 2004; Gerlach et al., 2005). Although it may seem logical that harder running surfaces would generate larger GRFs, this has not been found. When encountering surfaces of different stiffness, runners typically make individual adjustments in running kinematics that tend to maintain GRFs at a constant level (Dixon, Collop, & Batt, 2000).

Since the GRF is an external force acting on the human body, its magnitude and direction have implications for performance in many sporting events. In the high jump, for example, skilled performers are moving with a large horizontal velocity and a slight downwardly directed vertical velocity at the beginning

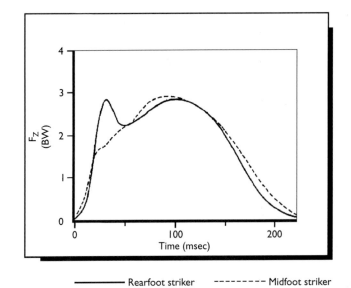

——— Rearfoot striker   ------- Midfoot striker

Figure 6.8 Typical ground reaction forces for rearfoot strikers and midfoot strikers.

of the stride before takeoff. The GRF reduces the jumper's horizontal velocity and creates an upwardly directed vertical velocity (Figure 6.9). Better jumpers not only enter the takeoff phase of the jump with high horizontal velocities but also effectively use the GRF to convert horizontal velocity to upward vertical velocity (Dapena, 1984).

Another external force that can change the motion of the human body is the force of **friction.** Friction acts at the interface of surfaces in contact in the direction opposite the direction of motion or impending motion. The size of the friction force is the product of the coefficient of friction (μ) and the normal (perpendicular) reaction force (R). The **coefficient of friction** is a number indicating the relative ease of sliding, or the amount of mechanical and molecular interaction between two surfaces in contact. Factors influencing the value of μ are the relative roughness and hardness of the surfaces in contact and the type of molecular interaction between the surfaces. The greater the mechanical and molecular interaction, the greater is the value of μ. For example, the coefficient of friction between two blocks covered with rough sandpaper is larger than the coefficient of friction between a skate and a smooth surface of ice. The coefficient of friction describes the interaction between two surfaces in contact and is not descriptive of either surface alone. The coefficient of friction for the blade of an ice skate in contact with ice is different from that for the blade of the same skate in contact with concrete or wood.

The **normal reaction force** (R) is the sum of all acting vertical forces, which most commonly is simply a body's weight. The magnitude of R can sometimes be intentionally altered to increase or decrease the amount of friction acting. When a football coach

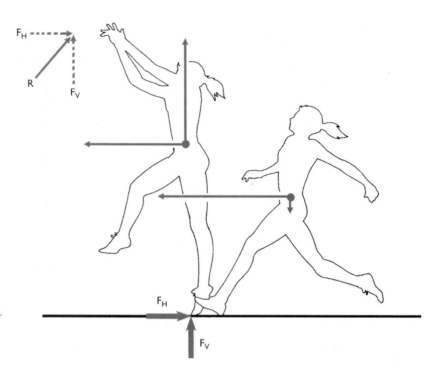

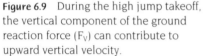

Figure 6.9 During the high jump takeoff, the vertical component of the ground reaction force (F_V) can contribute to upward vertical velocity.

stands on the back of a tackling sled, the normal reaction force exerted by the ground on the sled is increased, with a concurrent increase in the amount of friction generated, making it more difficult for a tackler to move the sled. Alternatively, if the magnitude of R is decreased, friction is decreased and it is easier to initiate motion.

How can the normal reaction force be decreased? Suppose you need to rearrange the furniture in a room. Is it easier to push or pull an object such as a desk to move it? When a desk is pushed, the force exerted is typically directed diagonally downward. In contrast, force is usually directed diagonally upward when a desk is pulled. The vertical component of the push or pull either adds to or subtracts from the magnitude of the normal reaction force, thus influencing the magnitude of the friction force generated and the relative ease of moving the desk (Figure 6.10).

The amount of friction present between two surfaces can also be changed by altering the coefficient of friction between the surfaces. For example, the use of gloves in sports such as golf and racquetball increases the coefficient of friction between the hand and the grip of the club or racquet. The application of a thin, smooth coat of wax to the bottom of cross-country skis is designed to decrease the coefficient of friction between the skis and the snow, with different waxes used for various snow conditions.

Friction exerts an important influence during many daily activities. Walking depends on a proper

coefficient of friction between a person's shoes and the supporting surface. If the coefficient of friction is too low, as when a person with smooth-soled shoes walks on a patch of ice, slippage will occur. The bottom of a wet bathtub or shower stall should provide a coefficient of friction with the soles of bare feet that is sufficiently large to prevent slippage.

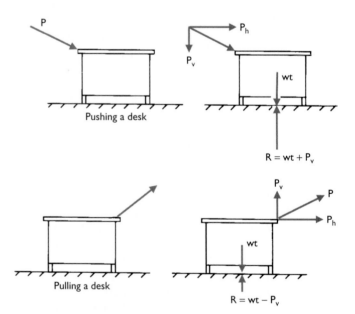

Figure 6.10 Pulling on an object such as a desk tends to decrease the magnitude of the normal reaction force (R) and friction (F), whereas pushing tends to increase R and F.

Another factor that affects the outcome of interactions between two bodies is **momentum,** a mechanical quantity that is particularly important in collisions. Momentum (M) is generally defined as the quantity of motion that an object possesses. More specifically, **linear momentum** is the product of an object's mass and its velocity. A body with zero velocity has no momentum; that is, its momentum equals 0. During performance of most weight training exercises, it is desirable for there to be zero momentum of the weight to help prevent injury at the joint range of motion end point. This translates to performing the exercises in a slow and controlled fashion.

A change in a body's momentum may be caused by either a change in the body's mass or a change in its velocity. In most human movement situations, changes in linear momentum result from changes in velocity. When a head-on collision between two objects occurs, there is a tendency for both objects to continue moving in the direction of motion originally possessed by the object with greater momentum.

A body's momentum can also be changed by the action of an external force over a period of time. The product of force and time is termed **impulse.** It is impulse that causes change in momentum. At the beginning of a toboggan race, the crew members push the toboggan to get it moving as rapidly as possible before they climb in. In so doing, they are applying a force over a time interval to change the toboggan's momentum from zero to a maximal amount.

This relationship between impulse and momentum holds true for angular motion as well. **Angular momentum** can be defined as the quantity of angular motion that a body possesses. Whereas linear momentum is the product of the linear inertial property (mass) and linear velocity, angular momentum (H) is the product of the angular inertial property (moment of inertia) and angular velocity. As mass or angular velocity increases, angular momentum increases proportionally. The factor that most dramatically influences angular momentum, however, is the distribution of mass with respect to the axis of rotation because angular momentum is proportional to the square of the radius of gyration.

Angular impulse is the product of torque and the time interval over which the torque acts. It is angular impulse that generates a change in angular momentum. When a competitive diver takes off from a springboard or platform, the diver must attain sufficient linear momentum to reach the necessary height (and safe distance from the board or platform) and sufficient angular momentum to perform the required number of rotations. As shown in Figure 6.11,

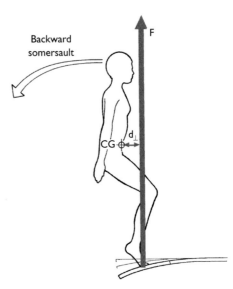

Figure 6.11 The product of the springboard reaction force (F) and its moment arm with respect to the diver's center of gravity ($d_\perp$) creates a torque, which generates the angular impulse that produces the diver's angular momentum at takeoff.

the angular momentum needed is produced by a torque from the diving board. For multiple-rotation, nontwisting platform dives, the angular momentum generated at takeoff increases as the rotational requirements of the dive increase. Angular momentum values as high as 66 kg m^2/s and 70 kg m^2/s have been reported for multiple gold medalist Greg Louganis during his back two and a half and forward three and a half springboard dives, respectively (Miller, Jones, & Pizzimenti, 1988).

Fluid Mechanics

Although in general conversation the term *fluid* is often used interchangeably with the term *liquid*, from a mechanical perspective a **fluid** is any substance that tends to flow or continuously deform when acted on by a shear force. Both gases and liquids are fluids with similar mechanical behaviors. Air and water are fluid mediums that exert forces on bodies moving through them. Some of these forces slow the progress of a moving body; others provide support or propulsion.

The ability of a body to float in a fluid medium depends on the relationship between the body's buoyancy and its weight. Buoyancy is a fluid force that acts vertically upward. In accordance with **Archimedes' principle**: the magnitude of the buoyant force is equal to the weight of the fluid displaced by the body. When weight and the buoyant force are the only two forces acting on a body and their magnitudes are equal, the body floats in a motionless

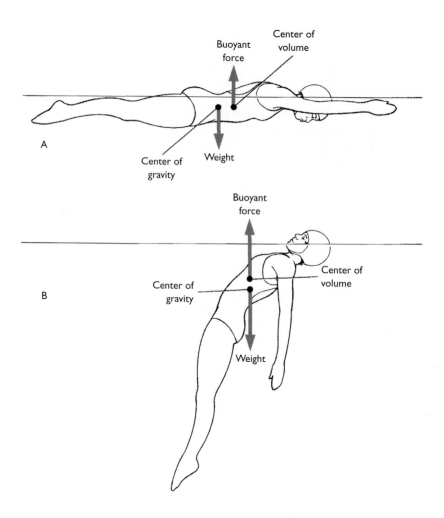

Figure 6.12 (a) A torque is created on a swimmer by body weight (acting at the center of gravity) and the buoyant force (acting at the center of volume). (b) When the center of gravity and center of volume are vertically aligned, this torque is eliminated.

state. If the magnitude of the weight is greater than that of the buoyant force, the body sinks, moving downward in the direction of the net force. Most objects float statically in a partially submerged position. The volume of a freely floating object needed to generate a buoyant force equal to the object's weight is the volume that is submerged.

In the study of biomechanics, buoyancy is of interest relative to the flotation of the human body in water. Some individuals cannot float in a motionless position, and others float with little effort. This difference in floatability is a function of body density. Since the density of bone and muscle is greater than the density of fat, individuals who are muscular and have little body fat have higher average body densities than individuals with less muscle, less dense bones, or more body fat. If two individuals have an identical body volume, the one with the higher body density weighs more. Alternatively, if two people have the same body weight, the person with the higher body density has a smaller body volume. For flotation to occur, the body volume must be large enough to create a buoyant force greater than or equal to body weight. Some individuals can float only when holding

a large volume of inspired air in the lungs, a tactic that increases body volume without practically altering body weight.

The orientation of the human body as it floats in water is determined by the relative position of the total body center of gravity relative to the total body center of volume. The **center of gravity** is the point around which the body's weight is balanced in all directions. The **center of volume** is the point around which a body's volume is balanced. The exact locations of the center of gravity and center of volume vary with anthropometric dimensions and body composition. Typically, the center of gravity is inferior to the center of volume due to the relatively large volume and relatively small weight of the lungs. Because weight acts at the center of gravity and buoyancy acts at the center of volume, a torque is created that rotates the body until it is positioned so that these two acting forces are vertically aligned and the torque ceases to exist (Figure 6.12).

Another important fluid force is drag. **Drag** is a resistance force that slows the motion of a body moving through a fluid. In accordance with the **theoretical square law,** the magnitude of the drag

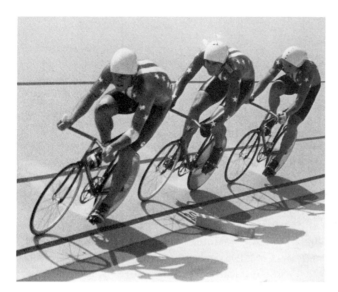

Cyclists drafting to minimize form drag.

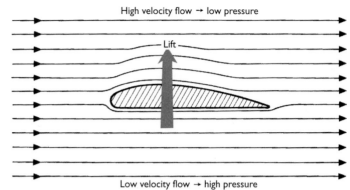

Figure 6.13 Lift force generated by a foil shape.

force increases approximately with the square of velocity. So if a cyclist's speed doubles, the drag force opposing the cyclist increases by a factor of four. There are three types of drag. **Skin friction,** or surface drag, is resistance derived from friction between adjacent layers of fluid near a body moving through a fluid. To minimize skin friction, athletes in racing events typically wear tight fitting attire made of an ultrasmooth fabric. Recent research shows that a water repellant swimsuit fabric improves swimming performance by reducing skin friction (Rogowski, Monteil, Legreneur, & Lanteri, 2006). **Form drag,** or profile drag, is resistance created by a pressure dif-

ferential between the lead and rear ends of a body moving through a fluid. Assuming a streamlined body position with the smallest possible area of the body oriented perpendicular to the fluid stream minimizes form drag. The third type of drag is **wave drag,** which is a resistance created by the generation of waves at the interface between two fluids, such as air and water. Minimizing up and down motion during swimming helps minimize the generation of a bow wave in front of a swimmer, thereby reducing wave drag.

Another type of fluid force acts perpendicular to the fluid flow. This force, known as lift, can be generated by a foil shape (Figure 6.13). Projectiles such as the discus, javelin, football, and Frisbee are shaped sufficiently like a foil that they can generate lift when oriented appropriately to the fluid flow. The human hand is also sufficiently foil shaped that it can generate lift force during swimming.

Other Topics

Myriad other topics are included in biomechanics textbooks. These typically include forms of motion, standard reference terminology, spatial reference systems, types of mechanical loading, vector algebra, projectile motion, relationships between linear and angular motion, impact, elasticity, work, power, energy, equilibrium, stability, centripetal force, and the biomechanical aspects of the major joints and tissues of the human body.

PROFESSIONAL ORGANIZATIONS

Several professional organizations focused on biomechanics offer student memberships as well as professional memberships. There are numerous advantages

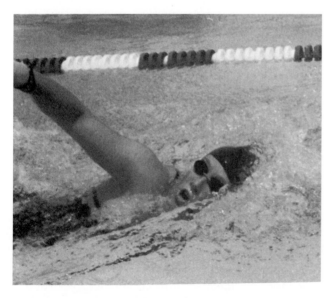

The bow wave generated by a competitive swimmer creates wave drag.

for student members of these organizations, particularly if the student is considering a career in biomechanics. These advantages typically include discounts on biomechanics journal subscriptions, discounts on conference fees, and funding for student research grants on a competitive basis. Most important, however, the biomechanics conferences hosted by these organizations provide opportunities for students to interact with professionals in the field in presenting and hearing the results of current research.

American Society of Biomechanics

The American Society of Biomechanics (ASB) was founded in 1977 "to encourage and foster the exchange of information and ideas among biomechanists working in different disciplines and fields of application, including biological sciences, exercise and sports science, health sciences, ergonomics and human factors, and engineering and applied science, and to facilitate the development of biomechanics as a basic and applied science" (ASB, n.d.). The organization hosts a scientific meeting each year and publishes a newsletter twice a year. Student members receive discounts on membership, conference fees, and journal subscriptions, and can participate in a program pairing them with faculty mentors. Graduate students can also compete for a grant-in-aid in support of research.

Canadian Society of Biomechanics

This organization was formed in 1973 to foster research and the interchange of information on the biomechanics of human physical activity. More specifically, the Canadian Society for Biomechanics (CSB) "is attempting to enhance interdisciplinary communication and thereby improve the quality of biomechanics research and facilitate application of findings by bringing together therapists, physicians, engineers, sport researchers, ergonomists and others who are using the same pool of basic biomechanics techniques but studying different human movement problems" (CSB, n.d.). The CSB organizes a biannual Scientific Conference held the years opposite those of the International Society of Biomechanics. Once every six years the meeting is held in association with the American Society of Biomechanics and is called the North American Congress on Biomechanics. The organization also publishes a periodic newsletter in web format. Student members receive discounts on membership, conference fees, and journal subscriptions. Graduate students can compete for travel awards to do research in another biomechanics laboratory and for a scholarship for students with disabilities.

European Society of Biomechanics

The European Society of Biomechanics (ESB) was founded in 1976 in a meeting in Brussels with 20 scientists from 11 countries. The primary goal of the ESB is "to encourage, foster, promote and develop research, progress and information concerning the science of Biomechanics" (ESB, n.d.). The organization defines biomechanics as "the study of forces acting on and generated within a body and of the effects of these forces on the tissues, fluids or materials used for diagnosis, treatment or research purposes" (ESB, n.d.). ESB meets biannually and holds workshop meetings on focused topics in the years that regular meetings are not held. Student members receive discounts on membership, conference fees, and journal subscriptions. Student membership also provides special access to information on biomechanics laboratories with ESB members, possible exchanges with other laboratories, available courses in biomechanics at different universities, job opportunities, and funding sources for research. Students can also participate in a mentoring program.

International Society of Biomechanics

The International Society of Biomechanics (ISB) was founded in 1973 to promote the study of all areas of biomechanics at the international level, although special emphasis is given to the biomechanics of human movement. The society encourages international contacts among scientists, promotes the dissemination of knowledge, and forms liaisons with national organizations. The society's membership includes scientists from a variety of disciplines including anatomy, physiology, engineering (mechanical, industrial aerospace, etc.), orthopedics, rehabilitation medicine, sport science and medicine, ergonomics, electro-physiological kinesiology, and others. Society activities include the organization of biannual international conferences, publication of congress proceedings and a biomechanics monograph series, distribution of a quarterly society newsletter, and sponsorship of scientific meetings related to biomechanics. The society also supports technical and working groups for the purpose of advancing knowledge in specialized areas within the field of biomechanics. The ISB sponsors BIOMCH-L (an Internet electronic discussion forum) and lecture tours for economically developing countries. Student members receive discounts on membership, conference fees, and journal subscriptions. The society offers a range of competitive funding opportunities for graduate student research.

International Society of Biomechanics in Sport

The International Society of Biomechanics in Sports (ISBS) is composed of members from all over the world with a common desire to study and understand human movement, especially as it relates to applied sport biomechanics. Members represent a wide range of academic backgrounds, including exercise science, engineering, computer science, rehabilitation and medicine, among others. The first full-scale conference of the ISBS was held in 1982 in San Diego, California. Some of the first field-based research activities of ISBS were at the 1976 Olympic Games and 1978 Commonwealth Games, with numerous other research projects completed since that time. Additional activities of ISBS and its members include seminars, clinics, exhibits, technical lectures, periodic online newsletters, annual conferences, and published proceedings. Student members receive discounts on membership, conference fees, and journal subscriptions.

Multidisciplinary Organizations

A number of multidisciplinary professional organizations also include biomechanists. These organizations bring together scientists and clinicians or educators from a range of related fields. Two of these, the American College of Sports Medicine (ACSM) and the American Alliance for Health, Physical Education, Recreation and Dance (AAHPERD), are described in detail in Chapter 2. Within both of these large umbrella organizations are biomechanics interest groups that hold separate meetings during the annual ACSM and AAHPERD meetings.

CAREERS

Employment opportunities in biomechanics span the academic, clinical, military, and industry arenas. Because students in exercise science programs typically have only one or two courses in biomechanics, graduate degrees are most commonly required. Within academia, professors specializing in biomechanics may have training in exercise science, physical therapy, engineering, or zoology. Clinicians with expertise in biomechanics are among those who staff gait analysis laboratories and physical therapy clinics. All of the major sport equipment and apparel companies hire biomechanists to assist with product design and testing, and the major automobile companies hire biomechanists to assist with safety feature implementation and crash testing. The U.S. Department of Defense employs biomechanists to conduct research related to equipment and apparel design and testing for the armed forces. Biomechanists are also involved in the ergonomic design of workstations to maximize worker efficiency and comfort and minimize injury risks. Design of prosthetic devices for optimal function, comfort, and durability is another area of biomechanics.

Future work in biomechanics will be driven by the shifting demographics toward a larger older adult population, as well as by future technological advances. Dynamic magnetic resonance imaging (MRI) provides the capability to directly view what the musculoskeletal system is doing during movement. Once this technology is practically available there will be a significant leap forward in our ability to analyze human movement. Although biomechanists in the future will continue to study performance attributes, there will be an increasing body of work in the areas of degenerative disorders, as well as injury prevention and rehabilitation. Specific topics that are likely to receive increasing research attention in the near future include balance and falling in the elderly, osteoporosis in the aging population, bone loss in astronauts, osteoarthritis development and prevention, the neuropathic foot in diabetics, gait normalization in children with cerebral palsy and other movement disorders, and ACL rupture among athletes.

SUMMARY

Biomechanics is a multidisciplinary science involving the application of mechanics in the study of the structure and function of living organisms. Within the field of exercise science, the living organism most commonly of interest is the human body. Although scientific analysis of human motion has been of interest since the time of the early Greeks, biomechanics was not adopted as the name of this science until the early 1970s. Many of the giants in the history of science made foundational contributions to what was to become biomechanics. Included are Aristotle, Archimedes, Galen, daVinci, Galileo, and Newton. Italian physiologist and physicist Borelli is known as the father of biomechanics. The most significant breakthrough for modern day biomechanics came about in the mid-1970s with the advent of the personal computer. This set the stage for storage of data files containing three-dimensional coordinates of joint centers and other points of interest for subsequent calculation of biomechanical quantities of interest.

Biomechanists study kinematic and kinetic quantities. Kinematics involves the study of the size, sequencing, and timing of movement, without reference to the forces that cause or result from the motion.

Kinematic quantities of interest include linear and angular distance, displacement, speed, velocity, and acceleration. Biomechanists typically use high-speed cinematography or videography to perform quantitative kinematic analyses. Kinetics is the analysis of the actions of forces. Being a vector quantity, force is characterized by magnitude, direction, and point of application to a body. A force rarely acts in isolation, so it is important to recognize that the overall effect of many forces acting on a body is a function of the net force, which is the vector sum of all the acting forces. Within a fluid medium such as air or water, lift and drag forces can exert large influences on a moving body.

Employment opportunities in biomechanics span the academic, clinical, government, and industrial arenas. Because students in exercise science programs typically have only one or two courses in biomechanics, graduate degrees are most commonly required. A number of professional organizations are available for students and professionals in biomechanics. These include the American, Canadian, European, and International Societies of Biomechanics and the International Society of

Biomechanics in Sports. Multidisciplinary organizations such as the American College of Sports Medicine and the American Alliance for Health, Physical Education, Recreation and Dance also include biomechanics interest groups.

To find the latest information in the biomechanics research literature on any given topic, access one of the online databases. The most comprehensive of these is PubMed, at **http://www.ncbi.nlm.nih. gov/entrez/query.fcgi?DB=pubmed**. PubMed is a service of the National Library of Medicine and the National Institutes of Health. The first step in using PubMed is to set limits. On an optional basis, it is possible to set limits for things such as the time period over which to search, the types of articles of interest, the language of the papers, and the places in the papers for PubMed to search for one or more key words. The next step is to enter the key word(s). PubMed then generates a list of paper citations that fit the criteria entered. If the paper was published with an abstract, the abstract can be viewed to find out what the paper is about. Some citations also provide links to the full-length paper online.

■ Key Resources

Key Journals

American Journal of Sports Medicine
Applied Bionics and Biomechanics
British Journal of Sports Medicine
Clinical Biomechanics
Ergonomics
Exercise and Sport Sciences Reviews
Foot and Ankle International
Gait and Posture
Human Factors
Human Movement Science
International Journal of Sports Medicine
Journal of Applied Biomechanics

Journal of Biomechanical Engineering
Journal of Biomechanics
Journal of Bone and Joint Surgery
Journal of Electromyography & Kinesiology
Journal of Human Movement Studies
Journal of Orthopaedic and Sports Physical Therapy
Journal of Orthopaedic Research
Medicine and Science in Sports and Exercise
Physical Therapy
Research Quarterly for Exercise and Sport
Sports Biomechanics

Key Web Sites

American College of Sports Medicine (ACSM) (http://www. acsm.org)
American Society of Biomechanics (ASB) (http://www. asbweb.org/index.html)
Biomechanics Academy of NASPE, AAHPERD (http://www. aahperd.org/index.cfm)
Canadian Society for Biomechanics (CSB) (http://www. health.uottawa.ca/biomech/csb/)

European Society of Biomechanics (ESB) (http://www. esbiomech.org/Home)
International Society of Biomechanics (ISB) (http://isbweb. org/)
International Society of Biomechanics in Sport (ISBS) (http://www.twu.edu/biom/isbs/)

■ Review Questions

1. Define biomechanics and explain why it is a multidisciplinary field of study.
2. Who is known as the father of biomechanics and what were his contributions?

3. List examples from an exercise or other movement activity of five qualitative and five quantitative variables of interest.

4. List examples from a sport or other movement activity of three kinematic and three kinetic variables of interest.
5. Explain your strategy for varying stride length and stride rate during a 100-m race.
6. Explain how ground reaction forces can influence performance in a jumping event.
7. Explain how you would choose to move a heavy desk from one side of a room to the other to minimize your effort.
8. List three careers that require training in biomechanics.
9. What topics are biomechanists of the future likely to study?

■ References

American Society of Biomechanics. (n.d.). mission statement. Retrieved from http://www.asbweb.org/htm/history_mission/history_mission.htm

Canadian Society of Biomechanics. (n.d.). About CSB. Retrieved from http://www.health.uottawa.ca/biomech/csb/about.htm

Cavanagh, P. R., & Kram, R. (1985). The efficiency of human movement—a statement of the problem. *Medicine and Science in Sports and Exercise*, 17, 304.

Cavanagh, P. R., & Williams, K. R. (1982). The effect of stride length variation on oxygen uptake during distance running. *Medicine and Science in Sports and Exercise*, 14, 30.

Chow, J. W., & Hay, J. G. (2005). Computer simulation of the last support phase of the long jump, *Medicine and Science in Sports and Exercise*, 37, 115.

Conoboy, P., & Dyson, R. (2006). Effect of aging on the stride pattern of veteran marathon runners. *British Journal of Sports Medicine*, 40, 601.

Dapena, J. (1980). Mechanics of translation in the fosbury flop. *Medicine and Science in Sports and Exercise*, 12, 37.

Dapena, J. (1984). Biomechanics of elite high jumpers. In J. Terauds et al. (Ed.), *Sports biomechanics*. Del Mar, CA: Academic.

Dapena, J., & Chung, C. S. (1988). Vertical and radial motions of the body during the take-off phase of high jumping. *Medicine and Science in Sports and Exercise*, 20, 290.

Dempster, W. T. (1955). Space requirements of the seated operator. Technical.Report WADC-TR-55-159. Ohio: Wright Patterson Air Force Base.

Derrick, T. R., & Mercer, J. A. (2004). Ground/foot impacts: Measurement, attenuation, and consequences. *Medicine and Science in Sports and Exercise*, 36, 830.

Dillman, C. J. (1985). Overview of the United States Olympic Committee sports medicine biomechanics program. In N. K. Butts, T. T. Gushiken, & B. T. Zarins (Eds.), *The elite athlete*. New York: Spectrum.

Dixon, S. J., Collop, A. C., & Batt, M. E. (2000). Surface effects on ground reaction forces and lower extremity kinematics in running. *Medicine and Science in Sports and Exercise*, 32, 1919.

Elliott, B. C. (1989). Tennis strokes and equipment. In C. L. Vaughan (Ed.), *Biomechanics of sport*. Boca Raton, FL: CRC Press.

Escamilla, R. F., Fleisig, G. S., Barrentine, S. W., Zheng, N., & Andrews, J. R. (1998). Kinematic comparisons of throwing different types of baseball pitches. *Journal of Applied Biomechanics*, 14, 1.

European Society of Biomechanics. (n.d.). Retrieved from http://www.esbiomech.org

Fleisig, G. S., Barrentine, S. W., Zheng, N., Escamilla, R. F., & Andrews, J. R. (1999). Kinematic and kinetic comparison of baseball pitching among various levels of development. *Journal of Biomechanics*, 32, 1371.

Gerlach, K. E., White, S. C., Burton, H. W., Dorn, J. M., Leddy, J. J., & Horvath, P. J. (2005). Kinetic changes with fatigue and relationship to injury in female runners. *Medicine and Science in Sports and Exercise*, 37, 657.

Gutman, D. (1988, April). The physics of foul play. *Discover*, p. 70.

Hardin, E. C., van den Bogert, A. J., & Hamill, J. (2004). Kinematic adaptations during running: effects of footwear, surface, and duration. *Medicine and Science in Sports and Exercise*, 36, 838.

Hay, J. G. (1986). The biomechanics of the long jump. *Exercise and Sport Sciences Reviews*, 14, 401.

Haywood, K. M., & Getchell, N. (2001). *Life span motor development* (3rd ed.). Champaign, Il: Human Kinetics.

Hubbard, M., de Mestre, N. J., & Scott, J. (2001). Dependence of release variables in the shot put. *Journal.of Biomechics* 34, 449.

Konczak, J., & Dichgans, J. (1997). The development toward stereotypic arm kinematics during reaching in the first 3 years of life. *Experimental Brain Research* 117, 346. 1997.

Kyrolainen, H., et.al. (2000). Effects of marathon running on running economy and kinematics. *European Journal of Applied Physiology*, 82, 297.

Lange, G. W., Hintermeister, R. A., Schlegel, T., Dillman, C. J., & Steadman, J. R. (1996). Electromyographic and kinematic analysis of graded treadmill walking and the implications for knee rehabilitation. *Journal of Orthopaedic and Sports Physical Therapy*, 23, 294.

Linthorne, N. P. (2001). Optimum release angle in the shot put. *Journal Sports Science*, 19, 359.

McCaw, S. T., & Hoshizaki, T. B. (1987). A kinematic comparison of novice, intermediate, and elite ice skaters. In B. Jonsson.(Ed.), *Biomechanics X-B*. Champaign, I: Human Kinetics.

Miller, S., & Bartlett, R. (1996). The relationship between basketball shooting kinematics, distance and playing position. *Journal Sports Science*, 14, 243.

Miller, D. I., Jones, I. C., & Pizzimenti, M. A. (1988). Taking off: Greg Louganis' diving style. *Soma*, 2, 20.

Nelson, R. C. (1980). Biomechanics: Past and present. In J. M. Cooper & B. Haven (Eds.). *Proceedings of the Biomechanics Symposium*, Bloomington, IN.

Nilsson, J., Tveit, P., & Eikrehagen, O. (2004). Effects of speed on temporal patterns in classical style and freestyle cross-country skiing. *Sports Biomechanics*, 3, 85.

Paradisis, G. P., & Cooke, C. B. (2001). Kinematic and postural characteristics of spring running on sloping surfaces. *Journal of Sports Science*, 19, 149.

Ramos, E., Latash, M. P., Hurvitz, E. A., & Brown, S. H. (1997). Quantification of upper extremity function using kinematic analysis. *Archives of Physical Medicine and Rehabilitation*, 78, 491.

Rogowski, I., Monteil, K., Legreneur, P., & Lanteri, P. (2006). Influence of swimsuit design and fabric surface properties on the butterfly kinematics. *Journal Applied Biomechanics*, 22, 61.

Rojas, F. J., Cepero, M., Ona, A., & Guitierrez, M. (2000). Kinematic adjustments in basketball jump shot against an opponent. *Ergonomics*, 43, 1651.

Thompson, K. G., Haljand, R., & MacLaren, D. P. (2000). An analysis of selected kinematic variables in national and elite male and female 100-m and 200-m breaststroke swimmers. *Journal of Sports Science*, 18, 421.

Watanabe, K. (1989). Ski-jumping, alpine, cross-country, and nordic combination skiing. In C. L. Vaughan (Ed.), *Biomechanics of sport*. Boca Raton, FL: CRC Press.

Wilson, B. D., McDonald, M., & Neal, R. J. Roller skating sprint technique. In B. Jonsson (Ed.), *Biomechanics X-B*. Champaign, L: Human Kinetics.

Exploring Sports Medicine

CHAPTER 7
Athletic Training

Ray Castle, PhD, ATC, LAT, Louisiana State University

Athletic training is a highly specialized subdiscipline of exercise science that makes up the sports medicine knowledge component. It is an interdisciplinary area of study that combines exercise physiology, nutrition, motor behavior, biomechanics, and sport psychology in the injury prevention and rehabilitation of athletes. The certified athletic trainer undergoes an intense program of clinical education, and the field of athletic training has experienced tremendous growth in recent years. Part 5 describes the role of the certified athletic trainer not only in the prevention of athletic injuries but also in the evaluation and rehabilitation of the injured athlete. We also examine the training a student must undergo to become a certified athletic trainer, along with career opportunities for athletic trainers.

CHAPTER 7

Athletic Training

Ray Castle, PhD, ATC, LAT, Louisiana State University

■ Chapter Objectives

After reading this chapter, you should be able to:

1. Provide a brief overview of the history of the athletic training profession.

2. Define the term *athletic training* and discuss the knowledge and skills that make up the practice of athletic training.

3. Define the educational and professional qualifications required to practice as a certified athletic trainer (ATC).

4. Describe the educational content and other requirements necessary obtain and maintain a medical license to practice athletic training.

5. Identify the role, structure, and functions of the National Athletic Trainers' Association.

6. Explain the various professional career paths available for students upon completing a degree in athletic training and passing the national certification examination.

■ Key Terms

approved clinical instructor
Board of Certification, Inc.
certified athletic trainer (ATC)
clinical instructor
clinical proficiency

cognitive competencies
Commission on Accreditation
 of Athletic Training Education
 (CAATE)
consensus statement

continuing education unit (CEU)
official statement
position statement
psychomotor competencies
support statement

Athletic training is one of the most popular and fast growing health care professions in the United States (U.S. Department of Labor, Bureau of Labor Statistics, 2006). In fact, athletic training is ranked as the 16th fastest-growing profession (projected growth from 2004–2014) among all professions requiring a minimum of a bachelor's degree in the United States. This rapid growth is being fueled in part by the unique health care skill set that certified athletic trainers (ATC) possess and in part by the number of evolving opportunities, or "niches," within various industries that did not exist 15 to 20 years ago or were not considered possible career paths for athletic trainers. Traditionally, the athletic trainer was the health care expert primarily for athletic populations. With the emerging career opportunities today, this title is somewhat of a misnomer. The unique health care skill set of the certified athletic trainer has created a high demand for professionals to meet the needs of a wide variety of health care populations, including the military, the performing arts, exercise and fitness programs, and industrial training settings.

To practice as a **certified athletic trainer (ATC),** individuals must complete an extensive and diverse medical education program accredited by the Commission on Accreditation of Athletic Training Education (CAATE) and pass a national medical board examination administered by the Board of Certification, Inc. (BOC). The knowledge and skill base of the ATC involves an extensive understanding and application of clinical skills related to human anatomy and physiology, exercise physiology, biomechanics, injury/illness epidemiology, clinical research, medical specialty areas (orthopedics, internal medicine, neurology, maxillofacial, cardiovascular), physical rehabilitation/therapy, nutrition, and emergency medicine. Upon entry into the athletic training profession, all ATCs must complete professional development courses, known as **continuing education units (CEUs),** to maintain and enhance their knowledge and skill base to meet the constantly evolving demands of the profession.

Today, more than 30,000 ATCs worldwide are represented by the National Athletic Trainers' Association (NATA, 2006c). Certified athletic trainers are highly qualified health care professionals who specialize in preventing, recognizing, managing, and rehabilitating injuries that result from physical activity. Certified athletic trainers provide preventative and primary medical care to individuals across the life span. Clients include adolescent athletes, law enforcement agencies (Hunt, 2004; Hunt & DeCourcey, 2006), performing ballet company members, military personnel in training or combat zones (Kirkland, 2004), employees at an automobile assembly plant, professional athletes, and geriatric patients.

HISTORY OF THE ATHLETIC TRAINING PROFESSION

The athletic trainer in the United States has its origins in the late 1800s, and for many years it was a male-only profession (Ebel, 1999). With the rapid rise of team sports in the late 1800s and early 1900s, there was also a dramatic increase in serious injuries. The increase in serious injuries was so significant (18 deaths and 159 serious injuries) that in 1905 President Theodore Roosevelt threatened to abolish football as in intercollegiate sport.

Early Notable Persons in Athletic Training

The early athletic trainer was usually a physician or coach who was designated to provide medical care, which may have included stretching, taping, and injury evaluation and treatments to injured athletes (Ebel, 1999). The earliest documented athletic trainers were James Robinson, hired in 1881 by Harvard University, and Michael C. Murphy, who originally worked as a track coach and provided athletic training services at Yale University and the University of Pennsylvania until his death in 1913.

Another notable person is Dr. Samuel E. Bilik, who is considered by many to be the "father of athletic training" (Ebel, 1999). Bilik registered in the pre-med program at the University of Illinois in 1914, and to make money to support himself in school, he landed a part-time job as an "assistant trainer" (for only one dollar an afternoon!). By 1916, Bilik had published *Athletic Training,* and a short time later *The Trainers' Bible,* which is believed to be the first publication dedicated to the profession of athletic training. Over the next 30-plus years, Dr. Bilik held athletic training seminars, which eventually led him to bring together a small group of athletic trainers that would eventually form the Eastern Athletic Trainers' Association, which today comprises Districts 1 and 2 of the NATA.

THE CRAMER BROTHERS HELP MOVE A PROFESSION FORWARD Charles "Chuck" (pharmacist) and Frank Cramer, two brothers from Gardiner, Kansas, made their mark early in the evolution of the athletic training profession (Ebel, 1999; O'Shea, 1980), and even today their influence is still felt. In 1920 the two brothers formed Cramer Chemical Company (later renamed Cramer Products Co.), which produced liniment for athletic teams. Both brothers had a strong interest in athletic training; to learn more about the specific needs of the athletic trainer, they began to travel with a number of teams, including the 1932 U.S. Olympic team. Their quest for knowledge led to them create a number of

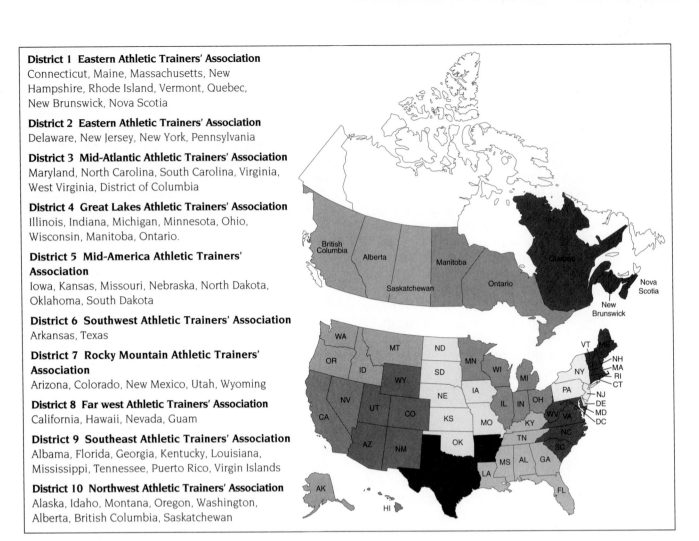

District 1 Eastern Athletic Trainers' Association
Connecticut, Maine, Massachusetts, New Hampshire, Rhode Island, Vermont, Quebec, New Brunswick, Nova Scotia

District 2 Eastern Athletic Trainers' Association
Delaware, New Jersey, New York, Pennsylvania

District 3 Mid-Atlantic Athletic Trainers' Association
Maryland, North Carolina, South Carolina, Virginia, West Virginia, District of Columbia

District 4 Great Lakes Athletic Trainers' Association
Illinois, Indiana, Michigan, Minnesota, Ohio, Wisconsin, Manitoba, Ontario.

District 5 Mid-America Athletic Trainers' Association
Iowa, Kansas, Missouri, Nebraska, North Dakota, Oklahoma, South Dakota

District 6 Southwest Athletic Trainers' Association
Arkansas, Texas

District 7 Rocky Mountain Athletic Trainers' Association
Arizona, Colorado, New Mexico, Utah, Wyoming

District 8 Far west Athletic Trainers' Association
California, Hawaii, Nevada, Guam

District 9 Southeast Athletic Trainers' Association
Albama, Florida, Georgia, Kentucky, Louisiana, Mississippi, Tennessee, Puerto Rico, Virgin Islands

District 10 Northwest Athletic Trainers' Association
Alaska, Idaho, Montana, Oregon, Washington, Alberta, British Columbia, Saskatchewan

Figure 7.1   National Athletic Trainers' Association district names with Web site links and region map.

Reprinted by permission of the National Athletic Trainers' Association.

workshops across the country, which were sponsored by their company, and they began publishing *The First Aider*. More than 85 years later, Cramer Products continues to be one the major supporters of the athletic training profession, sponsoring the NATA, *The First Aider*, and continuing to sponsor student athletic training workshops.

Athletic Trainers Unite to Form a National Organization

In 1938 the efforts of the Cramer brothers and Bill Frey of the University of Iowa (NATA, 2006b), as well as others, came to fruition when the first National Athletic Trainers' Association was formed. NATA grew slowly during the early years and struggled to stay alive as an organization during World War II (Ebel, 1999). After the war the association was reorganized at a meeting in June 1950 in Kansas City, Missouri, and it has been in existence ever since.

Today, the NATA is a highly structured organization with a member *Code of Ethics* (NATA, n.d.) and a well-defined internal governance structure to guide its

members and leaders. Since the rebirth of the NATA in 1950, the association has experienced significant growth and an increase in attendance at its annual symposia. Today athletic trainers are organized at the state level (state associations) and through NATA districts (Figure 7.1). More than 60 athletic training association meetings are held annually at the state, district, and national level. Attendance at NATA's Annual Meeting and Clinical Symposia has grown from approximately 125 in 1950 to over 11,000 today.

Membership and Gender Milestones in Athletic Training

For many years, even into the mid-1990s, the athletic training profession was predominantly a male profession and national association (Ebel, 1999). In 1966 Dotty Cohen, an Indiana University graduate student, became the NATA's first female member. Since that time the NATA has seen rapid growth to over 30,000 members (Figure 7.2). Of that number, 25,353 were ATCs in 2005, and women now account for approximately 48% of certified athletic trainers (Figure 7.3).

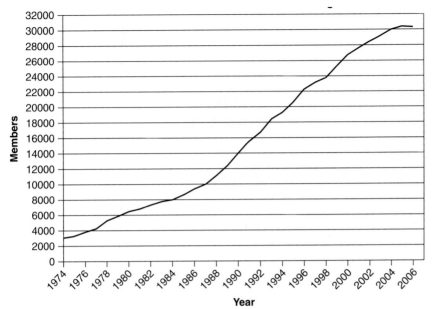

Figure 7.2 Membership in NATA, 1974–2006.

Reprinted by permission of the National Athletic Trainers' Association. Accessed on April 21, 2008 (http://www.nata.org).

Sharing Research and Clinical Evidence to Improve Health Care

The vast knowledge and clinical skill base that comprises today's ATC has created highly skilled health care providers, and they are leading other health care professions in improving injury prevention and patient care. As with other professions, evidence of theory and practice is validated through various professional publications, which are available to the public and to practitioners and other professionals. An extensive review process ensures that these publications are supported by current medical practice and internal (within the profession) and external (other professions or organizations) research. The professional peer-reviewed journals are the *Journal of Athletic Training* and the *Journal of Athletic Training Education*. In the profession of athletic training, a number of position statements, official statements related to specific health care issues, and consensus statements with other professional organizations outline the responsibilities of the athletic trainer.

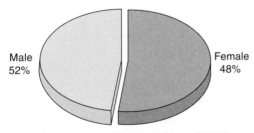

Total number of certified members = 25.353

Figure 7.3 NATA Members by gender that are BOC certified athletic trainers, December 31, 2005.

Reprinted by permission of the National Athletic Trainers' Association. Retrieved November 30, 2006, from http://www.nata.org

This information is not unique to athletic training; numerous professions utilize these information sources to create and share consistent, efficient, current health care practices across allied health care disciplines.

POSITION STATEMENTS Position statements are formal statements (can be considered a policy) related to specific topic areas in the profession that have been developed by experts in athletic training. These statements are based on extensive research data and clinical outcomes and provide the most immediate impact on the ATC's standards of professional practice. Position statements are available at the NATA Web site. Here are a few examples:

- Emergency Planning in Athletics (Anderson, Courson, Kleiner, & Mchoda, 2002)
- Exertional Heat Illnesses (Binkley, Beckett, Casa, Kleiner, & Plummer, 2002)
- Fluid Replacement in Athletics (Casa et al., 2000)
- Head-Down Contact and Spearing in Tackle Football (Heck, Clarke, Peterson, Torg, & Weis, 2004)
- Lightning Safety for Athletics and Recreation (Walsh et al., 2000; endorsed by the American Academy of Pediatrics)
- Management of Sport-Related Concussion (Guskiewicz et al., 2004)
- Management of Asthma in Athletes (Miller, Weiler, Baker, Collins, & D'Alonzo, 2005)

OFFICIAL STATEMENTS Official statements are issued by the NATA to address specific issues that may be affecting the professional practice of athletic training or patient health care practices. These official statements, which can be viewed on the NATA Web site, are not intended to change professional practice but rather support or refute specific issues that affect the practice of athletic training or patient care.

CONSENSUS STATEMENTS Similar to a position statement, a **consensus statement** is a comprehensive report that is completed through an extensive research process by various professional organizations. Like position statements, the consensus statement can create an immediate change in the ATC's standard of professional practice, as well as standards of practice for other professions. Here are a few examples:

- Appropriate Medical Care for Secondary School-age Athletes
- Executive Summary: Recommendations on Emergency Preparedness and Management of Cardiac Arrest in High School and College Athletic Programs
- Interassociation Task Force on Exertional Heat Illnesses
- Prehospital Care of the Spine-Injured Athlete

These statements and many others are available at the NATA Web site.

SUPPORT STATEMENTS In developing relationships with other professional organizations, an organization may receive a public comment, or **support statement,** related to the practice of another profession. Athletic trainers have received public support from major professional medical organizations (e.g., American Medical Association, American Academy of Orthopedic Surgeons) that relate to the practice of athletic training and NATA position statements.

PEER-REVIEWED PUBLICATIONS Specifically within the profession of athletic training, there are currently two peer-reviewed journals: *Journal of Athletic Training* and *Athletic Training Education Journal*. The *Journal of Athletic Training* (JAT) historically has been the primary source of peer-reviewed research and clinical case studies specifically related to the practice of athletic training. With the increased availability of quality research articles on the Internet, articles published in the JAT can be accessed through the following online databases: MEDLINE, PubMed Central, Focus on Sports Science & Medicine (subscription-based), Research Alert (subscription-based), Physical Education Index (subscription-based), SPORT Discus (subscription-based), CINAHL (subscription-based), PsychINFO (subscription-based), and EMBASE (subscription-based). With the increasing development of education programs over the last decade, the *Athletic Training Education Journal* (ATEJ) was created as a research publication partner to the *Journal of Athletic Training*. The ATEJ is an Internet-accessed, peer-reviewed journal

that publishes research related to educational practices within athletic training education.

CONTENT AREAS OF STUDY AND EDUCATIONAL PREPARATION

To become a certified athletic trainer, individuals must graduate from an undergraduate or graduate program in athletic training. The accreditation process for the 350-plus athletic training education programs is administered by the **Commission on Accreditation of Athletic Training Education (CAATE).** The following sections outline the process leading up to current accreditation standards that regulate the professional preparation of certified athletic trainers.

External Accreditation Process for Athletic Training Education Programs

In the 1980s, the NATA began forging critical relationships with other health care organizations, including the largest health care organization, the American Medical Association (AMA). In June 1990 the NATA and the athletic training profession received a major boost when the AMA formally recognized athletic training as an allied health profession (NATA, 1990).

The NATA also initiated discussions with the AMA to begin initial external accreditation of its athletic training education programs through the AMA's Committee on Allied Health Education and Accreditation (CAHEA). By 1990 the NATA had formed the Joint Review Committee on Educational Programs in Athletic Training (JRC-AT), which would oversee and organize input from external education "cosponsors" required for program accreditation by CAHEA. The AMA and NATA and the American Academy of Pediatrics and the American Academy of Family Physicians selected representatives to serve on the JRC-AT. The JRC-AT developed standards and guidelines that would govern the JRC-ATC and CAHEA accreditation process, which led to development of *Essentials and Guidelines for an Accredited Educational Program for the Athletic Trainer*, which was approved by the cooperating organizations and the AMA's Council on Medical Education on December 6, 1991 (NATA Professional Education Committee, 1991). This document, combined with *Competencies in Athletic Training*, originally developed by the NATA Professional Education Committee in 1983, served as the blueprint for development and implementation of CAHEA-accredited athletic training education programs.

In 1993 the NATA removed the curriculum approval process from the Professional Education Committee to the JRC-AT, and in February 1994 the first two entry-level athletic training education programs (Barry University, High Point University) received external accreditation by CAHEA. This accreditation process under CAHEA was eliminated by the AMA in 1994, and the AMA moved from a sponsor of accredited allied health care programs to a cosponsor role. A new independent agency, the Commission on Accreditation of Allied Health Education Programs (CAAHEP), was then formed to handle the accreditation process (JRC-AT, 1998).

The mid-2000s have brought about additional changes in accreditation of athletic training education programs. In 2006 the Commission on Accreditation of Athletic Training Education (CAATE) was formalized as an independent external accrediting agency that would take over the accreditation approval process that was being conducted by CAAHEP. All accredited programs must complete an extensive accreditation self-study review including an on-campus accreditation site visit by external reviewers every 5 years to maintain the institution's accreditation status by CAATE. A complete list of accreditation requirements and accredited degree programs can be accessed on the CAATE Web site.

PROFESSIONAL PREPARATION OF TODAY'S ATC

Today's ATC must complete an intensive medical education program that combines didactic (classroom) and clinical education components. The CAATE-accredited athletic training curriculum prepares individuals for a career by following a specific structure of sequential course progression. This sequential programming provides students with critical base knowledge and skills and structured clinical experiences under trained clinical instructors (**approved clinical instructors**) and other allied health care personnel (**clinical instructors**). As previously stated, a student must graduate from an accredited athletic training education program. Among the requirements of each program, athletic training students must have formal clinical experiences with a variety of health care settings and health care professionals for a minimum of 2 years.

The backbone of the CAATE accreditation is the *Athletic Training Educational Competencies* (NATA, 2006a), which outlines the knowledge and skills students must obtain in CAATE-accredited programs. The "Athletic Training Educational Competencies" is organized into two major areas: Foundational Behaviors of Professional Practice and Major Educational Content Areas.

Foundational Behaviors of Professional Practice

This area provides essential guidance to athletic training education programs and to students by linking the "Standards of Professional Practice" (BOC, 2008) and

the *Role Delineation Study* (BOC, 2004) with the overall outcomes of an athletic training education program, and ultimately, the common values of the profession. Upon completion of the CAATE-accredited athletic training education program, athletic training students should have developed the necessary skills and behaviors to perform as highly qualified health care professionals. The list of Foundational Behaviors of Professional Practice is inclusive (NATA, 2006a):

Primacy of the Patient

- Recognize sources of conflict of interest that can impact the patient's health.
- Know and apply the commonly accepted standards for patient confidentiality.
- Provide the best health care available for the patient.
- Advocate for the needs of the patient.

Teamed Approach to Practice

- Recognize the unique skills and abilities of other health care professionals.
- Understand the scope of other health care professionals.
- Understand and execute duties within the identified scope of practice for athletic trainers.
- Include the patient (and family, where appropriate) in the decision-making process.
- Demonstrate the ability to work with others in effecting positive patient outcomes.

Legal Practice

- Practice athletic training in a legally competent manner.
- Recognize the need to document compliance with the laws that govern athletic training.
- Understand the consequences of violating laws that govern athletic training.

Ethical Practice

- Understand and comply with the NATA's *Code of Ethics* and the BOC's *Standards of Practice*.
- Understand the consequences of violating NATA's *Code of Ethics* and BOC's *Standards of Practice*.
- Understand and comply with other codes of ethics, as applicable.

Advancing Knowledge

- Critically examine the body of knowledge in athletic training and related fields.
- Use evidence-based practice as a foundation for the delivery of care.
- Understand the connection between continuing education and the improvement of athletic training practice.

- Promote the value of research and scholarship in athletic training.
- Disseminate new knowledge in athletic training to fellow athletic trainers, patients, other health care professionals, and others as necessary.

Cultural Competence

- Understand the cultural differences of patients' attitudes and behaviors toward health care.
- Demonstrate knowledge, attitudes, behaviors, and skills necessary to achieve optimal health outcomes for diverse patient populations.
- Demonstrate knowledge, attitudes, behaviors, and skills necessary to work respectively and effectively with diverse populations and in a diverse work environment.

Professionalism

- Advocate for the profession.
- Demonstrate honesty and integrity.
- Exhibit compassion and empathy.
- Demonstrate effective interpersonal communication skills.

Major Educational Content Areas

The NATA Educational Competencies are organized under 12 major knowledge and skill areas, referred to as *content areas*. Within each content area are subcategories for **cognitive competencies** (knowledge) and **psychomotor competencies** (specific clinical skills). A critical aspect of any health care profession is the ability to synthesize or integrate the cognitive and psychomotor knowledge into clinical practice. This integration is referred to as **clinical proficiency.** The ability of the athletic training student to effectively and efficiently integrate knowledge and skills into daily health care practice is an essential aspect of any qualified health care provider. The 12 content areas outlined in the NATA Educational Competencies (NATA, 2006a) and identified for all CAATE-accredited athletic training education programs are as bollows:

- Risk management and injury prevention
- Pathology of injuries and illnesses
- Orthopedic clinical evaluation and diagnosis
- Medical conditions and diseases
- Acute care of injury and illness
- Therapeutic modalities
- Conditioning and rehabilitative exercise
- Pharmacology
- Psychosocial intervention and referral
- Nutritional aspects of injuries and illnesses
- Health care administration
- Professional development and responsibility

Upon successful completion of all educational requirements (cognitive, psychomotor, and clinical) set forth by CAATE, students are eligible to sit for the Board of Certification, Inc. (BOC) Certification Examination. Upon passing the BOC Certification Examination, a person is credentialed as a "BOC Certified Athletic Trainer" (ATC denotes the credential). The following section outlines in more detail the BOC and its role in regulating the profession of athletic training.

PROFESSIONAL CERTIFICATIONS FOR ATHLETIC TRAINERS

In the United States, health care professions are regulated by state regulatory practice laws and/or national regulatory boards. The **Board of Certification, Inc.,** commonly referred to as the BOC, serves as the regulatory board for the certified athletic trainer (ATC) on a national level and is the medical license/credential recognized by most state regulatory boards or legislative practice acts. The BOC serves as the national credentialing agency for athletic trainers and as a regulatory agency to protect the profession of athletic training. This "protection" occurs on several levels. First, it protects the ATC and the public by identifying individuals who are competent to practice the profession of athletic training (BOC, 2004). Second, the BOC guards the ATC's practice credential to protect against another profession's infringement on the scope and practice of the ATC. A third equally important protection aspect of the BOC is its work to regulate the profession against any unsafe practices that a person may (or may not perform) that could cause harm to the public.

State Regulation of Athletic Training

Most states have some form of regulation of credentialed health care providers, but the type of regulation varies among professions. States that regulate athletic training require qualified individuals to complete an extensive credential/background check and/or state-level administered examination through a designated regulatory agency. A current list of credentialing agencies in each state can be obtained through the Board of Certification, Inc. State laws that govern the practice of athletic training are structured to one of four regulation types: licensure, certification, registration, and exemption (Prentice, 2006; Ray, 2000). Understanding the structure of these laws is important for all health care providers as each type has its advantages and disadvantages.

Defining the Professional Practice of the BOC Certified Athletic Trainer

The BOC is a national credentialing agency that is separate from any professional organization, including the NATA. In regulating the practice of athletic training, the BOC uses several mechanisms to define and guide the practice of athletic training: *Role Delineation Study for the Entry-Level Certified Athletic Trainer*, BOC Standards of Professional Practice, and its credentialing examination.

BOC ROLE DELINEATION STUDY The roles and responsibilities of the certified athletic trainer are defined through the *Role Delineation Study for the Entry-Level Certified Athletic Trainer* (BOC, 2004). The *Role Delineation Study*, also referred to as the RDS, is now in its fifth edition and defines the major domains of professional practice for the entry-level ATC. The professional practice of athletic training consists of six domains that delineate the major responsibilities performed by the ATC:

- Prevention
- Clinical evaluation and diagnosis
- Immediate care
- Treatment, rehabilitation, and reconditioning
- Organization and administration
- Professional responsibility

The BOC conducts an extensive professional practice study (role delineation study) every 5 to 7 years that determines the scope of practice of the ATC, which ultimately provides the current and future ATC with a "guide" to define his or her professional abilities as well as the scope of practice to protect the public from harm.

BOC STANDARDS OF PROFESSIONAL PRACTICE The BOC (2008) also has developed the BOC *Standards of Professional Practice*, which provides additional direction for the ATC in his or her daily clinical practice as a competent health care provider. The objectives of any health care profession's standards of practice (also referred to as a "standard of care") are to help the public understand the type and level of care from an ATC, guide the ATC to effectively evaluate the level of patient care, and assist the ATC to understand his or her roles and responsibilities by possessing and representing the ATC credential.

BOC CERTIFICATION EXAMINATION To practice as a certified athletic trainer, individuals must successfully pass a credentialing examination administered by the BOC. The first credentialing examination for athletic trainers was conducted in 1969 (Ebel, 1999) and subsequently evolved into a three-part examination: written examination, written simulation examination, and practical examination. To sit for the BOC Certification Examination, a candidate must meet set criteria, including eligibility to graduate from an accredited degree program in athletic training. In 2007 the BOC eliminated the current certification examination format, instead implementing a two-part computerized testing format: written examination and simulation/scenario.

Professional Development for ATCs

MAINTAINING PROFESSIONAL COMPETENCE
The body of knowledge that comprises medicine is constantly under a state of change due in large part to research and advances in technology. The body of knowledge and skills required for today's athletic trainer fall under many subdisciplines of medicine, and ATCs need to maintain current competence as qualified health care providers. In most professions—and this is especially true in health care disciplines—the credentialed provider is required to document completion of professional development courses. These professional development courses, also referred to as continuing education units (CEUs) or continuing medical education, consist of attending and completing specific identified educational activities. The requirements for each profession vary and are dictated by the credential-granting agency, state or national regulatory boards, and/or regulations defined by state laws. Examples of how health care providers may show proof of completing professional development activities include, but are not limited to, attendance, participation, or presentation of a medicine-related topic at clinical symposia/workshops; completion of designated home-study continuing education courses; and writing a chapter in a textbook or acceptance of a research article in a journal.

The continuing education requirements for the ATC are dictated by the Board of Certification, Inc. and, if applicable, the state(s) in which the ATC holds a license to practice. It is important to keep in mind that the BOC grants the ATC credential, but each person must adhere to state or local regulations governing the practice of athletic training. Athletic trainers must submit appropriate documentation to each applicable credentialing/regulatory agency on a regular basis, which does vary from state to state. Most, if not all, state regulatory agencies for athletic training follow the continuing education requirements set forth by the BOC; the ATC can submit the same information to the BOC and other regulatory boards to meet his or her professional development requirements.

The BOC has a highly structured system for ATCs to follow to meet their professional development requirements (BOC, 2006). Completion of continuing education activities fall under one of four categories, and each category has specific limitations in terms of the total number of continuing education units (contact hours) and types of activities that are applicable.

Beginning January 1, 2006, the BOC mandated that all ATCs must complete a "CEU stagger"; that is, the ATC must complete a minimum of 25 contact hours of CEU in a defined year (corresponding to the year in which the first letter of their last name is identified), followed by a 3-year period in which ATCs must verify completion of 75 CEUs (BOC, 2006). The BOC Web site outlines the CEU reporting process in more detail.

ADVANCED DEGREES Upon successful completion of the BOC Certification Examination (now possessing the ATC credential), a person has the "key" that opens the door to numerous job opportunities in a variety of settings. Today it is extremely common for the entry-level ATC to pursue an advanced degree immediately following completion of an undergraduate athletic training education program. The graduate school route provides many entry-level ATCs with the opportunity to obtain valuable experiences under a more experienced ATC mentor while also expanding their education. Another driving force for many ATCs is career advancement in the workplace. More than 70% of all ATCs now possess an advanced degree (NATA, 2006d). Many ATCs pursue an advanced degree related to athletic training (e.g., exercise physiology, biomechanics, health education) or to job performance/advancement (e.g., management, health care administration).

One growing option for ATCs to significantly improve their knowledge and clinical skills is to pursue a master's degree from an NATA-approved graduate athletic training education program. ATCs can obtain a significant advantage by graduating from an NATA-approved graduate athletic training education program. The knowledge and skills addressed in these degree programs are highly advanced, and in most cases the schools have developed one of several "specialty tracks," or degree concentration areas, for the student to pursue. These specialty tracks provide ATCs with the opportunity to develop a high knowledge and clinical skill base, and upon completion of the degree they are usually highly recruited for top job positions. In terms of specialization in the profession, completion of these degree programs can be equated to any health care field in which minimal credentialing requirements (e.g., medical school) are followed by a specialization (e.g., a physician specializes in family practice residency/fellowship).

CAREER OPTIONS IN ATHLETIC TRAINING

Due to the extensive professional preparation and the knowledge and skill base of today's certified athletic trainer, it is easy to see why numerous career paths are open to the entry-level ATC. According to NATA statistics, more than 25,000 ATCs participate in a wide range of job settings (Table 7.1). In any job setting minimum performance criteria are determined by the employer and may include educational and experience background, expertise/specialty in a defined health care area, and credentials. A number of major career options available for ATCs, along with the minimum qualifications an ATC may need to obtain employment in the setting, are presented in the following sections.

Clinic Outreach

Certified athletic trainers in these positions work in an outpatient physical rehabilitation setting and provide medical coverage for high school sports, professional teams, recreational events, or some combination of these. Commonly, the ATC provides therapy services

TABLE 7.1 National Athletic Trainers' Association BOC Certified Athletic Trainers by Job Setting, December 31, 2005

Setting	% Of Members	Number of Members
College student	9%	2,266
University and college	19%	4,858
Clinic	19%	4,704
High school	16%	4,135
High school/Clinic	7%	1,836
Other professional	7%	1,803
Hospital	3%	868
Professional sports	4%	1,079
Unspecified	0%	67
Industrial	1%	172
Corporate	1%	150
Clinic/Industrial	4%	1,023
Junior college	2%	381
Unemployed	3%	696
Other	1%	378
Health/Fitness	1%	323
Middle school/ Junior high school	0%	122
Sales/marketing	1%	173
Retired	1%	319
Total Members		**25,353**

Reprinted by permission of the National Athletic Trainer's Association.

during a portion of the day and then performs event coverage in the local community. Minimum requirements for these positions are possessing the ATC credential, meeting state credentialing criteria, and graduating from a CAATE-accredited program.

Clinic

The certified athletic trainer works full-time in an inpatient or outpatient physical rehabilitation clinic (e.g., sports medicine clinic). The ATC conducts physical rehabilitation for patients across the life span with acute and nonacute physical conditions as prescribed by a licensed physician or collaboratively with a physical therapist or occupational therapist. Minimum requirements for these positions are possessing the ATC credential, meeting state credentialing criteria, and graduating from a CAATE-accredited program.

College or University

Colleges and universities are one of the largest employment sectors in athletic training.

ATHLETIC DEPARTMENT An ATC employed by an athletic department serves as the primary medical provider for its athletic teams. The ATC typically provides full-time event and practice medical coverage; travels with teams; establishes and coordinates a comprehensive health care delivery system consisting of physicians and other health care providers; establishes and implements medical records and insurance documentation systems and emergency planning protocols; and promotes injury/illness prevention programs such as nutritional assessments, conditioning programs, and drug-testing programs. Minimum requirements for these positions usually include the ATC credential, meeting state credentialing criteria, graduating from a CAATE-accredited program, and a minimum of a master's degree with 1 to 2 years experience as an ATC.

INSTRUCTOR Certified athletic trainers possess an extensive knowledge and skill base in health care and teach the areas outlined in the educational content areas required of athletic training education programs. ATCs also teach specialized courses such as human anatomy, human physiology, nutrition, health/wellness, exercise physiology, pharmacology, biomechanics, and health care administration, as well as technology-based and education courses unrelated to health care. Minimum requirements for these positions vary with institutional requirements but usually require a master's degree in the area of instruction. In an athletic training education program, the core athletic training courses of the curriculum must be instructed by an ATC or equally qualified health care professional to maintain accreditation requirements. As an example, a strength coach at a university is not qualified to teach physical reha-

bilitation courses, but these courses could be taught by either an ATC or a physical therapist as both professions have equal knowledge and skill related to physical rehabilitation and conditioning of injured patients.

PROFESSOR Similar to the instructor position, educational expertise is required to teach specific courses. Typically, professorial ranks at universities require a minimum of a doctoral degree (e.g., PhD, EdD). Most professorial positions are academic only, with no time allotted for coverage of athletic teams. Today most athletic training program directors possess a doctoral degree, and all possess the ATC credential. These faculty positions, along with other athletic training faculty positions, are given selected percentages of *release time* (time allotted to perform particular job-related activities) for program administration, teaching, service, and research per semester. Some faculty positions (as is the case with the author of this chapter) are referred to as "clinical faculty" or "professional practice" ranks. These positions allow for a blend of clinical activity, service, and teaching, and usually have no formal research responsibilities as is the case for tenure-track faculty positions.

INTRAMURAL/RECREATIONAL SPORTS A number of universities hire certified athletic trainers on a full-time basis or in graduate assistantship positions to provide on-site medical coverage of organized recreational campus sport activities, conduct injury evaluations, and provide physical rehabilitation to the general student population. Minimum requirements for these positions are possessing the ATC credential, meeting state credentialing criteria, and graduating from a CAATE-accredited program. Other specific requirements and additional duties may be involved with these positions depending on the institution's specific needs.

Corporate/Industrial

Certified athletic trainers are employed by companies such as General Motors and Chevron to provide on-site employee wellness programs, supervise workplace injury prevention training, organize emergency response programs, provide work-skill conditioning programs, and offer physical rehabilitation for injured employees.

Government

Various governmental agencies (local, state, federal) employ ATCs to provide comprehensive injury prevention, immediate care, and physical rehabilitation/conditioning to employees. Examples of governmental employers include the Las Vegas Police Department; U.S. Department of Homeland Security; Federal Bureau of Investigation; and NASA. All of these agencies employ individuals whose jobs require both extensive mental and physical training/conditioning, and a common by-product of these programs are job-related injuries. The ATC fulfills a unique position, providing multiple health care services that include emergency medicine, orthopedic and general medical assessment, physical rehabilitation and conditioning, risk management, and injury prevention skills. Minimum requirements for these positions are possessing the ATC credential and possibly other job requirement credentials/training, meeting state credentialing criteria, and graduating from a CAATE-accredited program. Educational level may vary (e.g., master's degree or doctoral degree) for these positions.

Military

The military is rapidly increasing its utilization of ATCs to provide a variety of health care services to its enlisted and officer personnel. The ATC is uniquely qualified to provide emergency medicine, injury/illness assessment, and physical rehabilitation and conditioning of troops either at physical training grounds or during military engagements. ATCs currently work with various military personnel at Navy SEAL training facilities, U.S. Navy ships at sea, and at Air Force bases to provide a variety of medical services. Minimum requirements for these positions are possessing the ATC credential and possibly other job requirement credentials/training, meeting state credentialing criteria, and graduating from a CAATE-accredited program. Educational level may vary (e.g., master's degree or doctoral degree) for these positions.

Performing Arts

The performing arts sector is an emerging job setting. ATCs have extensive training and skills related to providing care to competitive and highly conditioned performers. Many performing art companies are hiring ATCs to provide full-time primary medical care services to their members, which include injury evaluation and referral, physical rehabilitation and conditioning, and implementation of nutritional and psychological wellness programs. Minimum requirements for these positions are possessing the ATC credential and possibly other job requirement credentials/training, meeting state credentialing criteria, and graduating from a CAATE-accredited program. Educational level may vary (e.g., master's degree or doctoral degree) for these positions.

Physician Extender

Physicians and physician office administrators are rapidly seeing the advantages of utilizing an ATC in various patient care settings. The ATC can conduct initial patient interviews and assessment, educate the patient on home exercise/therapy programs upon completion of the physician visit, assist in splinting/

casting of injuries, and assist in surgeries. In a number of settings, the physician employs the ATC to assist in coverage of local high school sports in addition to his or her physician office duties. Minimum requirements for these positions are possessing the ATC credential and possibly other job requirement credentials/training, meeting state credentialing criteria, and graduating from a CAATE-accredited program. Educational level may vary (e.g., master's degree or doctoral degree) for these positions.

Professional Sports Teams

Professional teams at all levels utilize ATCs for duties similar to those outlined in the Athletic Department setting. These settings were traditionally viewed as male-only positions, but this is not the case. Some professional sports teams, such as the Pittsburgh Steelers of the National Football League, employ a female ATC for their team, and almost half of the head athletic trainers for NFL-Europa teams are female. The increase in female professional sports teams, such as the WNBA and professional women's soccer and softball leagues, has also helped to increase the number of opportunities for females in professional settings.

Secondary School Athletic Trainer

The secondary school setting is currently a major employment sector for students to consider as a future career path. School systems are hiring ATCs to be the primary on-site health care provider or a combination of ATC and teacher. In the combination position, the ATC teaches classes during the day and provides and coordinates medical coverage for extracurricular activities after school (game and practice). For combination positions, it is a common practice for the school system to pay the ATC a full-time teaching salary and supplement that salary for coverage of extracurricular activities. Minimum requirements for these positions are possessing the ATC credential and possibly other job requirement credentials/training such as a teaching credential, meeting state credentialing criteria, and graduating from a CAATE-accredited program. The minimum educational level for these positions is usually a bachelor's degree; however, each position is unique to the needs of the school system.

United States Olympic Committee

A number of ATCs are employed by the USOC to provide full-time medical coverage to its athletes at one of the four U.S. Olympic Training Centers (Chula Vista, CA; Colorado Springs, CO; Marquette, MI; Lake Placid, NY). In addition to these full-time positions, the USOC also utilizes 1-year fellowship programs and a "volunteer" program for ATCs. The volunteer program is a feeder selection program to recruit and utilize

ATCs to cover various U.S. teams during the year and also at major events (e.g., Pan American Games, World Championships, Winter and Summer Olympics). After completing a 2-week rotation at one of the U.S. Olympic Training Centers, ATCs are evaluated on their ability to interact with athletes, coaches, and peers; their work ethic; quality of health care provided; and many other attributes. This evaluation process may result in the ATC being invited to serve as a medical staff member for travel with a team to a major athletic event or on competition tours. Minimum requirements for these positions are possessing the ATC credential and possibly other job requirement credentials/training. Educational level may vary (e.g., master's degree or doctoral degree) for these positions, but for the volunteer position the USOC requires a minimum of 2 years' experience as an ATC prior to application.

Medical Sales

Certified athletic trainers also gain employment in various medical sales areas. The ATC's extensive medical background and experience in communicating with various health care professionals provides a unique skill set for employers. ATCs are employed by major companies as sales personnel for durable goods medical equipment (e.g., bracing, therapy equipment) and for surgical hardware sales and training. These positions may require the person to possess the ATC credential, but this is usually not a requirement at time of hiring. Educational level and past sales experience may vary for these positions.

SUMMARY

Athletic trainers work under the direction of licensed physicians to provide essential health care services to patients across the life span. The ATC is the one health care provider who has the opportunity (depending on job setting) to see the patient from initial injury through full recovery. This process may involve applying emergency medicine skills in the initial injury management of the patient's condition, having the ability to make a medical diagnosis of the injury/condition, making appropriate and efficient referral to other health care specialists if needed, and directing and supervising the patient's physical rehabilitation to full recovery. The patient may be an adolescent athlete, a NASCAR driver, a Marine injured in combat, a professional football player, or an elderly patient who has sustained a heart attack.

The profession of athletic training has evolved, and ATCs are highly skilled and respected health care providers. This evolution has occurred over many years through the efforts of many individuals to enhance the quality of care provided to patients. Today the profession of athletic training is represented by the NATA, which fosters collaboration with other highly respected professional organizations such as the AMA, the American College of Sports Medicine (ACSM), the American Academy or Orthopedic Surgeons, the American Academy of Family Physicians, and the NCAA to enhance the quality and delivery of patient health care.

Since January 1, 2004, persons desiring to become athletic trainers must graduate from a comprehensive degree program in athletic training that has been accredited by CAATE. The evolution of the breadth of knowledge and skills required of the ATC has drastically increased job opportunities in athletic training and related fields. Numerous career options are available for athletic trainers, which include employment in secondary schools, medical sales/training, sports medicine clinics, physician offices, military branches, professional sport teams, and corporate/industrial settings, just to name a few.

■ Key Resources

Key Journals
Athletic Training Education Journal
Journal of Athletic Training

Key Web sites
Athletic Training Education Journal (www.nataej.org)
Board of Certification, Inc. (www.bocatc.org)
Commission on Accreditation of Athletic Training Education (www.caate.net)
Journal of Athletic Training (www.nata.org/jat)
NATA *District Web Sites*
District 1: Connecticut, Maine, Massachusetts, New Hampshire, Rhode Island, Vermont, Quebec, New Brunswick, Nova Scotia (www.eatald1.org)
District 2: Delaware, New Jersey, New York, Pennsylvania (www.natad2.org)

NATA *News* (association-based monthly publication)

District 3: Maryland, North Carolina, South Carolina, Virginia, West Virginia, District of Columbia (www.maata.org)
District 4: Illinois, Indiana, Michigan, Minnesota, Ohio, Wisconsin, Manitoba, Ontario (www.glata.org)
District 5: Iowa, Kansas, Missouri, Nebraska, North Dakota, Oklahoma, South Dakota (www.maata.net)
District 6: Arkansas, Texas (www.swata.com)
District 7: Arizona, Colorado, New Mexico, Utah, Wyoming (www.rwata.org)
District 8: California, Hawaii, Nevada, Guam (www.fwata.org)

District 9: Alabama, Florida, Georgia, Kentucky, Louisiana, Mississippi, Tennessee, Puerto Rico, Virgin Islands (www.seata.org)

District 10: Alaska, Idaho, Montana, Oregon, Washington, Alberta, British Columbia, Sas Katchewar (www.nwata.net)

NATA Education Council (www.nataec.org)

National Athletic Trainers' Association (www.nata.org)

■ Review Questions

1. Define athletic training as a field of study.
2. Explain the process by which a person becomes an entry-level BOC-certified athletic trainer (ATC).
3. Explain the importance of completion of continuing education units (CEU) to the professional practice and development of the certified athletic trainer.
4. Explain the differences between position statements, official statements, and consensus statements.
5. Explain how standards of professional practice direct the actions of an allied health care professional.

6. Identify the six professional practice domains in the profession of athletic training.
7. Distinguish between the different types of continuing education activities a certified athletic trainer may complete to maintain his or her professional credential.
8. Summarize the 12 content areas identified in the NATA Educational Competencies that define the educational requirements of students in entry-level athletic training education programs.

■ References

Anderson, J. C., Courson, R. W., Kleiner, D. M., & McLoda, T. A. (2002). National Athletic Trainers' Association position statement: Emergency planning in athletics. *Journal of Athletic Training, 37*(1), 99–104.

Binkley, H. M., Beckett, J., Casa, D. J., Kleiner, D. M., & Plummer, P. E. (2002). National Athletic Trainers' Association position statement: Exertional heat illnesses. *Journal of Athletic Training, 37*(3), 329–343.

Board of Certification, Inc. (2004). *Role delineation study for the entry-level certified athletic trainer* (5th ed). Omaha, NE: Author.

Board of Certification, Inc. (2006). *Recertification requirements (2006–2011)*. Retrieved from http://bocatc.org/images/stories/athletic.trainers/recertificationrequirements2006-2011.pdf

Board of Certification, Inc. (2008). BOC *standards of professional practice*. Retrieved from http://bocatc.org/images/stories/multiple-references/standardsprofessionalpractice.pdf

Casa, D. J., Armstrong, L. E., Hillman, S. K., Montain, S. J., Reiff, R. V., Rich, B. S. E., Roberts, W. O., & Stone, J. A. (2000). National Athletic Trainers' Association position statement: Fluid replacement for athletes. *Journal of Athletic Training, 37*(3), 329–343.

Ebel, R. (1999). *Far beyond the shoe box: Fifty years of the National Athletic Trainers' Association*. Dallas, TX: National Athletic Trainers' Association.

Guskiewicz, K. M., Bruce, S. L., Cantu, R. C., Ferrara, M. S., Kelly, J. P., McCrea, M., Putukian, M., & McLeod, T. C. V. (2004). National Athletic Trainers' Association position statement: Management of sport-related concussion. *Journal of Athletic Training, 39*(3), 280–297.

Heck, J. F., Clarke, K. S., Peterson, T. R., Torg, J. S., & Weis, M. P. (2004). National Athletic Trainers' Association position statement: Head-down contact and spearing in tackle football. *Journal of Athletic Training, 39*(1), 101–111.

Hunt, V. (2004, August). Athletic trainers boost homeland security. NATA *News*.

Hunt, V., & DeCourcey, B. (2006, October). Athletic training in law enforcement: Serving those who protect & serve. NATA *News*.

Joint Review Committee on Educational Programs in Athletic Training. (1998, Spring). JRC-AT *News*.

Kirkland, M. (2004, October). COE working to increase, enhance ATC employment. NATA *News*.

Miller, M. G., Weiler, J. M., Baker, R., Collins, J., & D'Alonzo, G. D. (2005). National Athletic Trainers' Association position statement: Management of asthma in athletes. *Journal of Athletic Training, 40*(3), 224–245.

National Athletic Trainers' Association. (1990, September). AMA endorses athletic training as allied health profession. NATA *News*, P. 4.

National Athletic Trainers' Association. (2006a). *Athletic training educational competencies* (4th ed.). Dallas, TX: Author.

National Athletic Trainers' Association. (2006b, February.). Voices from the past: How the NATA and athletic training grew. NATA *News*.

National Athletic Trainers Association. (2006c). *What is an athletic trainer*. Retrieved December 28, 2006, from http://www.nata.org/about_AT/whatisat.htm

National Athletic Trainers' Association. (2006d). [Data Sheet]. Retrieved December 28, 2006, from http://www.nata.org/membership/MembStats/2006_10.htm

National Athletic Trainers' Association. (n.d.) *Code of ethics*. Retrieved November 28, 2006, from http://www.nata.org/codeofethics/index.htm

National Athletic Trainers' Association Professional Education Committee. (1991). *Athletic Training Education Newsletter*. Dallas, TX: Author.

O'Shea, M. (1980). A *history of the National Athletic Trainers' Association*. Dallas, TX: National Athletic Trainers' Association.

Prentice, W. (2006). Arnheim's principles of athletic training: A competency-based approach (12th ed.). New York: McGraw-Hill.

Ray, R. (2000). Management strategies in athletic training (2nd ed.). Champaign, IL: Human Kinetics.

U.S. Department of Labor, Bureau of Labor Statistics (2006). Occupational information. Retrieved December 19, 2006, from www.careerinfonet.org

Walsh, K. M., Bennett, B., Cooper, M. A., Holle, R. L., Kithill, R., & Lopez, R. E. (2000). National Athletic Trainers' Association position statement: Lightning safety for athletics and recreation. *Journal of Athletic Training, 35*(4), 471–477.

PART 6

Exploring the Social Science

CHAPTER 8
Sociology of Physical Activity
Mary McElroy, PhD, Kansas State University

CHAPTER 9
History of Exercise and Sport
William Harper, PhD, Purdue University

We often think of exercise science as a discipline devoted to an examination of the physiological processes associated with exercise, but it is important to look at exercise in both its societal and historical contexts as well. It is essential to know how the discipline got its start, and the historical influences that shaped the field. Exercise science has deep historical roots dating back in this country to its earliest inhabitants. Furthermore, societal influences help to shape both physical activity patterns and attitudes about sports and exercise. In Part 6 we look at the historical influences that have shaped exercise behavior in the United States and how exercise and sport have influenced society as a whole. Chapter 8 focuses on the sociology of physical activity, and Chapter 9 discusses the history of exercise and sport in the United States.

Sociology of Physical Activity

Mary McElroy, PhD, Kansas State University

■ Chapter Objectives

After reading this chapter, you should be able to:

1. Appreciate what is meant by a sociological imagination and relate its significance to understanding the various forms of physical activity.

2. Provide a brief overview of the history of the sociology of physical activity, including the key events in the last half century that served as the impetus for the evolution of the academic discipline.

3. Describe the typical course content taught in most sociology of physical activity courses.

4. Recognize some of the scientific journals that publish research findings in the sociology of physical activity.

5. Identify the various professional societies that focus on the sociology of physical activity.

6. Identify the various career options for students with training in the sociology of physical activity.

■ Key Terms

community capacity
community competence
daily living activities
ecological models
gender roles
health inequity framework
health-related physical activity

occupational physical activity
organized sport
personal attributes
recentering social institutions
sense of community
social class
social environments

social mobility
socializing agents
socializing situations
sociological imagination
sociology
Title IX, Education Amendments
  Act of 1972

Organized sport and other forms of physical activity permeate American society so thoroughly that we cannot avoid their influence. As best-selling authors James Michener (1976) noted, whether watching sporting contests or participating in local fun runs, these activities have their grip on the American audience. Physical activity dominates much of our conversation, reading material, and leisure pursuits. Whether discussing the results of the World Cup (soccer), the Wimbledon Championships (tennis), the Masters (golf), the World Series (baseball), or even your participation in the local softball or bowling league, organized physical activity (sport) dominates American culture.

For many of us, our indoctrination began early in life. For many boys, and more recently girls, participation in organized sporting activities originates with T-ball, Little League, or a youth soccer program. For many teenagers, participation on high school and college teams is a central part of their educational experience. While interest shifts to a spectator role as one grows older, many adults still find organized sport and other forms of physical activity significant in their everyday lives. Today, organized sport is as popular as ever and has catapulted into a multibillion dollar enterprise. The total annual revenue of the U.S. sports industry tops more than $213 billion. Television networks bid billions of dollars for multiyear rights to televise college basketball tournaments, professional sports, and the Olympic games (Coakley, 2006). The Super Bowl remains the number-one televised event, and advertisers are willing to spend more than $2.6 million for a 30-second spot (Elliott, 2007).

It is likely that your life has been affected in some way by physical activity due to the highly touted fitness and exercise craze. The proliferation of exercise equipment and fitness facilities and the emergence of the personal trainer and home gym have generated a whole new vocabulary of fitness terms and a greater public awareness of the importance of health-related physical activity (Bryant & McElroy, 1997). At the same time, many health professionals are questioning the actual activity habits of most Americans. Less than half of all Americans participate in an appropriate amount of physical activity (Macera et al., 2005). In fact, physical inactivity was felt to be such a large public health problem the U.S. Surgeon General released a landmark report, *Physical Activity and Health: A Report of the Surgeon General*, hoping to reverse the trends of physical inactivity among most Americans (U.S. Department of Health and Human Services, 1996). More than 10 years later the trends have not been reversed.

The consequences of a sedentary lifestyle have raised concerns for the growing number of people dealing with obesity (Hill & Trowbridge, 1998). The "obesity epidemic" has received considerable attention from mass media and numerous scientific organizations. One of the leading medical authorities, *the Journal of the American Medical Association*, reported that poor diet and physical inactivity are responsible for more than 400,000 deaths in the United States, accounting for 16.6% of all deaths (Mokdad, Marks, Stroup, & Gerbending, 2004). The incidence of childhood obesity is also rising rapidly. The annual National Health and Nutrition Examination Survey by the Centers for Disease Control and Prevention found nearly 20% of U.S. children are overweight and many more are at risk of becoming overweight (Ogden et al., 2006). The number of obese children has quadrupled over the last several decades, raising significant concerns regarding the development of chronic diseases in adulthood.

This chapter examines some of the key issues concerning physical activity as a social phenomenon. **Sociology,** a term coined by Auguste Comte (1798–1857), is the systematic study of human social life. It is a systematic study because sociologists apply both theoretical perspectives and research methods to examinations of social behavior. A sociological perspective is based on the concept that people are by nature social beings; that is, they are products of their social environments. As pointed out by sociologist Peter Berger (1963), society not only controls our movements but shapes our identity, our thoughts, and our emotions. Sociologists who study sport and physical activity are interested in the connection of these activities to the social and cultural contexts in which they exist.

A sociological perspective is often used to understand social issues that emerge in organized sport and to provide a "critical view" regarding practices in sport and other physical activity programs. Although physical activity has been part of the American scene for centuries, sociologists have only more recently accepted these activities as a legitimate topic for academic inquiry. Sociologists historically have focused on organized sporting practices, but during the 1990s a growing interest has developed in examining physical activity as part of a healthy lifestyle. The underlying assumption of the sociological study of physical activity is that organized sporting practices and other forms of physical activity are crucial to understanding the deeper meaning of experiences in American society.

BRIEF HISTORY OF THE SOCIOLOGY OF PHYSICAL ACTIVITY

The sociological study of physical activity is one of several subdisciplines within physical education as set out by Franklin M. Henry in his position paper, "Physical Education: An Academic Discipline," in

1964. Europeans took the early lead in developing the academic study of physical activity. As a result of a working session held in Geneva, a committee consisting of representatives from both physical education and the social sciences was formed as an outgrowth of the International Council for Sport and Physical Education (ICSPE). The first scholarly association to study the sociology of physical activity, the International Committee of Sport Sociology, was formed in 1964, and the first scholarly journal, *International Review of Sport Sociology*, emerged in 1966.

Academic interest in the sociology of physical activity began to take shape in North America in the 1970s with publication of two popular books. Jack Scott's (1970) *The Athletic Revolution* and Harry Edwards's (1970) *The Revolt of the Black Athlete* were both highly critical of the sport establishment, particularly the National Collegiate Athletic Association (NCAA). Gerald Kenyon, a faculty member in physical education at the University of Wisconsin, was also quite influential in bringing attention to the growing interest in the sociological study of sport. Kenyon, along with his student John Loy, published the groundbreaking article "Toward a Sociology of Sport" (1969), which is considered to be the first programmatic statement for the need for a sociology of sport. Loy and Kenyon (1969) also edited the first reader on the sociology of physical activity, titled *Sport, Culture and Society*. Throughout the late 1960s and 1970s sessions on the sociology of physical activity were held at major conferences in physical education and sociology throughout North America. The first major conference on the subject was attended by member schools from the Big Ten universities. The symposium was held at the University of Wisconsin in November 1968. In addition to sponsorship by professional physical education associations, the sociology of physical activity—particularly with a focus on organized sport—emerged as a legitimate topic for discussion at meetings of the American Sociological Association (ASA). From its start as discussion to a roundtable luncheon session in 1968, ASA members have expanded their many timely issues in sport and physical activity at both national and regional meetings.

Acceleration of research and writing on the sociology of physical activity in Canada and the United States created a demand for scholarly journals on the topic, and the *Review of Sport and Leisure* was first published in North America in 1976. Soon thereafter Arena, the Institute for Sport and Social Analysis, began publication of the Arena newsletter and the *Journal of Sport and Social Issues* (1976). Perhaps the most influential organization to address the sociology of physical activity in North America was the North American Society for the Sociology of Sport (NASSS), formed in 1978. NASSS held its first annual conference in 1980 and began publishing the *Sociology of Sport Journal* in 1984. Today, the organization continues to publish the journal 4 times a year, holds an annual conference, and manages a very useful Web site.

By the 1990s scholars had expanded their interests to include topics related to a *social critical paradigm*. The social critical perspective assumes practices associated with physical activity are interwoven in a social structure that reinforces the subordination and oppression of disadvantaged groups. Issues related to gender roles, discrimination, racism, and other examples of social inequities were incorporated into discussions related to organized sport and other forms of physical activity.

Significant interest in the sociology of physical activity from a health perspective did not emerge until the mid-1990s, coinciding with the publication of several high profile reports such as the surgeon general's report titled *Physical Activity and Health* (U.S. Department of Health and Human Services, 1996) and *Healthy People 2010* (U.S. Department of Health and Human Services, 2000), which highlighted the health consequences of a sedentary lifestyle. By the end of the 20th century, several nationwide campaigns brought attention to the social issues associated with getting people to adopt healthy habits of physical activity. Medical sociologists such as Robert Crawford (1980) argued for a sociological basis for understanding the difficulties in creating a social structure more conducive to a healthier society. Robert Putnam's *Bowling Alone* (2000) provided insight into why many Americans have disengaged not only from health promoting lifestyles but from their communities as well. Mary McElroy (2002) published one of the first in-depth analyses of the current epidemic of sedentary living from a sociological perspective. In *Resistance to Exercise: A Social Analysis of Inactivity* McElroy addressed the question of whether it is possible to transform contemporary American society into a more physically active society. More recently, the Institute of Medicine (2004) outlined specific actions for families, schools, industry, communities, and government necessary to address the epidemic of childhood obesity. The American Public Health Association (APHA) identified lifestyle issues as a major health problem and devoted a significant part of its 2005 meeting to issues related to promoting physical activity.

COURSE CONTENT

Key topics in the sociology of physical activity are related to the forms of physical activity, particularly *sport* (organized, competitive) and *health-related exercise* (motivated to improve health). Physical activity that is incorporated into daily living also is an important area of inquiry. Many sociology courses focus primarily on issues related to organized sport and are taught in sociology, exercise science, physical education, or kinesiology departments. Topics in a traditional sociology of sport course vary according to the interest of the instructor but typically include the following:

Organized sport and social class

Organized sport and social institutions (family, education, corporate sport, religion)

Professional sport

Gender and organized sport

Race/ethnicity in organized sport

Politics in organized sport

Economics of organized sport

Organized sport and social problems (crime, violence, deviance, drugs)

Youth in organized sport

Recently, attention given to the consequences of physical inactivity in contemporary society and a nationwide concern regarding the health consequences of sedentary living have opened up new topics for a sociological inquiry. As a result, a growing number of sociology of physical activity classes that had emphasized organized sport now have expanded their format to include issues related to health and exercise. Topics covered might include the following:

Physical activity and health

Role of sedentary pursuits (television, video games, computers)

Obesity epidemic

Social inequities and physical inactivity

Building physically active communities

The business of fitness

Disorder eating in contemporary society

Cultural competency and the exercise profession

Creating a physically active society

Using a "Sociological Imagination"

Before examining a number of interesting issues related to sport and physical activity, we first need to appreciate what is meant by a sociological perspective. In understanding human social behavior, the sociologist steps back and examines social forces operating outside the individual. In so doing, the sociologist uses a **sociological imagination,** a concept first articulated by C. Wright Mills (1959), which refers to the ability to see the interconnections between individual experiences and broader social forces. A sociological imagination helps us distinguish between personal troubles and social (public) issues. Personal troubles are private problems of individuals and can

be resolved by individuals within their immediate social setting. Public issues are matters beyond the control of an individual and are produced by circumstances at the societal level. We can extend Mills's thinking to the causes of unhealthy habits associated with living in contemporary society. If unhealthy behaviors such as eating a poor diet or engaging in inadequate amounts of physical activity are confined to only a few individuals, these lifestyle behaviors can be seen as personal troubles. The effective remedy under these circumstances would be to enact physical activity programming and other health promotion programs targeting individuals directly. However, when the problems of poor nutrition and inadequate physical activity are so pervasive that they contribute to a high rate of sedentary living and obesity, physical inactivity takes on the character of a public problem. A sociological imagination suggests that significant improvements in physical activity for so many Americans require us to look beyond individuals to the factors in society that lie beyond their control.

Classifying Forms of Physical Activity

The term *physical activity* encompasses many different forms of activity. In attempting to classify the potentially overwhelming number of roles associated with physical activity, social scientists have identified four broad categories.

Organized sport is characterized by physical exertion and complex physical skills exhibited by participants within a framework of formal rules and structure. Organized sport is driven by intrinsic factors related to competition such as defeating opponents and winning championships. It is influenced highly by extrinsic factors from the social environment such as fans, media, and economic impact. Many sports can be viewed as a major production effort. The production of sport can be further classified into three groupings: *primary producers* (the actual event participants), *secondary producers* (coaches, officials, etc.) whose responsibility directly influences whether the contests are won or lost, and *tertiary producers* (the media, fans, etc.) who are necessary to complete the event successfully but have no significant impact on the scoreboard (Bryant & McElroy, 1997).

Health-related physical activity contributes to the individual's overall physical and mental state. Activities designed to improve an individual's ability to maintain a healthy lifestyle include aerobic activities such as running, hiking, and biking. Health-related physical activity also includes measures of physical activity designed to restore the body to a healthy state, such as cardiac rehabilitation exercise programs and strength training programs associated with injury. The American College of Sports Medicine and the Centers for Disease Control and Prevention have jointly issued guidelines for improving health through physical activity (U.S. Department of Health and Human Services, 1996). These guidelines are based on time devoted to the physical activity (at least 30 minutes), the days performed (at least 5 days a week) and intensity level (moderate > 4 METS). These guidelines are designed to help the general public understand the minimum amount of physical activity necessary for good health (see Chapter 2). The goals of health-related exercise may be to return an injured athlete to the game or an accident victim to normal functioning capacity.

Daily living activities consist of ordinary, everyday physical activities such as walking to and from classes and completing household chores. Shopping is a good example of a daily living physical activity. Studies of physical activity have often underestimated the amount of physical activity performed particularly by women and seniors because activities of daily living are not considered.

Physical activity can also be categorized as **occupational physical activity;** that is, physical activity relative to work requirements. The physical and energy requirements of some blue-collar and unskilled labor occupations are greater than traditional forms of health-related exercise. On the other hand, the reliance on machinery and technology has created office and other work-related positions that can easily be classified as sedentary jobs.

Socialization Into Physical Activity Roles

Fitting into physical activity roles is a complex process, and no two individuals experience the same process. Predicting whether an individual is likely to participate in any of the forms of physical activity is best understood by utilizing a social learning approach. Gerald Kenyon and Barry McPherson (1973) introduced a framework for consolidating the overwhelming number of factors that play a role in an individual's likelihood of participation in an organized sport or other physical activity. Drawing on general theories of social learning, predictors of participation in physical activity roles can be categorized into three groups: personal attributes, socializing agents, and socializing situations.

Personal attributes are any descriptive features that characterize the individual. They include the physical dimensions (height, weight, age, physical condition) the psychological dimension (personality, competitiveness, psychological maturation) and the social psychological dimensions (coping skills, social interaction skills). **Socializing agents** are significant persons in one's life who provide social influence. The family is considered the most significant socializing agent for all age groups, but particularly for children.

Social support, whether from family members or friends, is an important factor in whether people start and continue participation in sport and other forms of physical activity. Social support takes a variety of forms. It may consist of accompanying someone to an exercise class, calling someone to see how a program is going, or providing information about new programs. The third grouping, **socializing situations,** consists of individuals' unique blend of opportunities and life experiences. The social class of a family, for example, affect socializing in physically active roles. Health risk factors, such as low levels of physical activity, are related to social position. That is, the causes of a sedentary lifestyle differ with the socioeconomic status of particular groups. Physical activity participation is known to be related to both culture and gender. Among U.S. adults, physical activity is lower for African Americans than for Caucasians, and this difference is particularly pronounced in women (Crespo, Keteyian, Heath, & Sempos, 1996). Similar patterns have been observed in U.S. high school students: only 47.8% of African American girls met current guidelines for participating in vigorous physical activity compared to 59.8% of Caucasian girls (Centers for Disease Control and Prevention [CDC], 2002). Physical environment also plays a major part in socialization. Growing up in sunbelt regions such as Florida and Arizona certainly affects physical activity differently from life in snowbelt areas.

This social learning framework can help us understand why some individuals do not choose to participate in physical activity. The personal attribute of being female predicts a low likelihood of participation in an organized football league. A junior high school boy who has not reached his height potential may be drawn away from the high school basketball team. This model is useful in describing the barriers adults face in developing a physically active lifestyle as well. As mentioned previously, the lack of social support from socializing agents can play a crucial role in the failure to develop an active physical lifestyle.

Dynamics of Social Class and Social Mobility

Sociologists examine the social groups that make up a society and seek to determine how inequalities are structured and persist over time. American society has a hierarchical arrangement, with **social classes** based on level of education, occupational prestige, and income (Blau & Duncan, 1967). The social class structure in American society can help us define the type and amount of participation in many forms of sport and physical activity. Those in the upper classes have the material wealth, monetary resources, and time to engage in a variety of physical activities. They comprise a large portion of the fitness boom participants. The middle class participates in structured team sports and, to a lesser extent, in structured fitness programs both in the community and in the workplace. Contrary to popular belief regarding using sport as a way to move out of the lower social class, members of the lower social class have the lowest participation rate of all groups. African Americans and Hispanics are least likely to participate in regular physical activity (Crespo, 2000). Health-related exercise, such as joining a fitness club or participating at the worksite fitness center, is largely a middle- or upper-class phenomenon that accompanied the rise of living standards in the United States over the last century and the increasing separation of work from physical activity in a postindustrial, technological society (McElroy, 2002).

Social class position is directly related to health. As people's economic status increases so does their health status. Those who are wealthy, well educated, and have higher paying jobs are much more likely to be healthy than are poor people. The poor have shorter life spans and are at greater risk for chronic illness such as diabetes, heart disease, and cancer. Max Weber (1922/1968) used the term *life chances* to refer to the extent individuals have access to important societal resources such as food, clothing, shelter, education, and health care. More affluent people typically have better life chances than the less affluent because they have greater access to quality education, safe neighborhoods, and high-quality nutrition and physical activity programming. In contrast, persons from the lower social classes have limited access to these resources.

Importance of the Built and Social Environments

Physical activity takes place in specific geographical areas. Physical environments, also known as the *built environment*, conducive to physical activity provide the infrastructure that contributes to substantial increases in physical activity opportunities (Papas et al., 2007). The possibility of including physical activity as part of one's daily routine varies depending on circumstances related to one's job, amount of free time, availability of space or facilities, and the physical characteristic of the neighborhood, workplace, and school setting. Several promising studies support the idea that small modifications to the built environment can have a positive impact on physical activity behavior. Adding signs to increase stair use, providing showers and changing rooms for employees, and increasing access to trails in rural communities are examples of changes to the built environment that have been shown to increase physical activity levels.

Social environments consist of the nonphysical products of human interaction, which include the ideas shared by members of a particular group as well as the ways individuals come together to participate.

Social connectedness is important in matters of good health including participation in physical activity. Building on the work of Berkman and Syme (1979), a number of studies have suggested that social relationships also enhance positive health behaviors. In these studies, social connection has been associated with improvement in behavioral health factors such as smoking cessation, control of diet, and physical activity (Kawachi, Kennedy, & Glass, 1999).

Race/Ethnicity Issues and Sport

A commonly held belief in contemporary America is that sport participation is the ticket for members of racial minorities to escape their impoverished conditions. The highly visible presence of African Americans in professional sports such as football and basketball and Hispanics in baseball has certainly contributed to this thinking. Visible African American athletes such as Barry Bonds, Kobe Bryant, and Shaquille O'Neal command multimillion-dollar player contracts. Child phenoms such as tennis sisters Venice and Serena Williams have widened the eyes of many African American youngsters. The emergence of Tiger Woods on the professional golf scene, in particular, has created a heightened perception of mobility opportunities among ethnic minorities.

Social mobility is movement or change in lifestyle accompanied by specific changes in occupation, education, and income. The lifestyles of many professional athletes, as depicted in the media, make a professional sports career a highly desirable goal. Sociologists have attempted to quantify the odds of making it to the professional ranks. Based on the number of available positions and the number of active participants, a professional sports career is remote.

Many social scientists argue that this belief in sport as a social mobility escalator is counterproductive to ethnic minorities. African American leaders point to the unrealistic time allocated to sport involvement and the unrealistic expectations associated with social advancement through sport. Dreams of a professional sports career can be counterproductive to the extent that they distract individuals from pursuing more realistic opportunities.

One of the ongoing controversies in the sporting world is the use of American Indian names and mascots for sport teams. A well-known example is the Cleveland Indians and their mascot, Chief Wahoo. Critics of the sport teams who adopt American Indian imagery argue that such representations create false and degrading images of American Indians and believe that the rituals carried out by teams or fans show disrespect for Indian culture. A number of schools, including Cornell, Dartmouth, Marquette, Stanford, and Syracuse, have changed their team names and mascots. Others, and some professional sports teams such as the Cleveland Indians, Washington Redskins, and Atlanta Braves, have not changed their names.

Physical Activity and Health Disparities

One of the major goals of the national health objectives for the year 2010 is a reduction in the health disparities between the general population and racial and ethnic minorities. The objectives make a special point to address reducing the disparity in physical activity differences among these groups. Racial and ethnic minority health disparities became a public policy issue in the United States following the publication of the Department of Health and Human Services Secretary's Task Force Report in 1985, called the Heckler Report after then DHHS Secretary Margaret Heckler. The report acknowledged that the health status of the U.S. population as a whole had improved significantly since the beginning of the 20th century but concluded that "persistent, significant health inequities exist for minority Americans."

Twenty years after the Heckler Report, the *Third National Healthcare Disparities Report* (Agency for Healthcare Research and Quality, 2005) concluded that disparities related to race, ethnicity, and socioeconomic status still exist in the American health care system. The changing demographics of American society point to the need to address the physical inactivity problem with different race and ethnic groups in mind. According to the U.S. Census Bureau (2007), the two fastest-growing population groups are Asian and Hispanic, with the Asian population growing 16% between 2000 and 2004, and the Hispanic population growing 17% during the same period. Of the 100 million Americans added to the population since 1967, 53% are recent immigrants or their descendants. These trends clearly show that the United States is a diverse society. Health interventions and programs to get people from all social categories to participate in more health-related physical activity must be responsive to this diversity. Being responsive to diversity means taking a look at these differences sociologically. The general experience of discrimination, social exclusion, lack of access to resources, and higher prevalence of poverty are just a few factors sociologists can connect to risky health behaviors such as physical inactivity. Populations that have experienced disproportionate poverty may be less accustomed to some of the lifestyle patterns that have become commonplace among wealthier groups in American society.

The sociologist uses a **health inequity framework** to focus on the effect of social inequalities and racial discrimination and to explain low participation rates in physical activity (Hogue, Hargreaves, & Scott Collins, 2000). Physical activity rates among people of color, particularly African Americans and Hispanics, are significantly lower than their white counterparts. This is in contrast to the perception resulting from their visibility in sport that members of minority groups are fit and active. In reality, members of many minority populations have a higher incidence of cancer and cardiovascular diseases (Institute of Medicine, 2003). Members of these groups are at risk for early death caused by poor nutrition and physical inactivity. The low physical activity participation rates among racial and ethnic minorities were confirmed in the National Health and Nutrition Examination (Crespo, 2000). A central theme of *Healthy People 2010* (U.S. Department of Health and Human Services, 2000) emphasizes that improving the physical activity levels among minority populations cannot be accomplished without addressing their socioeconomic circumstances. Without economic equity, physical activity increases are unlikely.

Gender Roles and Sport Participation

Males and females differ in both biological and sociological factors. Biological difference are based on factors such as physical strength, height, cardiovascular endurance, and reproductive capabilities. Sociological differences are fixed in socialization such as the role of significant others, socialization situations, and socializing institutions. Although biological sex differences are important, most are actually socially constructed gender differences. The sociologists who study **gender roles** in sport and other forms of physical activity recognize the presence of biological differences while emphasizing the culturally prescribed values or gender roles that influence aspects of the sport and exercise experience. American society still clings to vestiges of a patriarchal society, a dominant value orientation that defines society by male standards and identified appropriate masculine and feminine behaviors. Not surprisingly, sport and other forms of physical activity embody many of the same social ills, problems, and inequities.

The advances of women in sport, particularly since the mid-1970s and the enactment of Title IX legislation, have been significant. **Title IX, Education Amendments Act of 1972,** opened doorways of opportunity for girls and women. Although slow to get off the ground, it has been responsible for a steady growth in the number of sport teams for girls and women at all levels of participation—youth sport, high school, college, and club sport. Inroads have not come easily or without strong attempts to discourage women's active participation in sport. The court system has contributed to significant changes in women's participation in organized sport. A school is in compliance with Title IX if it meets any one of three conditions:

> *Proportionality test:* The school must demonstrate that sport participation opportunities for each

gender are substantially proportionate to its full-time undergraduate enrollment.

History of progress test: The school must show that it has a history and continuing practice of expanding its women's athletic programs.

Accommodation of interest test: The school must show that its programs and teams have fully accommodated the interests and ability of members of the underrepresented gender.

More girls are engaged in sport today than at any other time in history, but other areas remain virtually closed to them such as administrative positions as athletic directors and fitness center directors. Entrance into the exercise professions also has been slow and gradual. Although more female physicians practice sports medicine than in the past, men still outnumber women significantly in roles such as team doctor, athletic trainer, and orthopedic surgeon.

Society places expectations on women that can foster health problems. The increased emphasis on exercise for women during the last several decades has focused much attention on topics related to dysfunctional eating patterns, or eating disorders. Anorexia nervosa, a disorder characterized by starvation, and bulimia, an eating disorder characterized by binging and purging, have reached epidemic proportions, particularly in young women. A contributing factor to eating problems is the cultural gender-role expectations of thinness. The strong cultural expectations for a lean body can lead to disorders related to a distorted body image and an obsession for thinness. Characteristics associated with success in sport—highly competitive, achievement-oriented, self-sacrificing—coupled with society's expectations of a thin body make female athletes a particularly vulnerable group for developing eating disorders. Explanations regarding the relationship between gender and eating problems must take into account a complex array of social factors including gender socialization and societal expectations concerning women's body image.

Physical Inactivity and Childhood Obesity

Over the past 20 years, obesity rates in U.S. children and youth have escalated. Among children ages 6 to 11, 15.8% are overweight and 31.2% are overweight or at risk for overweight. Among adolescents ages 12 to 19, 16.1 to 30.9% are overweight or at risk for overweight, and 20% of children and youth in the United States will be obese by 2010 (Institute of Medicine, 2004). These trends are particularly troubling because youth obesity starts young people on the path to health problems such as diabetes, high blood pressure, and heart disease that were once confined to adults. Sociologists have pointed to two major social institutions as being responsible for failing the health needs of children—the family and the school (McElroy, 2002). The family is fundamental to children's socialization into physical activity habits. Families teach skills and reinforce beliefs that can help to shape important attitudes and behaviors associated with participation in physical activity. Children typically remain within the family unit for up to 18 years during their formative years. Families can help develop the appropriate attitudes in children so they will remain physically active for a lifetime. Sociologists offer two approaches to explaining the role parents play in transferring to their children the necessary values and habits for a lifelong commitment to participation in physical activity. The first focuses on parents' modeling positive physical activity habits, and the second focuses on the importance of instilling perceptions of competency in their children (McElroy, 2002). The rapid increase in the prevalence of childhood obesity is coupled with other disturbing trends at school. Between 1991 and 2003, enrollment of high school students in daily physical education decreased from 41.6% to 28.4% (Pate et al., 2006). Physically active transport to and from school has significantly declined from previous generations. Even recess has been reduced or eliminated in some elementary schools. Many physical education organizations have recommended that schools adopt policies that require daily PE, elementary school recess, and physical activity opportunities before, during, and after school. School-based programs are critical for the development of healthy behaviors, but many physical education classes do not teach the skills necessary to increase activity outside of class or to maintain physical activity over the lifetime (Corbin, 1987).

Changing Sedentary Lifestyles: A Sociological Perspective

Particularly during the 1970s a growing body of research established a strong case that many health problems could be traced to the living habits of individuals. This position was well chronicled in an essay by John Knowles (1977) who proclaimed that "the greatest enemy to the health of the individual is the individual." Such thinking would lay the groundwork for the health movement of the 1980s and would unite health promotion with the goal of changing risk behaviors of individuals. In recent years sociologists have questioned the wisdom behind emphasizing good health through individual lifestyle changes (Minkler, 2000). Social scientists do not claim that individual behaviors are unimportant. Unlike the exercise psychologist, who uses behavior change strategies to get people to participate in physical activity, the sociologist's interest lies in how the social structure of society presents significant challenges to the adoption of behaviors to maintain a physically active lifestyle.

Social epidemiologists Leonard Syme and Linda Balfour (1998) offer several reasons strategies focused on changing individual behaviors are likely not to work. First, they point to the fact that previous health promotion strategies aimed at changing individual behaviors have not worked. The second reason is that the health conditions of today, such as cardiovascular disease, diabetes, and cancer, involve such large numbers of people that it is impossible to prevent such diseases by simply changing the behavior of individuals one at a time. Finally, and perhaps crucial to an understanding of the disappointing results of health promotion efforts, targeting the behaviors of individuals directly, they point to how individual approaches do little to address the social conditions that have contributed to the problem. Even if individual health habits are changed, if the wider social and cultural context in which these behaviors occur is not altered, the next generation of people will suffer from the same adverse social conditions.

Social Ecological Approaches to the Study of Physical Activity

Models of human behavior that focus attention on environmental factors, also known as **ecological models,** have been widely recognized for their importance in increasing health promoting behaviors such as physical activity (Stokols, 1996). The ecological approach assumes that appropriate changes in the social environment will produce changes in individuals. Sociologists who study health-related physical activity have increased their attention on identifying strategies that promote physical activity through environmental and policy changes (French, Story, & Jeffrey, 2001). Environmental and policy approaches may be particularly effective because they can benefit all people exposed to the environment rather than focusing on changing the behavior of individuals one person at a time. Examples of environmental and policy approaches to increase physical activity include accessible walking and bike trails, zoning and land use, and building construction that encourages activity policies.

A number of related constructs may be helpful in enhancing our understanding of how changing social environments may promote increases in physical activity. For example, sense of community is an important social environment variable when examining physical activity. **Sense of community** measures the extent to which individuals have developed feelings of belonging to their community and the extent to which they engage with community members to create changes in their community (Putnam, 2000). Other social environment factors including **community competence,** in which community members are able to collaborate effectively to identify problems and needs, and **community capacity,** or characteristics of communities that affect their ability to mobilize and address social and public health issues, are also important for promoting physical activity habits of individuals.

Changing Social Institutions to Create a Physically Active Society

The current status of our social institutions has a distinct bearing on how and even whether we participate in physical activity. As discussed previously, society relies on social institutions such as the family and school to pass on to succeeding generations a set of values, expectations, and solutions individuals can draw on when making their way through life. Unfortunately, many of our key social institutions fail to relay the importance of a physically active lifestyle. McElroy (2002) offered a framework known as **recentering social institutions** to structure a meaningful change toward a society that is fully engaged in physical activity. A major portion of this model focuses on how social institutions of family, education, work, and health care actually create obstacles to participation in physical activity. McElroy argued that to achieve a healthy and physically active society individuals and the organization structures to which they belong need to change. The focus on changing levels of physical activity must be combined with efforts directed at changing the value systems associated with our social institutions. Strategies of changes to our social institutions must promote norms of active living, social equity, and collaboration. Efforts to promote a physically active society will not succeed unless individuals take an active role in changing their own health behaviors (personal control over health), but they must also take an equally active role in changing value structures within social institutions (citizenship skills). Such an approach may finally provide the impetus to transform contemporary American society into a physically active society.

CAREERS IN SOCIOLOGY OF PHYSICAL ACTIVITY

Countless studies have concluded that a college degree in any major is an asset in many ways later in life. Sociology provides new ways of approaching problems and making decisions in everyday life. For this reason, people with a knowledge of sociology are employed in a variety of fields that apply sociological insights to everyday life. Students with an emphasis in the sociological study of physical activity can pursue a host of employment areas. Many of these jobs would require additional undergraduate or graduate work. City, state, and community agencies are actively looking for well-trained individuals who can develop programs to promote healthy living including increasing participation in physical activity. You may want to consider working in the following areas:

Public health physical activity specialist

Personal training

Sports and health journalism

High school or college athletic director

Business and sport, planning and consulting

Lecturing and research

Health promotion

Leisure management

Sports promotion and public relations

Sports clothing retail and production

Sports medicine

Coaching

Sports administration

Public health specialist

Community health specialist

Health advocacy

Nonprofit organizations

SUMMARY

During the last several decades, social scientists have begun to appreciate that physical activity in its variety of forms possesses rich potential to explain and analyze human social organization, behavior, and social life. Organized sport and other forms of physical activity are such pervasive elements of American life that virtually every individual is touched by them. A sociological perspective helps us gain a better understanding of ourselves and our social world. The values and behaviors we observe in society are often readily observable in the context of our own physical activity practices. The many forms of physical activity discussed in this chapter serve as a mirror, or microcosm, of American social life. Attention to the low levels of physical activity of many Americans reinforces the importance for social change.

Although sociologists historically have focused on organized sporting practices, during the last decade, in particular, there has been a growing interest in examining health-related physical activity. Changing the sedentary behaviors of most Americans requires serious attention to developing interventions aimed at society's social structure. The interest in changing the behaviors of individuals stems from the belief among health professionals that changing individual risk factors is easier than tackling the many social problems plaguing society today. There is also a growing understanding that organized sport and other forms of physical activity are linked to the social relations of everyday life that underlie social class inequality, sexism, racism, and other forms of discrimination. Changing the sedentary behaviors of most Americans requires serious attention to developing interventions aimed at society's social structure. Students with an emphasis in the sociological study of physical activity are well prepared to enter a wide variety of careers. Sociologists of physical activity are usually faculty members in colleges or universities and teach classes, offer related professional services, and engage in research. Students with training in the sociological perspective should be able to find jobs with local public health agencies and nonprofit organizations focused on addressing social and health conditions in American society.

■ Key People

Peter Berger	Gerald Kenyon	C. Wright Mills
Auguste Comte	John Knowles	Meredith Minkler
Robert Crawford	John Loy	Robert Putnam
Harry Edwards	Mary McElroy	Jack Scott

■ Key Resources

Key Professional Organizations
American College of Sports Medicine
American Public Health Association

International Society for Sociology of Sport
North American Society for the Study of Sport Sociology

Key Journals
Adapted Physical Activity Quarterly
American Journal of Public Health
International Journal of Sport Sociology
Journal of Behavioral Medicine
Journal of Gender, Culture and Health
Journal of Health and Social Behavior
Journal of Physical Activity and Health
Journal of Sport and Exercise Psychology

Journal of Sport Management
Journal of Sport and Social Issues
Pediatric Exercise Science
Quest
Research Quarterly for Exercise and Sport
Sociology of Health and Illness
Sociology of Sport Journal

Key Web Sites

American Alliance for Health, Physical Education, Recreation and Dance (www.aahperd.org)

American Council on Exercise (www.ace.org)

American Public Health Association (www.apha.org)

American Sport Educational Program (www.asep.co)

Association of Black Sociologists (www.blacksociologists.org)

Association for Women in Sports Media (www.awsmonline.org)

Black Women in Sport Association (www.blackwomeninsport.org)

Blue Cross and Blue Shield of Massachusetts (www.ahealthyme.com)

Center for the Study of Sport in Society (www.sportsinsociety.org)

International Olympic Committee (www.olympic.org)

NASLIN Directory of Scholarly Sport Sites (www.ucalgary.ca/library/ssportsite/)

National Collegiate Athletic Association (www.ncaa.org)

National Youth Sports Safety Foundation (www.nyssf.org)

Native American Sports Council (www.nacsports.org)

North American Society for the Sociology of Sport (www.nasss.org)

North American Society for the Sociology of Sport—listserv (www.nasslistserv.bc.edu)

United States Olympic Committee (www.usoc.org)

Women's Sports Foundation (www.womenssportsfoundation.org)

Women's Sports Wire (www.womensportswire.com)

■ Review Questions

1. What is meant by a sociological imagination?
2. What are some examples of the pervasiveness of physical activity in contemporary society?
3. What are the three categories of the social learning framework used to predict participation in physical activity?
4. Identify characteristics associated with physical activity at the upper, middle, working, and lower social classes.
5. What is the difference between gender and biological sex?
6. What is meant by the term *health inequality*?
7. According to a sociological perspective, why are health promotion programs that focus on changing individual behaviors limiting?
8. What is meant by an ecological approach to promoting physical activity?
9. What are the key elements of the recentering social institutions framework?
10. What kinds of careers are available to individuals with training in the sociology of physical activity?

■ References

Agency for Healthcare Research and Quality. (2005). *Third national healthcare disparities report*. Rockville, MD: Author.

Berger, P. (1963). *Invitation to sociology*. New York: Anchor Books.

Berkman, L., & Syme, S. (1979). Social networks, host Resistance, and mortality. A nine year follow-up study of Alameda County residents. *American Journal of Epidemiology*, 109, 186–204.

Blau, P., & Duncan, O. (1967). *The American occupational structure*. New York: Wiley & Sons.

Bryant, J., & McElroy, M. (1997). *Sociological dynamics of sport and exercise*. Englewood, CA: Morton Press.

Centers for Disease Control and Prevention. (2002). Youth risk behavior surveillance—US 2001 *Morbidity and Mortality Weekly Report*, 52(33), 785–788.

Coakley, J. (2006). *Sport in society: Issues & controversies*. New York: McGraw Hill.

Corbin, C. (1987). Physical fitness in the K–12 curriculum: Some defensible solutions to perennial problems. *Journal of Physical Education, Recreation and Dance*, 58, 49–54.

Crawford, R. (1980). Healthism and the medicalization of everyday life. *International Journal of Health Services* 10, 365–388.

Crespo, C. (2000). Encouraging physical activity in minorities. *Physician and Sports Medicine*, 28, 36–51.

Crespo, C., Keteyian, S., Heath, G., & Sempos, C. (1996). Leisure-time physical activity among US adults: Results from the Third National Health and Nutrition Examination Survey. *Archives of Internal Medicine*, 156, 93–98.

Edwards, H. (1970). *The revolt of the black athlete*. New York: Free Press.

Elliott, S. (2007, January 26). Multiplying the payoffs from a superbowl spot. *New York Times*, p. 2.

French, S., Story, M., & Jeffrey, R. (2001). Environmental influences on eating and physical activity. *Annual Review of Public Health*, 22, 309–335.

Henry, F. M. (1964). Physical education: An academic discipline. *Journal of Health, Physical Education, Recreation*, 35, 32–33, 69.

Hill, J., & Trowbridge, F. (1998). Childhood obesity: Future directions and research priorities. *Pediatrics*, 101, 570–574.

Hogue, C., Hargraves, M., & Scott Collins, K. (2000). *Minority health in America*. Baltimore, MD: Johns Hopkins University.

Institute of Medicine. (2003). *Unequal treatment: Confronting racial and ethnic disparities in health care*. Washinton DC. National Academy Press.

Institute of Medicine. (2004). *Preventing childhood obesity: Health in the balance*. Washington, D C. The National Academy Press.

Kawachi, L., Kennedy, B., & Glass, R. (1999). Social capital and self related health: A contextual analysis. *American Journal of Public Health*, 89, 1187–1193.

Kenyon, G. S., & McPherson, B. D. (1973). Becoming involved in physical activity and sport: A process of socialization. In R. G. Lawrence (Ed.). *Physical activity: Human growth and development* (pp. 303–332). New York: Academic Press.

Knowles, J. (1977). The responsibility of the individual. *Daedalus*, 106, 57–80.

Loy, J., & Kenyon, G. (1969). (Eds.) *Sport, culture, and society: A reader on the sociology of sport*. New York: Macmillan.

Macera, C., Ham, S., Yore, M., Jones, D., Ainsworth, B., Kimsey, D., & Kohl, H. (2005) *Preventing Chronic Disease* 2(2). [serial online]. Retrieved from htpp://www.cdc.gov/pcd/issues/2005/apr/04 00114.htm

McElroy, M. (2002). *Resistance to exercise: A social analysis of inactivity*. Champaign, IL: Human Kinetics.

McLeroy, K., Biveau, D., Steckler, A., & Glanz, K. (1988). An ecological perspective on health promotion programs. *Health Education Quarterly*, 15, 351–377.

Michener, J. (1976). *Sports in America*. New York: Random House.

Mills, C. (1959). *The sociological imagination*. New York: Oxford University Press.

Minkler, M. (2000). Personal responsibility for health: Contexts and controversies. In D. Callahan (Ed.), *Promoting healthy behavior: How much freedom? Whose responsibility?* Washington, DC: Georgetown University Press.

Mokdad, A., Marks, J., Stroup, D., & Gerberding, J. (2004). Actual causes of death in the United States 2000. *Journal of the American Medical Association*, 291(10) 1238–1245.

Ogden, C., Carroll, M., Curtin, L., McDowell, M., Tabak, C., & Flegal, K. (2006) Prevalence of overweight and obesity in the United States, 1999–2004. *Journal of the American Medical Association*, 295(13) 1549–1555.

Papas, M., Alberg, A., Ewing, R., Helzlsouer, K., Gary, T., & Klassen, A. (2007). The built environment and obesity. *Epidemiologic Review*, 29, 129–143.

Pate, R., Davis, M., Robinson, T., Stone, E., McKenzie, T., & Young, J. (2006). Promoting physical activity in children and youth: A leadership role for schools. *Circulation*, 114, 1214–1224.

Putnam. R. (2000). *Bowling alone: Collapse and revival of American community*. New York: Simon & Schuster.

Scott, J. (1970). *The athletic revolution*. New York: Free Press.

Stokols, D. (1996). Translating social ecological theory into guidelines for community health promotion. *American Journal of Health Promotion*, 10, 282–298.

Syme, S., & Balfour, J. (1998). Social determinants of disease. In R. Wallace (Ed.), *Maxcy-Rosenau-Last public health and preventive medicine.* (pp. 795–810). Stamford, CT: Appleton & Lange.

U.S. Census Bureau. (2007). *The population profile of the United States: Dynamic version*. Retrieved from www.census.gov/population/www/pop-profile/dynamic.html

U.S. Department.of Health and Human Services. (1985). *Report of the Department of Health and Human Services and Human Services Secretary 's Task Force on Black and Minority Health Vol.1 Executive Summary*. Washington, DC: Author.

U.S. Department of Health and Human Services. (1996). *Physical activity and health: A report of the surgeon general*. Atlanta: Centers for Disease Control.

U.S. Department of Health and Human Services. (2000). *Healthy people 2010: Objectives for improving health*. Washington, D.C. U.S. Government Printing Office.

Weber, M. (1968). *Economy and society: An outline of interpretive sociology*. Trans. G. Roth and G. Wittich. New York: Bedminister. (Originally published 1922).

CHAPTER 9

History of Exercise and Sport

William Harper, PhD, Purdue University

■ Chapter Objectives

After reading this chapter, you should be able to:

1. Define the phrase *exercise and sport history* and relate its significance in the exercise science curriculum.

2. Provide a brief overview of the history of exercise and sport history, including the key events in the 1800s and 1900s that gave rise to the gradual evolution of exercise and sport history as an academic discipline.

3. Describe the typical course content taught in many exercise and sport history classes.

4. Recognize some of the journals and book series that publish academic exercise and sport history scholarship.

5. Identify the various scholarly and popular exercise and sport history organizations and associations germane to the discipline.

6. Describe the variety of careers and professional opportunities associated with the study of exercise and sport from a historical perspective.

■ Key Terms

assimilation
blood sports
Blue Laws
color line
exercise systems
frontier thesis
Golden Age of sport
gouging contests

hegemony
journalizing
muscular Christianity
Negro leagues
new physical education
North American Society for Sport
 History (NASSH)
pedestrianism

popular press
soft Americans
social safety valve
Title IX

On one hand, defining what we mean by exercise and sport history is obvious. Simply put, this story is the story of humans at play. On the other hand, there is no generally accepted meaning of what constitutes exercise or sport, and these concepts have been defined variously as recreation, elite competition, fitness, leisure activities, physical diversions, games, and contests. When you combine the variety of meanings of exercise and sport with the number of civilizations that over time have engaged in these play forms, it is easy to become overwhelmed when trying to teach or learn the history of exercise and sport.

As an academic field of study, historians of exercise and sport nevertheless do define what they do in quite practical terms. Like any scholarly field, these historians narrow the subject of their inquiry by following a question that arises out of their research interest: It might be the history of a certain exercise practice or sport in a fixed period of time; the prevalence or absence of an exercise work ethic in a particular era; the impact of specific social legislation on individual access to exercise or fitness facilities or competitive teams; or the role of a single individual in the development of a unique technique or practice.

In a typical program in the exercise sciences, courses in exercise and sport history often focus on American social and competitive exercise and sports from the 19th century into modern times. Other exercise and sport history courses focus on the story of exercise and physical activity in the educational systems of the day, including on-campus physical fitness and education programs and interscholastic and intercollegiate athletics in the 20th century. It is preferred that students have a good background in the history of North America for either approach to the discipline, but prerequisite courses are not usually required for a course in history of exercise and sport. Most history of exercise and sport courses are upper-level courses because 2 years of general or liberal education can enrich the nature and significance of whatever exercise or sporting era or people are being studied.

BRIEF HISTORY OF EXERCISE AND SPORT HISTORY

In briefly summarizing the development of the discipline of exercise and sport history, our focus will be on North America. Thus we have already intentionally excluded the history of exercise and sport in many different ages and cultures. Such delimitation cuts us off from the larger story of exercise and sport history—for example, the early history of the Olympic games, the health and exercise practices of China, or the origins of soccer as a world phenomenon. This restriction is both convenient and germane to our discussion of the evolution of American exercise and sport history. One other necessary distinction is that there are basically two subdisciplines roughly paralleling one another: exercise and sport history and physical education and health history.

Exercise and Sport History

The earliest historians in this field were not academicians; they were popular writers. Beginning in the early 1800s, immigrants from England, Ireland, and Scotland not only brought their exercise and sports with them but helped begin the practice of exercise and sporting participants **journalizing** their experiences. In the late 1820s and 1830s, several such publications appeared, including the *American Turf Register and Sporting Magazine* (1829) and the *Spirit of the Times* (1831). As America gradually became more urban and less rural towards the end of the 19th century, big city newspapers looking for commercial profits added sports and recreation pages and hired writers who could contribute news to them. By the turn of the 20th century, an expanding **popular press** gave rise to sports sections in such legendary newspapers as Joseph Pulitzer's *New York World*, James Gordon Bennett's *New York Herald*, and William Randolph Hearst's *New York Journal*.

As American newspapers and their writers chronicled the extraordinary growth of American exercise and sport in the early 1900s, it was inevitable that some of these writers would publish lengthier pieces in magazines and journals. Their copy appeared in such magazines as *Colliers Weekly*, *American Magazine*, *Outing*, *McClure's*, and *Country Life*. Famous writers like Grantland Rice eventually became wordier as they published full-length books, usually the history of a specific sport or pastime or biographies of famous athletes. One additional reason it is possible to point to these early writers as the first wave of the evolution of the discipline of exercise and sport history is that these first-person writings became primary sources for the future wave of academicians and scholars (Harper, 1999).

In time Americans would become both participants in health-related activities and watchers of exercise and sport. Popular writers began serving up exercise and sporting literature for a hungry public. Although not necessarily trained as historians, writers after World War I, for example, produced an incredible amount of print on the heroes and heroics of the **Golden Age of sports** in the 1920s. Because of these busy typewriters and telegraph keys, college and professional athletes and coaches became household names: Jim Thorpe, Ty Cobb, Jack Dempsey, Gertrude Ederle, Helen Wills, Amos Alonzo Stagg, Knute Rockne, Babe Didrikson, and, of course, the other Babe, who was more famous than them all, Babe Ruth.

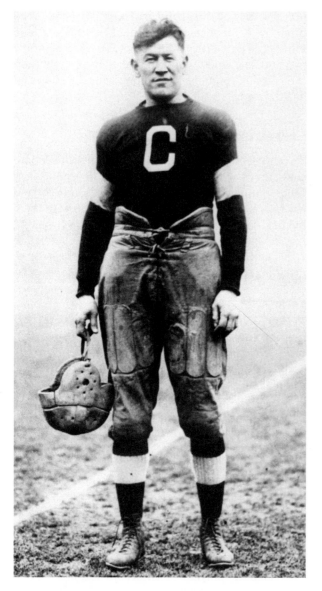

Native American James "Jim" Thorpe seen here in uniform as star football player for Carlisle (Pennsylvania) Indian School. Thorpe won the pentathlon and decathlon in the 1912 Olympic Games, and later played major league baseball and professional football.

the time Betts's work was published posthumously in book form in the early 1970s, exercise and sport was no longer taken as mere frivolity, and the historical study of it was growing in respectability. It was clear to Betts that modern exercise and sport arose from at least three intersecting social forces: the closing of the Western frontier, the growth of cities and urban centers, and the growing sophistication of industrial technology. In other words, exercise and sport was evolving into an American institution (Betts, 1974; Massengale & Swanson, 1997).

The history of the exercise and sport subdiscipline came of age in the 1980s. Until then, and except for the occasional academic maverick, the story of exercise and sport was told by voices that were male, white, and middle class. Consequently, this version of the story of exercise and sport was functionally disconnected from the everyday lives of the diverse masses of Americans of different economic circumstances, ages, genders, religions, ethnicities, races, and physical talents and limitations. Exercise and sport was no longer seen as primarily escape, as a **social safety valve,** or as a mirror of America's popular culture. Instead, historians began critically exploring the human experience of exercise and sport, especially within such cultural contexts as **assimilation,** power, **hegemony** (domination), and consumption. The newest academic approaches to the history of exercise and sport reinforce the idea that it is the study of the dynamic interaction between exercise/sport and society—for better and for worse—and that ultimately this will determine the richness of the future of the field of history of exercise and sport (Pope, 1997).

Physical Education and Health History

Another history of the discipline must also briefly be told if the history of exercise and sport is to be complete. The history of public and private school programs of physical education, health, fitness, exercise, and interschool sporting contests provide yet another facet of this story. For the most part, this physical education and history was recorded not by historians but by educational leaders in the field. Many of these early educational leaders were themselves trained in the health fields, primarily in medicine.

Consequently, most of the early writing chronicling the historical development of the field of physical education was health-promotion material. By around 1850 in America, a number of **systems of exercise,** physical training, and callisthenic gymnastics were competing for popular attention. Many of these approaches to health were European based. The supposed foundation of all of these educational programs was physical movement, and those who wrote about

But it was not until shortly after World War II that exercise and sport was recognized as a possible bona fide subject of academic study. One good and early example of such work was the 1951 dissertation, "Organized Sport in Industrialized America," by John Richard Betts (1951). This scholarly study ushered in the beginning of a serious social history of American exercise and sport. Betts argued that by the mid-19th century American exercise and sport was not only growing in popularity, but that the origins and directions of this popularity deserved the attention of professional historians. Most academics had considered exercise and sport little more than a diversion or escape from the stress and pressures of ordinary daily life, and hence unworthy of serious scholarship. By

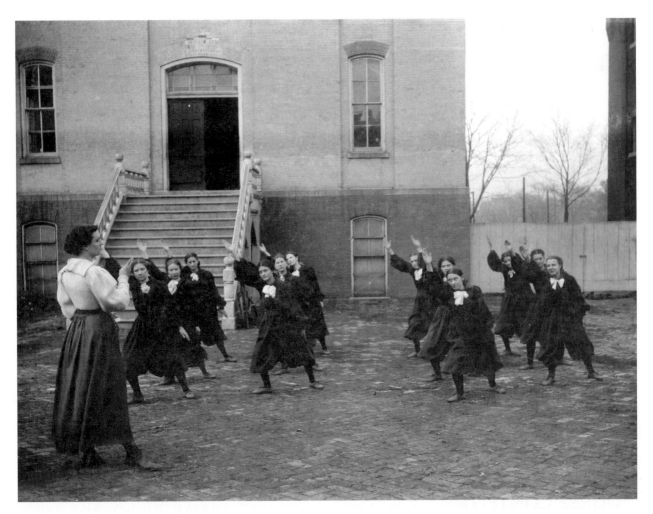

Young women earnestly engaged in light exercises in a physical education class led by their female exercise director in their schoolyard at the turn of the 20th century.

a particular exercise approach—whether strenuous or light weight—basically espoused the virtues of their preferred vehicle to good health: Charles Follen, Charles Beck, and Francis Lieber pushed Germany's Friedrich Jahn's apparatus gymnastics; Catherine Beecher (sister to Harriet Beecher Stowe) wrote on her system of lightweight exercises, posture activities, and exercise and sports for the sake of beauty and health in girls; Dio Lewis lectured on his compromise between the German immigrants' and Beecher's approaches, using bean bags, social games, dance, and music; and Edward Hitchcock, MD, promoted his quasimilitary exercise and training program at Amherst College.

By the turn of the 20th century, these various philosophies of physical education and health were promoted and cultivated in a variety of publications: *Mind and Body* (1894), *The American Physical Education Review* (1896), and *Physical Training* (1903). So the early written history of physical education and health turns out to be much like the earliest era of the writers journalizing their firsthand witnessing of physical activities and

sports. Neither group professed to be historians, but both groups did indeed profess.

Even as the professing eventually led to the creation of a profession of physical education and health, making history still outweighed the writing of it. For example, college sports in the early 1900s had only recently been taken out of the hands of college students by faculty, then by administrators; and playing sports in the public schools was not historically interesting. So it would be a few decades later before anything resembling an integration of exercise and physical education occurred in educational institutions. This **new physical education,** as it was called, gave birth to another generation of writers, most of whom attempted to propose ways in which exercise could be both physical and yet defensibly educational at the same time: Thomas D. Wood, Charles H. McCoy, Jesse Fairing Williams, Luther Gluck, Clark Hetherington, Dolphin Hanna, R. Taut McKenzie, Ethel Perrin, and Amy Morris Humans (Freeman, 2001).

By the 1960s, however, much of the relevant historical writing in physical education and health had something of an edge to it. So many social issues were in flux at the time that the profession seemed to be perpetually on the defensive: defending the educational values of the field to academic critics; defending the legitimacy of various state requirements for physical education and health in the schools; defending itself against the many attacks on the commercialism of intercollegiate athletics; or even defending the indefensible—the slow response to including women and minorities in educational programs of study and college sports either as players or coaches.

The profession created an academic outlet for the historical study of exercise and sport in the 1960s by way of a study section in the College Physical Education Association (shortly thereafter the CPEA was renamed the National College Physical Education Association for Men). This led quite naturally to integrating both the practicing exercise and sport historians and the physical education and health historians into a new professional society, the **North American Society for Sport History (NASSH),** created in 1973. From this point on and into the present, the scholarly activity on exercise and sport history has redoubled, and a genuine disciplinary field of study was born (Massengale, 1997). Integration of these two scholarly interests has culminated in their representation in the curricular field of exercise science, and this history is well worth exploring.

COURSE CONTENT

The general course content for studying the history of exercise and sport is defined variously. Typically, however, and no matter the breadth or narrowness of the course itself, the content is approached chronologically. The common denominator in courses in the history of exercise and sport is (or should be) to learn and understand the remarkable continuity over time of the urge for human beings to play. William James (1907), the American psychologist/philosopher, once wrote that the humanistic value of almost any subject will be self-evident if the subject is taught historically. "Geology, economics, and mechanics are humanities," James wrote, "when taught with reference to successive achievements of the geniuses to which these sciences owe their being." He went on to say that "not taught thus, literature remains grammar, art a catalogue, history a list of dates, and natural science a sheet of formulas and weights and measure." No less is true of the subject of exercise and sport. Not mere dates but the human story line itself becomes the proper general course content of exercise and sport history.

But what story line to tell? The teachers of exercise and sport history usually focus their courses this way or that depending on the integration of the course into the larger curriculum, and maybe even into the overall philosophy of the academic department or college/school in which the course resides. For the most part, however, typical discipline-based American exercise and sport history textbooks and courses develop their content along the following historical time line, which are roughly consistent with significant dates in American history:

- 1600–1776
- 1776–1850
- 1850–1896
- 1896–1950
- 1950–present

By any account, this approach is not the only way to study the discipline of exercise and sport history. Much like other exercise science disciplines, sometimes general survey courses precede more specialized courses or advanced study. For example, some programs of study might include Olympic Games history in a survey course on American exercise and sports, whereas others might set aside the Olympic Games as a historical course worthy of study on its own. Perhaps a more global approach is taken in a survey course—including, for example, an overview of exercise and sports and games from the early ancient cultures through European influences, and then into modern global exercise and sport. This is followed by a course specific to modern 20th century American exercise and sport. A further specialization is to create a course around a single sport history, as is sometimes the case with the fascinating history of America's so-called national pastime—baseball—or around the social history of women and exercise pursuits.

Since it is more commonly the case that exercise and sport history courses follow the chronological time line, a brief overview of the content of a typical course follows based on that structure.

1600-1776

Imagine the difficulty of making brief but accurate generalizations about 200 years of American history. Yet when we try to outline the development of exercise and sport between 1600 and 1776, that is exactly what we do. For the most part, what today we might call modern exercise and sport simply did not exist in colonial America.

What we see in these early years is essentially a transplanted European version of exercise and sportlike festivities, celebrations, and games. At least these were the playful temperaments gradually brought over from Europe. Already on the North American continent by this time, of course, were the Native Americans, the vast tribes of Indians who had established tribal structures, rituals, and loyalties.

Early strains of lacrosse, polo (on horseback, not in water), basketball-like ball games, shinny (like field hockey), horse riding and racing, games of chance and skill, and warlike competitions were well under way before the Anglos arrived in small groups, and later in mass (Oxendine, 1988).

The mostly white immigrants who settled along the eastern seaboard in these 200 years of our history didn't have much time for frivolity, however. There was work to be done, and settlements needed to be built. Survival needs for food, shelter, and clothing took precedence over the more human needs of artistic expression, dance, education, social diversions, physical activity, and cultural diversification. This was especially so in the New England Atlantic colonies where we find both religious and social prohibitions imposed on carryings-on that might have suggested time wasting, individualism, or sinful indulgences. As the more Puritan-leaning early villages took root, local laws were often enacted restricting games and play on the Sabbath; these so-called **Blue Laws** tried to put an end to Sunday frolics of any kind. Remnants of these laws remain in parts of the Midwest, where selling automobiles (they used to be driven for essentially recreational purposes) or alcohol or playing high school sports are still strictly forbidden on Sundays.

In spite of various discouragements, these early European immigrants managed to find time for physical activity, games, and celebrations. In the northern colonies, settlers engaged in tavern gambling games and contests, golflike stick and ball games, boat racing, shooting competition, rassling, running races, soccerlike football games, fishing, hunting, and throwing feats. The taverns and pubs in both the North and the South were the primary social and recreation centers of the day.

In the southern colonies, more degrees of playful freedom were the rule as the stern religious prohibitions slowed from Virginia to parts further south. Instead, what did rear its ugly head in the South was social exclusion. Indentured servants were numerous in the North, but it was the South that became the new home of hundreds of thousands of African slaves. Southern plantation owners did their best to imitate the wealthy in England itself, who used land ownership as a social and economic wedge between the rich and the poor. The poorest of the poor were essentially the southern slaves upon whose backs the plantation owners sustained their extravagant lifestyle. This practice rather quickly created upper-class play forms that were frowned on in the more conservative North, but lively in the South: horse racing, fisticuffs (boxing), fencing, duels, fox hunting, and a variety of other activities associated with the exercise and sporting life, including competitions staged between plantations. Another category of popular diversion were blood exercise and sports; these were the animal cruelty "sports" such as

bull baiting or cock fighting. **Blood sports,** and the gambling that was the main justification for them, attracted both the upper and the lower classes. Gambling, too, was at the core of early American interest in horse racing. In fact, if we were asked what popular activity was the first organized American exercise and sport—whether in the North or the South—the answer would be horse and harness racing. Most of the racing was privately promoted and conducted as public horse racing was largely illegal until the 1820s (Rader, 2004).

1776–1850

For the most part, prior to the Revolutionary War, early American immigrants and settlers lived up and down the Atlantic coast, east of the Appalachians. But by 1800 the itch to move west was beginning to be scratched in great numbers. Partly due to perceived crowding, and partly due to tired agricultural land and increasing scarcity of game to hunt, immigrants and settlers suddenly became pioneers and frontier folks. According to the historian Frederick Jackson Turner, it was this westward expansion that exaggerated certain characteristics in these pioneers that created distinctive American traits: adventuresome, violent, resourceful, practical, hard working, and wasteful. This **frontier thesis,** as it came to be called, explained that it was the actual experience of settling the West that reformed what had been mostly Europeans into Americans. By the time gold was discovered in the far west in 1848, Americans were settling in from coast to coast (Harper, 1999).

Nearer the Atlantic, and in the original colonies, exercise and sports were on the rise. Some historians date the beginning of modern American sport with the 1823 horse race between the best horse from the South and the best horse from the North. Nearly 100,000 spectators came from afar, pouring into the Long Island race course to see Sir Henry, the southern entry, face the northern horse Eclipse in the best of three 4-mile heats. In the end, Eclipse won, signaling both the beginning of sport and of sectional rivalry that would result in the War Between the States 40 years later.

Other exercise and sports continued to attract public interest, including the blood sports, boxing, running races, and rowing. One early boxer, Tom Molyneux, was a Virginia slave who was given his freedom because he was such a good bare-fisted fighter. Molyneux eventually fought the British Champion, Tom Cribb, in 1810. The fight went 44 "rounds" and lasted nearly an hour. Rounds were determined by knockdowns, and Cribb won. The earliest running contests were referred to as **pedestrianism.** These races varied in length from as short as a quarter of a mile to as many as 30 or 40 miles. The runners were called "peds," and they would often go from town to town, challenging the

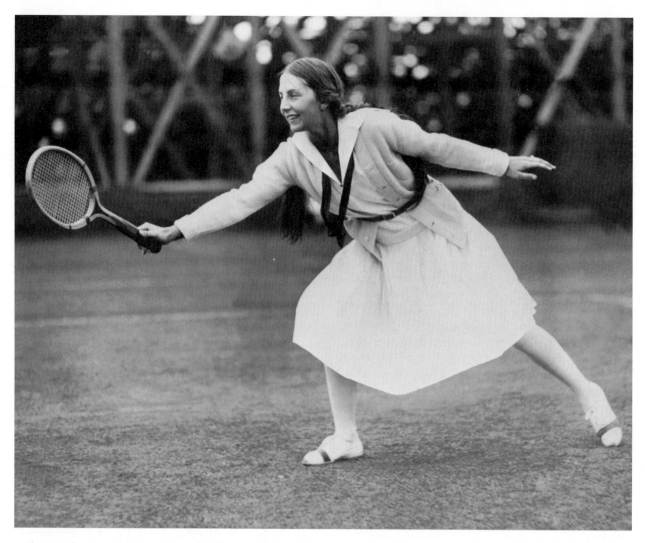

In these early years, there were occasional opportunities for women to play recreational sports, primarily for social interaction and health improvement, but not for competition.

locals to a race. Rowing, on the other hand, grew by way of competitions between our early colleges. Yale, for instance, started the first college boat club in 1843. And in 1852 Yale rowed against Harvard in the first intercollegiate crew race. It wasn't long before college crew races drew as many as 50,000 spectators.

Out west (from western Pennsylvania and beyond the Mississippi River), given smaller populations in the towns and the distance between the farms and ranches, exercise and sports were more for diversion and recreation. Hunting and fishing were popular, both for the exercise and sport of it and for sustenance. The taverns and saloons were the sites for shooting contests; gouging matches were common as well. **Gouging contests** were basically free-for-all fights, no rules. Most of the informal and spontaneous contests and competitions revolved around the physical skills necessary to staying alive, such as tests of stamina, strength, speed, and endurance.

Opportunities for physical activities for girls and women in this era were few and far between. The most

visible organized activities were to be found in the early schools and colleges. Those few colleges or academies for women provided limited physical exercise and activity in the form light calisthenics; most certainly they were not invited to engage in competitive sports. In the men's colleges, the European systems of gymnastic exercise dominated. It was the rare college that allowed competitive sports; if sports like football or wrestling were available at all, students organized them themselves. Outside of the colleges men were the primary custodians of physically active play and contests, but there is some evidence that women were active too, just not visibly so. "For certain, colonial and early national women participated in recreational forms, although not always in full view of contemporary chroniclers" (Struna, 1995, p. 24).

1850–1896

If we consider the history of exercise and sport to be the story of the evolution of modern exercise and sport, then the period between 1850 and 1896 can be considered a genuine growth spurt. Before this time Americans were certainly interested in physical tests and contests, not to mention some early forays into health and fitness, but the rapid social and technological changes after 1850 produced surprisingly modern exercise and sporting possibilities and promotions. The bottom line, of course, was the discovery that American sport could mean business. In time, exercise and fitness would mean business too.

Consider the remarkable timing of so many social and economic forces coming together after 1850: rapidly growing cities, closing of the Western frontier, increasing numbers of remarkable industrial inventions and discoveries, weakening of the religious objections to exercise and sport, colleges beginning to see the positive values associated with exercise and sport participation, and especially the growing sense that sport itself could generate income and profit. For example, there was a direct connection between technology and physical activity in the form of sport. Invention meant that physical activity and sporting news could be quickly spread through newspapers by way of telegraphy; teams and fans could be transported by railroads; penny printing presses could disseminate exercise and sporting news; exercise and sports equipment could be standardized in factories; sewing machines could be used for uniforms; the incandescent bulb made it possible for evening competitions; and even the invention of the bicycle multiplied opportunities for exercise, leisure outings, and competitions. This last invention, the bicycle, turned out to be especially helpful in advancing the cause of women's slow progress toward social, political, and economic equality (Harper, 1999).

By 1850 baseball was already on its way to becoming America's national game. In New York in 1845, Alexander Cartwright organized a voluntary group of bank clerks and other middle-class professionals to form the New York Knickerbockers Base Ball Club. Standardizing the rules of the game attracted other New Yorkers to form clubs, and the game spread quickly. However well-rooted the belief that Abner Doubleday invented baseball at Cooperstown, New York, in 1839 (hence, the 1939 celebration of the "invention" the game by locating the Baseball Hall of Fame in Cooperstown), there is no truth to the story (Adelman, 1990).

The War Between the States in the early 1860s turned out to be therapeutic to the spread of most physical activity and sports, and especially baseball. The Union soldiers who were prisoners in the Confederate stockades played the game. Southerners picked it up, and postwar fence-mending was accelerated by North and South competing in healthier alternatives to war, like baseball. The game also moved west, motivated in part by the desire for cities to put themselves on the map by way of urban rivalries. In 1869 the Cincinnati Red Stockings became the first all-salaried baseball team. The eight-team National League was created in 1876, followed 5 years later by the six-team American Association. By the turn of the 20th century, professional and semiprofessional baseball was played by thousands and watched by millions.

Other exercise and sports were growing in popularity at the same time. The creation of athletic clubs, college teams, immigrant sporting competitions, and promotions by the wealthy all added to the sporting and physical activity calendar that now included tennis, golf, basketball, wrestling, and track and field. Newspapers increased their coverage of these activities, adding to America's longstanding fascination with rowing, horse racing, and prizefighting. Boxing, in particular, still represented then to America what America represented to its people: opportunity. Fighting an image problem—given its early association with gambling, mob mentality, alcohol, prostitution, bigotry, and fight-fixing scandals—the sport of boxing gradually became more respectable, which is to say, legal. The Boston Strong Boy, James L. Sullivan, won the heavyweight championship in 1882 and held onto it for 10 years, eventually losing to James J. Corbett in 1892. Sullivan is considered the first national sports hero, and some scholars mark the beginning of commercialized sports with his loss to Corbett given that the fight was so highly publicized and followed (Rader, 2004).

In this same time period, the advance of the sciences ignited increasing interest in the relationship between health and exercise. Evolutionary theory contributed to the notion that physical health improvements could translate into successful adaptation and progress of the human race in the face of change. This was especially so when the topic of women and their so-called nervous systems were at issue. The common assumption was that women were frail by nature, and any decision to mess with women's physical constitution had to be cautious and guided by the medical profession—conservative by its nature. Whether for college women or men, the exercise programs that developed were based on anatomical and anthropometric measurements, quasi-scientific biases, and various callisthenic regimens largely imported from Europe.

Given the inherent limitations of larger cities to provide healthy outdoor physical outlets such as those associated with rural America, adult-managed youth programs sprang up. The Young Men's Christian Association (YMCA), in particular, represented another call for increasing exercise opportunity. The YMCAs perpetuated what had earlier been called **muscular Christianity,** the view that vigorous physical expression was not incompatible with spiritual life. Also, there was the view that young urban boys, in particular, needed socializing to become real, not effeminate, men. Even more, physical health achieved by way of being a muscular Christian was also a condition of a successful life. Luther Halsey Gulick, for example, in his role in the YMCA, and later as founder of the Pubic Schools Athletic League in New York City, helped sell the idea of the strenuous life to American youth; he also believed strongly in the social and democratic benefits of play. Besides healthy exercise, he welcomed adding sports to these nonschool programs. In 1887 Gulick became an instructor in the Department of Physical Training at the YMCA International Training School, later named Springfield College.

However popular exercise and sporting activities were becoming by the end of the 19th century, they were for whites only. Even in the otherwise well-intentioned health and exercise programs for men, women, and children promoted by colleges, schools, or public agencies, the population they benefited was white, and mostly middle or upper class. The goals for most of these programs were to upgrade the opportunities for success for the class, race/ethnicity, and gender the programs themselves were designed to serve. "No need to apply" was the disappointing message delivered to the increasing numbers of immigrants pouring into urban centers, most of whom were poor, all colors of the rainbow, and frequently judged to be of questionable character.

Even in the sporting worlds, all-comers were not welcome. Oddly enough, there was more opportunity for African Americans and whites to compete with and against one another before the War Between the States than after the war. Although not overwhelming in numbers, prior to the 1860s there are accounts of integration in such sports as horse racing, boxing, baseball, football, and bicycle racing. But by the 1880s, the **color line** was being drawn. For instance, in his 10-year reign as heavyweight champion, John L. Sullivan refused to fight an African American. By 1887 organized baseball refused to allow participation by blacks. And by 1896 the Supreme Court of the United States legalized a separate but "equal" (it never was) arrangement for the entire nation, thereby effectively eliminating integrated physical activity and sport for the next 60 years. So while opportunity was what America represented to its people, this representation was sadly conditional. The incredible growth of American exercise and sport in the 20th century was to be big business, and big business depended on pleasing the majority at the expense of the minorities.

1896–1950

It would have been impossible to live through the first half of the 20th century in America and not notice that sport was becoming a permanent institution. A world war, a major scandal in baseball, the stock market crash, followed by the Great Depression, and then another world war should have been enough to kill it off. But to think that is to underestimate how central and resilient the exercise and sporting life was, and how strongly it was tied to the vitality of American life.

In the first two decades of the 20th century, a relatively quiet time compared to the roar of the 1920s, baseball began to take on its modern form with the first World Series played in 1903. College football was increasing in popularity in spite of the growing complaints that the sport was too violent. The American Olympic teams were competitive and dominated the earliest competitions in Athens (1896), Paris (1900), St. Louis (1904), and London (1908). Jim Thorpe won the Pentathlon and Decathlon at the 1912 Olympics at Stockholm. Many other sports were also in the early stages of organizing themselves, including tennis, golf, wrestling, and track and field. The organizing bodies were increasing in number, including the AAU, NCAA, and even the YMCA and YWCA—both of which increased their sponsorship of sporting competitions. Despite the interruption of World War I, the stage was set for a most remarkable decade in physical activity and sport history, an era that has since come to be called the Golden Age of sports.

The 1919 White Sox World Series "fix" scandalized the baseball world. Eight Chicago White Sox players were said to have "laid down" in their games against the Cincinnati Red Stockings. Although there is still a good deal of confusion even today about exactly what happened, the eventual upshot was that the new (and first) Commissioner of Baseball, Kenesaw Mountain Landis, banned all eight players from the game of baseball for life. Within the baseball world, game throwing certainly wasn't news—baseball history is full of pre-1919 examples of attempts by professional gamblers to guarantee the outcome before the games were played—but for the world at large, even the possibility that baseball could be crooked was stunning news. The world of sport was one world where everything was supposed to be on the up-and-up, or so it was rather naively believed (Harper, 1999).

It would take something or someone really big to help American baseball fans recover from their collective depression over the scandal. It turned out to be someone. He was called the "Babe." George Herman Ruth, largely abandoned by his parents at an early age, grew up in a home for wayward boys. By the time he was 19, he was playing professional baseball, first for the Baltimore Orioles, then the Boston Red Sox, and in 1920 he was a New York Yankee. That year he belted 54 home runs in a single season. By 1923, in Babe Ruth's first appearance in the brand spanking new three-decker Yankee Stadium—the house that Ruth built—he blasted a low line drive home run that by then was already his 198th career round tripper and the first ever hit out of that park (he had already hit 59 home runs in the 1921 season and would hit 60 in 1927) (Harper, 1999, pp. 321–322). Throughout the 1920s, Babe Ruth's bat would help everyone forget the baseball scandal; his oversized 52-inch bat would also be the symbol of the incredible growth of health, physical activity, recreation, exercise, and sports in the golden decade of the 1920s. It was possible, Ruth's mighty swing said, that anyone could be a success no matter their upbringing; Ruth's bat was proof enough that the American Dream was alive and well.

It didn't much matter where one looked in the 1920s; sporting heroes and fawning fans combined to drive up the commercial value of modern sport. The ever-expanding newspaper coverage led to wildly successful radio play-by-play broadcasting. Throughout the country Americans invited the legends of sport into their living rooms: Jack Dempsey (boxing), Bobby Jones (golf), Bill Tilden (tennis), Suzanne Lenglen (tennis), the Four Horsemen of Notre Dame (football), Mildred Babe Didrikson (everything), and even the horse, Man O'War, who won 20 out of 21 races between 1919 and 1920.

While the 1920s certainly were flush times for the continued growth of American exercise and sport, it was the next couple of decades—the decades of the Great Depression and World War II—that actually served to cement the love affair between the American people and their recreation and sports. Although professional and elite amateur sports took a significant downturn, what actually propped up sports was the recognition that games and play could do more than provide entertainment (Spears & Swanson, 1978). Massive unemployment meant an increase in available free time for the masses. Informal sport, youth exercise and sports, and public recreation suddenly increased in popularity. Federal agencies such as the Works Progress Administration (WPA) and the Civilian Conservation Corps (CCC) became employment agencies for those out of work. Armed with this sizable and willing workforce, these and other agencies built swimming pools, baseball fields, gymnasiums, stadiums, and exercise and sport facilities. Colleges and universities also began investing in recreational and physical education facilities. Oddly enough, it took both a national crisis and a world war to make more available to the public so many of the sports that a decade earlier they had largely followed as spectators.

Another turn of events in this era demonstrated not just the staying power of sports but the basic power of sports itself. The year was 1938; the place

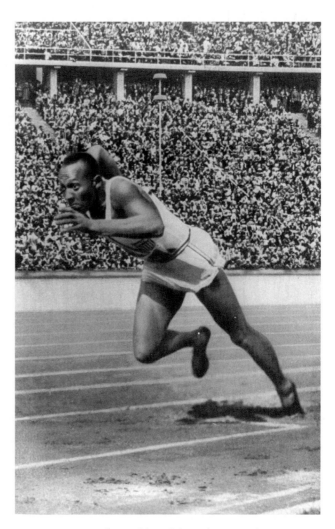

Jesse Owens wins four gold medals at the 1936 Olympic Games in Berlin, Germany, practically singlehandedly refuting Hitler's claim of the supremacy of the Aryan race.

was Yankee Stadium. The event was the second bout between two heavyweight world champions, African American Joe Louis and the then current heavyweight champion from Germany, Max Schmeling. Louis had lost his crown to Schmeling 2 years earlier, also in New York, when Louis had been a 10 to 1 favorite and hadn't taken the fight seriously—the only time Louis had ever lost a fight. This first fight took place only 2 months before the 1936 Olympic Games in Berlin, Germany. Schmeling's victory fed Hitler's ideology of the supremacy of the Ayran race. But it would be the remarkable feat of Jesse Owens's four gold medals in the Berlin Games that seriously weakened the supremacist claims of Hitler's regime. The second Louis and Schmeling fight in 1938 became a real showdown. This time, however, Louis trained. The live gate was around 70,000. Worldwide, over 100 million at-a-distance fight followers would hear the radio broadcasts—the "largest audience in the history of *anything*" (Margolick, 2005, p. 5). This

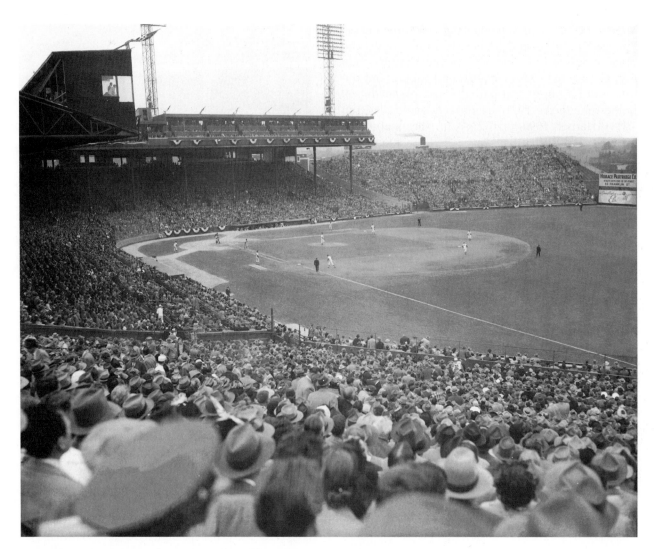

Baseball was recovering in the years immediately following World War II. There is standing room only at Braves Field, home of the Boston Braves (1915–1952), for the 1948 World Series between Boston and the Cleveland Indians.

second fight represented so many other intangibles besides the fight itself: black versus white, freedom versus fascism, youth versus age (Louis was 24 and Schmeling was 33), and even the United States versus Hitler's Germany (within a few short years they would be at war). The fight itself was short by any standard. Joe Louis landed 41 blows to Schmeling's 2 and the fight was over in the first round (Margolick, 2005). Mirroring the shortness of the fight, one newspaper, the *Charlotte News*, ran this headline: BLOW-BY-BLOW STORY OF FIGHT. The story itself was one word: "Bang!" (Margolick, 2005).

The real shooting began a few years later as the world entered into its second war in hardly 20 years. Once again, conventional sport took it on the chin. Also once again, the war was somewhat therapeutic in regard to creating new exercise, physical activity, and sporting opportunities. As more and more women stepped up to replace conscripted male soldiers by working in the defense-related

factories, women also found new sporting opportunities. Softball was already an incredibly popular participatory sport in this era; it was especially popular with women (Rader, 2004). When the professional baseball owners feared the collapse of their men's leagues, Philip Wrigley, the owner of the Chicago Cubs, proposed the idea of a women's professional baseball league. The All-American Girls Baseball League took the fields in a number of Midwest cities in 1943. To its credit, the teams drew nearly 1 million fans a year; the league hung on until 1954. To its discredit, this league sold feminine beauty first, playing skills second, and like its male counterparts, the teams also drew the color line: No blacks need bother to show up.

The equal rights and civil rights movements in schools and in popular sports were several decades away, but by the end of World War II the reality of both could be seen as inevitable. The so-called **Negro baseball leagues,** now with a 20-year history, rivaled their white counterparts in popularity

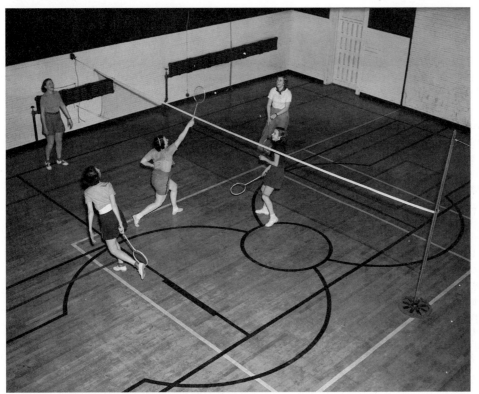

By the mid-20th century, there were greater opportunities for women to compete in more vigorous recreational and competitive activities.

and skill. The era of separate but equal, codified by the 1896 Supreme Court, was wearing down. Accommodation was difficult to justify when so many African Americans fought so gallantly in the war and this in spite of the troops being separated by race there, too. By mid-century women in increasing numbers were also stepping out of their stereotypical gender roles, becoming a force in the workplace. The long history of sports promotion in the industrial leagues (going back to the 1920s) also contributed to the increasing sense of new possibilities for women. By the 1950s both blacks and women were poised to create another and newer history of American sport opportunities.

1950-Present

One year before Babe Ruth's death in 1948, Jackie Robinson played his first professional baseball game with the Brooklyn Dodgers. Branch Rickey's "social experiment" formally opened the door a crack for other black baseball players to slowly begin joining the white leagues. Jackie Robinson's talent, comportment, and character made the experiment a successful one; Robinson was even named the 1947 Rookie of the Year. Within 10 years, many other American professional team sports followed baseball's lead. However right and long overdue integration in professional sports was, in reality the bottom line for it was the bottom line from it. Franchise expansion and the promise of ever more ticket sales combined to make the decision to be more inclusive a good business decision.

There is little question that the longer history of American life is the history of human events, sporting or otherwise; but human events are often influenced or even determined by the developing nonhuman technology. By mid-century, one technological development was rapidly gaining traction and would forever change physical activity habits of the typical American (we got lazier), not to mention the delivery of sports and entertainment: television. Historian Benjamin Rader (2004) argues that television has significantly shaped not just the delivery of sports but the very way we attend to them.

In the early days of fixed camera locations, boxing, wrestling, and roller derby fit the television bill. In time, the television networks realized that increasing sports programming meant increasing visibility and revenue. It wasn't long before TV cameras were mobile and could be aimed from anywhere and at anything on the fields of play—and sometimes off the fields of play—for most of the major revenue-producing sports, including baseball, football, basketball, ice hockey, golf, tennis, and even the Olympic Games. But television would not be just a mechanical, passive eyewitness. It would eventually be an active change agent in the presentation of sports themselves. To facilitate television viewing, sports accepted playing season adjustments, game start time coordination, scheduled time outs, tape delays, and even rules changes. As the sporting television markets expanded, national audiences multiplied exponentially. Newspaper sportswriters and radio broadcasters suddenly were not the sole purveyors of what was happening in sports venues across America. Television viewers could see for themselves what was going on and didn't rely on the traditional press surrogates as much anymore. Gone were the days when reporters and broadcasters could enliven what they were covering through hyperbole and exaggeration. In time, however, television substituted its own brands of hyperbole and exaggeration as the presentation of sports met the voracious needs of the entertainment industry.

It is difficult to separate sports from politics, or for that matter, politics from sports. Long ago, the word *politic* meant judicious, wise, and prudential. It meant the promotion of public welfare. This is what John F. Kennedy had in mind in his two essays in *Sports Illustrated* in the early 1960s (Kennedy, 1960, 1962). Kennedy believed that America was getting **soft,** and at a time when we could least afford to do so. He believed that physical fitness, exercise, and athletic prowess were essential in nation building. He pointed out that "we face in the Soviet Union a powerful and implacable adversary determined to show the world that only the Communist system possesses the vigor and determination to satisfy awakening aspirations for progress and the elimination of poverty and want" (Kennedy, 1960, p. 16). Kennedy's wordy competitive challenge was prompted in part by the face-to-face competitions between the two superpowers in the Olympic Games. The Soviets had not competed in the Games until 1952 (as Russia, they competed in 1908 and 1912). However, once entered, they outclassed the entire field in total medals won; between 1952 and their last competition as the USSR in 1988, the Soviets placed first in seven of their nine appearances in total medals won. They placed second in the other two appearances (they did not compete in 1984).

This international competition for bragging rights between two countries with entirely different political systems rallied the American sporting spirits. In particular, these years produced remarkable competitive responses from our African American women athletes. In the main, women physical educators were not especially focused on promoting intercollegiate or international women's athletics; the educators did not approve of the men's model of athletics, the win-at-all-costs nature of it, and the tendency to cultivate spectators of elite athletes instead of participants in a variety of health-giving and socially positive exercise and sports experiences. But male coaches of women's sports thought otherwise.

Many southern and historically black high schools and colleges created and promoted track and field and basketball for their women students. Ed Temple, for example, created a female track and field powerhouse at Tennessee State where he coached for 44 years. His Tigerbelle athletes produced 23 medals in Olympic track and field competition (Spears & Swanson, 1978).

It wasn't until the early 1980s that women began finding financial and moral support for their latent physical activity and sports interests. The early pioneer competitors, such as Mildred "Babe" Didrikson, helped point the way; but it wasn't until the 1972 passage of **Title IX** of the Educational Amendments Act that women were given some semblance of entitlement to competitive athletics. It took 10 more years before the institutional expectations were fully defined to provide equity, and since then compliance has gradually gained some momentum. If there was a single female who might qualify as the modern crusader for gender equity in sport, it would have to be tennis player Billie Jean King. She not only democratized the sport of tennis, but she became a spokesperson against sexism in the world of sport and for greater opportunity for women's sporting rights (Rader, 2004).

In the years since the 1980s, American sports have grown in popularity, access, complexity, diversity, age span appeal, and financial impact. Club exercise and sports competition opportunities now exist for the interested practically from the womb to the tomb. Interscholastic and intercollegiate sports are prepared for and played year-round. The number of individual and team professional and semi-professional sports players has grown exponentially throughout the sporting alphabet, from archery to yachting. Like a rock dropped in still waters, the ripple effect of this explosion of exercise and sporting opportunities has created careers for millions of others, whether coaches and teachers, trainers, exercise and sports medicine staff, strength and conditioning experts, promoters, administrators, reporters and broadcasters, photographers and camera men and women, television personnel, team or franchise owners, investors, lawyers and agents, referees and umpires, rules and regulatory bodies, national organization and committee members, marketing and licensing specialists, commercial vendors, facilities construction and operations, technical and electronic support, and, to be inclusive, even the oddsmakers and gamblers.

The innate human impulse to play has in modern times cultivated institutions, industry, and technology that challenge our ability to fully understand and control. On one hand, good exercise habits and sport participation provide inspiring experiences that help

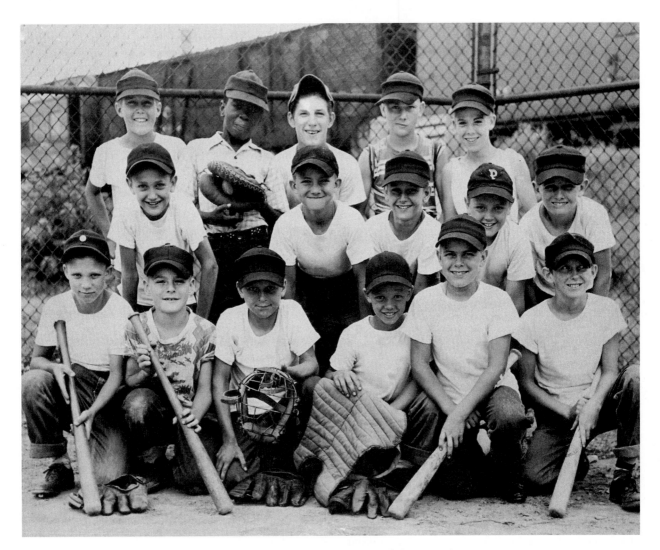

From the mid-20th century until modern times, sport and exercise gradually became what it was always capable of becoming—democratized. Minorities, women, and the young finally were given opportunities to play.

us all find meaning in our lives. Exercise and sport can help reconcile a series of living paradoxes that define the human condition, experiences that require a comfortable balance between security and adventure, necessity and freedom, stability and change, order and serendipity. On the other hand, the field of exercise and sport can and often does degenerate into conduct that reveals the lowest forms of human behavior, whether instanced in bigotry, greed, selfishness, dishonesty, violence, or hate. It is the responsibility of every generation in this field of study and practice to perpetuate the best in us and to minimize the worst in us.

When the physicist Richard Feynman (1918–1988) traveled to Hawaii, he visited a Buddhist temple and a monk told him, "I am going to tell you something that you will never forget." And then he told Feynman, "To every man is given the key to the gates of heaven. The same key opens the gates of hell" (Feynman, 1998, p. 6). For those of us choosing a profession related in a direct way to exercise and sport, the question we all need to ask ourselves is, "Which lock will we open?"

PROFESSIONAL ORGANIZATIONS

The primary scholarly organization for the study of exercise, physical activity, and sport history is the North American Society for Sport History (NASSH). Established in 1973, the organization's mission is to stimulate and support the scholarly study of exercise and sport; it publishes the *Journal of Sport History* and has done so since 1974. This organization has attracted scholars from around the world. The scope of its history-related topics of study is wide-ranging and includes research in both physical education and exercise and sport studies. NASSH encourages the participation of graduate students in its annual programs.

Given the global nature of exercise and sports, and exercise and sports studies, it should be no surprise that many other countries have founded history of exercise and sport scholarly societies and organizations. There are active international exercise and sport history associations, for example, in Great Britain, Australia, Brazil, Finland, Norway, France, Canada, and Japan. Naturally they also publish historical research and scholarship. One of the more international tending journals, for example, is *Sport History Review*, published in the United States by Human Kinetics since 1991. Conversations within and between these various organizations and their publications is regular and vibrant.

If the notion of history of exercise and sport organizations is broadened to include more popular venues, there are innumerable sports archives, exhibitions, libraries, bookshops, conferences, and memorabilia collections. Perhaps the largest sport history collection in North America is housed in the Paul Ziffren Sports Resource Center at the Amateur Athletic Foundation (AAF) of Los Angeles. AAF was created from proceeds Los Angeles generated by hosting of the 1984 Olympic Games. Ziffren (1913–1991) was chairman of the Los Angeles Olympic Committee for the 1984 Games. In addition to a vast numbers of books, journals, and periodicals, the resource center includes an extensive video and photography collection. Other prominent international organizations that focus on exercise and sport history include the British Society of Sport History, the International Society for the History of Physical Education and Sport, the International Society of Olympic Historians, the Australian Society for Sport History, and the International Association for Museums and Halls of Fame.

Last but not least in importance are the myriad organizations and societies devoted to individual exercise and sport histories. Almost every American exercise and sport has one kind of association or organization or another that is responsible for preserving the past, either through a hall of fame, a museum collection, or an archive. One prominent example of a single history is in the sport of baseball. The Society for American Baseball Research was established in 1971 in the Hall of Fame Library at Cooperstown, New York. The society has regional chapter meetings and sponsors any number of baseball history-related projects, including a lending library, research grants, electronic forums, conferences, oral history interviews, and book publishing. They also publish two journals, *The Baseball Research Journal* and *The National Pastime*.

CAREERS IN EXERCISE AND SPORT HISTORY

Any number of careers are founded on the direct use of exercise and sport history studies and education. There are also many professional opportunities in which knowledge of exercise and sport history can significantly contribute to career success.

Careers Directly Connected to Exercise and Sport History

Higher education academic teaching and research in history of exercise and sport

Archivist in libraries with collections related to exercise and sport

Historian in sporting Halls of Fame

Curator in museums

Exercise and sports journal or magazine editor

Producer of documentaries and/or features for television or movies

Sports statistician or record keeper

Resident historian for exercise and sporting organization or associations

Translator for exercise and sporting texts into other languages

Fiction writer with sport history as backdrop for stories

Biographer of significant exercise and sporting individuals

Professional Opportunities Indirectly Tied to Exercise and Sport History

Broadcasting

Newspaper writer or editor

Sports magazine writer or columnist

Photographer of sports or popular physical activities

Videography

Athletic director

Sports information director

Career in sports organizations (e.g., NCAA or USOC)

Sporting event promoter, coordinator, or manager

Corporate positions tied to exercise and sports sponsorship

Exercise or fitness business entrepreneur

Marketing and sales in exercise facilities or equipment sales

Promoters for sports programs, franchises,
or teams

Web site development

Fund-raising and development in both profit
and nonprofit sectors

Freelance writing on exercise and sports-related
topics

Teachers and coaches

Sports law or sports agent

Motional picture production

Artistic endeavors related to exercise and sport
(music, painting, sculpture)

Youth development worker in nonprofits

SUMMARY

Exercise and sport history is typically defined as the study of the human at play. For focus and convenience, American exercise and sport history is usually defined as the study of exercise and sport from the colonial days to the present. As an academic field of inquiry, exercise and sport history didn't surface in higher education institutions until after World War II. The coming of age of this discipline occurred in the 1980s. Both the institution of exercise and sport in and out of colleges and universities and the profession of physical education are studied by historians. The typical course content for most history courses in the exercise science curriculum follows a chronological time line from around 1600 until the modern day.

Since the earliest days of the colonies, Americans played. But given the basic survival needs of the times, there were a considerable number of restrictions on the kinds of folk games played and the amount of time that should be given to them. By the time of the Republic, there was growing interest in ball games, horse racing, boxing, and other physical activities. The early colleges and universities also provided student-organized exercise and sports and some educational programming. After 1850, the combination of the closing of the Western frontier, the rise of industrial technology, and the growth of urban centers gave 19th century Americans a wide variety of competitive exercise and sports to enjoy, including baseball, bicycle tours and racing, and club exercise and sports such as golf, tennis, yachting, and track and field.

In the 20th century, the first signs of the commercial possibilities for exercise and sport appeared. Exercise and sport attracted supporters, fans, and business investors. Women and minorities were given ever more opportunities to play as the 1950s approached. Since that time, exercise and sport has boomed. One result of the popularity of exercise and sports is the development of academic and popular scholarly organizations. In addition, an increasing number of careers and professional opportunities are connected to studying the history of modern exercise and sport, including work in academic settings, museums and halls of fame, magazine and journal writing, and documentary research and production.

■ Review Questions

1. What kinds of people became the earliest historians of exercise and sport?
2. When did serious social history of exercise and sport begin?
3. Discuss some of the earliest European exercise systems brought to America.
4. When did the profession create an academic outlet for the historical study of exercise and sport?
5. What kinds of physical activity were engaged in by the early American colonists along the eastern seaboard?
6. How did the northern colonies differ from the southern colonies with regard to their physical activity preferences between 1600 and 1776?
7. What is Frederick Jackson Turner's frontier thesis, and how does it relate to the growth of exercise and sports?
8. What kinds of physical activity opportunities were available to girls and women in the early 1800s?
9. Briefly discuss the relationship between industrialism after 1850 and the growth of American exercise and sports.
10. Did the Civil War facilitate or inhibit the growth of exercise and sport in America? Why?
11. What arguments were used to discourage the development of physical activity for girls and women in the late 1800s?
12. What was the role of the YMCAs and the YWCAs in the promotion of exercise and physical activity for youth by the end of the 19th century?
13. When was the color line drawn and why?
14. What was the overall impact of the 1919 White Sox World Series "fix"?
15. What role did the early 20th century sports heroes play with regard to the commercial value of sports?
16. What was the impact of World War II on the conduct of American sports?
17. When was American sports formally racially integrated by law?
18. What was the impact of early television on the growth of sports?
19. Discuss Title IX and its impact on girls and women's collegiate sports.
20. Name some primary organizations devoted to professional and scholarly activities in the area of exercise and sport history.

References

Adelman, M. A. (1990). *A sporting time: New York City and the rise of modern athletics, 1820–1870*. Urbana, IL: University of Illinois Press.

Betts, J. R. (1951). *Organized sport in industrial America*. Unpublished doctoral dissertation. Columbia University.

Betts, J. R. (1974). *America's sporting heritage, 1850–1950*. Reading, MA: Addison-Wesley.

Feynman, R. P. (1998). *The meaning of it all: Thoughts of a citizen scientist*. Reading, MA: Perseus Books. (2001).

Freeman, W. H. (2001). *Physical education and sport in a changing society* (6th ed.). Boston: Allyn & Bacon.

Harper, W. A. (1999). *How you played the game*. Columbia, MO: University of Missouri Press.

James, W. (1907). *The social value of the college-bred*. Address delivered at Radcliff College, November 7, 1907.

Kennedy, J. F. (1960, December 26). The soft American. *Sports Illustrated*, pp. 15–17.

Kennedy, J. F. (1962, July 16). The vigor we need. *Sports Illustrated*, pp. 12–14.

Margolick, D. (2005). *Beyond glory: Joe Louis vs. Max Schmelling, and a world on the brink*. New York: Alfred A. Knopf.

Massengale, J. D., & Swanson, R. A. (1997). *The history of exercise and sport science*. Champaign, IL: Human Kinetics.

Oxendine, J. B. (1988). *American Indian sports heritage*. Champaign, IL: Human Kinetics.

Pope, S. W. (Ed.). (1997). *The new American sport history*. Urbana, IL: University of Illinois Press.

Rader, B. G. (2004). *American sports from the age of folk games to the age of televised exercise and sports* (5th ed.). Upper Saddle River, NJ: Prentice Hall.

Spears, B., & Swanson, R. A. (1978). *History of sport and physical activity in the United States*. Dubuque, IA: Wm. C. Brown.

Struna, N. L. (1995). Gender and sporting practice in early America, 1750–1810. In D. K. Wiggens (Ed.), *Sport in America*. Champaign, IL: Human Kinetics.

PART 7

Exploring the Context and Future of Exercise Science

Exercise science is a multifaceted discipline affected by many specialty areas beyond the subdisciplines already discussed. This section provides an overview of some of these varied areas: societal health-trends, epidemiology, legal and ethical issues that affect the exercise scientist, and future trends in research and applied science. Chapter 10 explores current societal health trends in the United States and how such factors as sedentary lifestyles influence the need for exercise programs. Physical activity epidemiology is the focus of Chapter 11. Epidemiology is the study of health events in a population, and this chapter explores the rate of physical activity and its affect on the health status of Americans. Legal and ethical discussions are important to any field of study, and the exercise scientist is faced with such questions each day. Chapter 12 explores those areas of law that directly affect the exercise scientist, such as tort liability. Chapter 13 discusses a variety of salient ethical considerations important in today's society including the use of performance-enhancing substances in sports. Finally, Chapter 14 explores future trends in the exciting and vibrant field of exercise science as interest in preventive medicine and public health initiatives continue to grow.

CHAPTER 10

Current Societal Health Trends

Lynn Penland, PhD, University of Evansville

■ Chapter Objectives

After reading this chapter, you should be able to:

1. Explain why exercise science is important in improving the health status of the nation today.
2. List two commonly used statistics that illustrate the changes in population health over the past 100 years.
3. Describe the general change in leading causes of death over the past 100 years.
4. Explain why exercise was not understood as an important factor for health 100 years ago.
5. Describe two health revolutions that have taken place in the past century.

6. Identify two current major demographic trends that will have an impact on U.S. population health in the future.
7. Describe the categories of health determinants.
8. Explain why health behavior is such an important health determinant.
9. List the 10 leading health indicators identified in the *Healthy People* 2010 project.
10. Describe major health benefits of physical activity.

■ Key Terms

chronic and degenerative diseases
communicable disease
demographic trend
health determinant

health revolution
infant mortality
leading health indicator
life expectancy

maternal mortality
mortality
pharmacological revolution

An examination of current societal health trends provides a context for understanding the importance of exercise science in improving and maintaining population health in the United States. Exercise science is a relatively new academic discipline because, historically, lack of exercise was not a concern.

A century ago physical inactivity was not a contributing factor to any of the major health problems experienced by the populace of the United States. The physical demands of normal daily living—such as work and household tasks—provided significant physical activity. Walking was, of necessity, a major mode of transportation, as the automobile was in its early infancy and not yet available to the general public. In addition, more people were involved in physically demanding daily activities. Women, usually working in the home, did not have the benefit of labor-saving devices commonly in use today. In the workforce in 1900 nearly half of the workers were in the physically demanding occupations of farming and labor. Less than 10% were employed in typically sedentary positions such as clerical personnel, professionals, or managers. One hundred years later, these percentages are nearly reversed (Carter et al., 2006).

This chapter chronicles a dramatic shift in the types of health problems experienced by people in this country over the past century. Comparing the causes of illness in the past with those of today explains why exercise science, unheard of 100 years ago, assumes preeminence in any serious consideration of prevention of illness and optimization of wellness for the 21st century populace.

HISTORICAL CONTEXT FOR HEALTH IN THE UNITED STATES

Life in general was different in many ways 100 years ago. In 1900 the majority of Americans heated with wood stoves, used gas or candles for lighting, drew their water with a hand pump from a well outside their home, and depended on outdoor facilities for sanitation. Conveniences of electricity, running water, indoor plumbing, and central heating were enjoyed by a minority of the population. Families were larger, they lived in smaller homes, and the general standard of living was significantly lower than it is today. At the turn of the 20th century, the gross domestic product, the most widely used measure of the material standard of living, was approximately 3% of its 21st century level (Carter et al., 2006; Maddison, 2003; U.S. Census Bureau, 2002).

The health of the population was also significantly different 100 years ago. There are many ways to describe the health of a population. One common way is to use **mortality** statistics. The mortality rate indicates the number of people who die in a given number of people. In 1900 approximately 100 babies out of every 1,000 live births died within the first year of life; that is, the **infant mortality** rate was 100 per 1,000 live births. The **maternal mortality** rate, the number of women who died because of pregnancy-related conditions, was 6 to 9 per 1,000 live births ("Achievements," 1999).

Another way to measure the health of a population is through **life expectancy** statistics. In the year 1900 a baby born in the United States had an average life expectancy of 47.3 years. Although low, this compared favorably to the average life expectancy of the world population, which was 31 years at that time (Maddison, 2003).

A third way to understand the health of a population is to study of the causes of mortality. In the year 1900 people could expect to die from an infectious disease. Infectious diseases, also called **communicable diseases,** are those that can be transmitted from one person to another through bacteria, viruses, or other infectious agents. Communicable diseases such as pneumonia, influenza, tuberculosis, and dysentery—a common and serious digestive tract infection—were the top causes of mortality in 1900.

HEALTH OF THE U.S. POPULATION TODAY

The health of the population has changed dramatically over the past century. In many ways it has improved; people are definitely, living longer. Today the

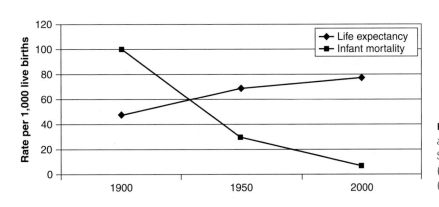

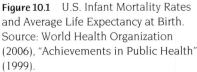

Figure 10.1 U.S. Infant Mortality Rates and Average Life Expectancy at Birth. Source: World Health Organization (2006), "Achievements in Public Health" (1999).

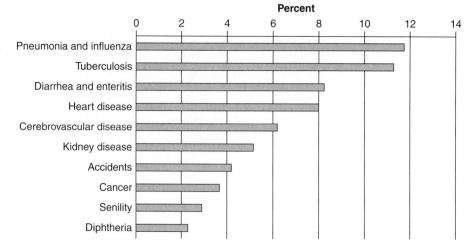

Percent

Pneumonia and influenza
Tuberculosis
Diarrhea and enteritis
Heart disease
Cerebrovascular disease
Kidney disease
Accidents
Cancer
Senility
Diphtheria

Figure 10.2 Leading Causes of Death by Percentage of Total Deaths, 1900.
Source: National Office of Vital statistics 1947.

TABLE 10.1 Leading Causes of Death in the United States, 1900 and 2004	
1900	**2004**
1 Pneumonia and influenza	Heart disease
2 Tuberculosis	Cancer
3 Diarrhea and enteritis	Cerebrovascular disease
4 Heart disease	Chronic lower respiratory disease
5 Cerebrovascular disease	Accidents
6 Kidney disease	Diabetes
7 Accidents	Alzheimer's disease
8 Cancer	Pneumonia and influenza
9 Senility	Kidney disease
10 Diphtheria	Septicemia

Source: DHHS (2007), National Office of Vital Statistics (1947).

life expectancy of a baby born in the United States is an average of 77.5 years, up more than 30 years over the past 100 years (Department of Health and Human Services [DHHS], 2007; Hoyert, Heron, Murphy, & Kung, 2006). Infant mortality at the beginning of the 21st century is 6.9 per 1,000 live births, down from 100 per 1,000 live births in 1900 (DHHS, 2007). This is a decrease of more than 90%. Figure 10.1 shows the change in both infant mortality and average life expectancy from the beginning of the 20th century to the beginning of the 21st century.

In addition to having longer life spans, today's Americans have very different mortality patterns from their predecessors of a century ago. Today very few people die from the infectious diseases that raged in 1900. Instead, most people can expect to die from some type of noncommunicable, chronic, degenerative disease such as heart disease, cancer, cerebrovascular disease, or respiratory disease. Table 10.1 shows the leading causes of death in 1900 and those in 2004, in order of decreasing frequency. The relative percentages of total deaths attributed to each cause in 1900 and in 2004 are illustrated graphically in Figures 10.2 and 10.3.

Among the top 10 leading causes of death in the early 2000s only two are infectious: pneumonia/influenza ranks number 8, accounting for under 2% of the country's mortality, and septicemia (generalized infection) ranks number 10, accounting for approximately 1%. In 1900 all top 3 causes of mortality were infectious diseases: pneumonia/ influenza, tuberculosis, and diarrhea/enteritis (DHHS, 2000, 2007). The death rates from infectious diseases dropped 93% over the last 100 years, from approximately 800 per 100,000 at the beginning of the 20th century to approximately 60 per 100,000 by the end of the century (Armstrong, Conn, & Pinner, 1999).

There have been several reasons for the change in the health of the population over the past century. One major reason was a cluster of factors that occurred in the early 1900s and created an improved health environment for people. Among those factors were improvements in general standard of living, nutrition, basic sanitation, hygiene, and water quality. Because these factors caused massive improvements in the well-being of the population, they are sometimes referred to as the country's first **health revolution.** The result of this revolution was a marked decrease in morbidity and mortality due to communicable diseases. Disease-causing organisms had thrived because of poor sanitation in the 1800s, but safe water supplies, usually piped directly

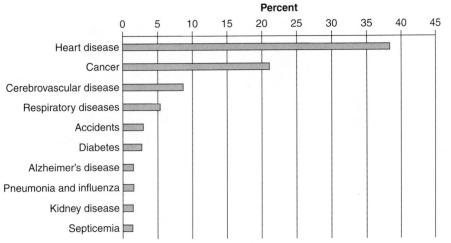

Figure 10.3 Leading Causes of Death by Percentage of Total Deaths, 2004.
Source: DHHS (2007).

into people's homes, and improved sanitation in the 1900s limited the ease with which disease-causing organisms could thrive and spread from person to person. Improved public health measures prevented much disease by reducing exposure to the causative agents. In addition, as the general standard of living rose, people had healthier living conditions and their diet improved. Thus they had better general health and were less likely to be susceptible to infectious agents (Porter, 1996).

The second major reason for change in population health came in the mid-20th-century as a result of advances in medicine. These advances created another health revolution, sometimes referred to as the **pharmacological revolution.** In 1928 Alexander Fleming discovered that penicillin was an effective antibiotic, able to kill disease-causing microorganisms. Sulfa drugs followed in the 1930s, streptomycin in the 1940s, and many other antibiotics soon became widely available. These medicines came into use following the time of improved nutrition and public health and were successful in further reducing mortality from influenza and pneumonia, tuberculosis, and dysentery—the top causes of death in 1900. In addition, the increasingly widespread use of vaccines made it possible to prevent communicable diseases such as smallpox, polio, tuberculosis, diphtheria, and measles (Harding, 2000; Porter, 1996).

The health changes of the past century have brought us to the health situation of today. Many of the dreaded communicable diseases of 100 years ago have been brought under control and, in some cases, are completely eliminated. It is unlikely that additional simple pharmacologic, medical, or public health breakthroughs will dramatically affect population health. The major health challenges of today are **chronic and degenerative diseases,** for which causation is multifactorial and for which solutions depend at least as much on personal decisions and lifestyle choices as on public health and medical or pharmaceutical interventions. Application of principles of exercise science and other wellness behaviors assume significant importance in improving population health when the major problems are chronic, noncommunicable conditions.

Current Influences on Population Health

The United States has been experiencing two major **demographic trends** that increasingly are affecting the health of the nation. First, the population is becoming more diverse. In 1900 the U.S. Census indicated that 1 out of 8 people was of a race other than white. By the year 2000, the nonwhite proportion had increased to 1 out of 4 (Hobbs & Stoops, 2002). The Census Bureau projects that by 2020 the U.S. nonwhite population will be approximately 50%. All racial groups other than white/not Hispanic are projected to increase between now and 2050 (U.S. Census Bureau, 2004). Figure 10.4 shows the percentage of the U.S. population in the white/non-Hispanic category and in the other (nonwhite) category in the past and projected into the future.

Different racial, ethnic, and cultural groups have different rates of prevalence for individual diseases and illnesses. They also have varying health beliefs that affect prevention or treatment of health conditions. For instance, there are marked differences in the amount of physical activity of different racial-ethnic groups. The percentage of people who report no leisure time physical activity varies from approximately 40% in some racial-ethnic groups down to just over 20% in other groups (DHHS, 2005). The increased diversity of the population means that improving the health of the entire nation will require careful attention to specific illnesses, health beliefs, health behaviors, and health indicators found in different segments of the population. It will mean that health care and wellness service providers must gain

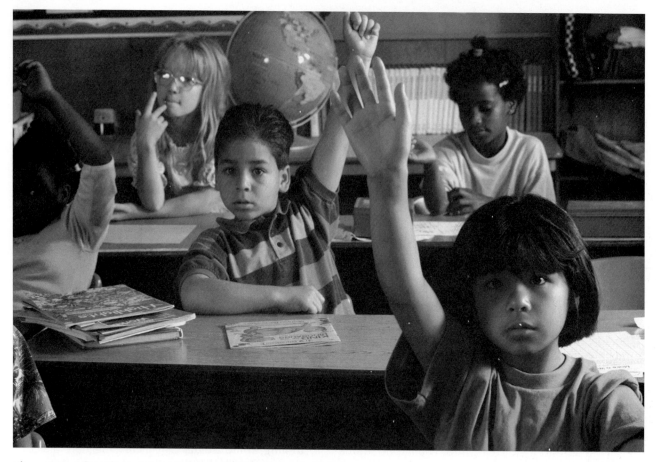

Classrooms reflect the country's increasingly diverse population.

skill at providing culturally competent care and that providers, educators, and policymakers concerned with improving population health must be attentive to access issues and to cultural, lifestyle, and genetic factors in different segments of the population.

The second demographic trend that will affect the health of the nation is the aging of the population. The percent of the total population in the 65-plus age group was only 4% in 1900 (Hobbs & Stoops, 2002); however, the U.S. Census Bureau (2004) projects that the 65-plus age group will increase to over 20% of the population by 2050. Likewise, the 75-plus age group has been growing. Just over 1% of the population in 1900, the 75-plus population is projected to reach 12%, or about 1 in 8 Americans, by 2050 (Hobbs & Stoops, 2002; DHHS, 2007). Figure 10.5 illustrates the

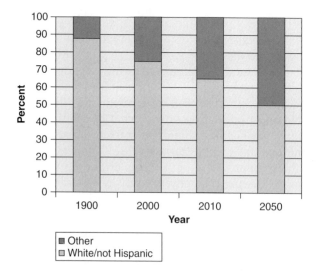

Figure 10.4 Percentage of U.S. Population in White/Not Hispanic and Other (Nonwhite) Groups.
Source: U.S. Census Bureau (2004).

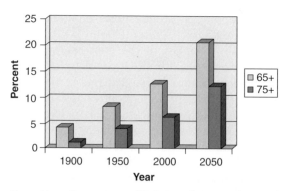

Figure 10.5 Percentage of U.S. Population in the 65-plus and 75-plus Age Groups, 1900 to 2050.
Source: DHHS (2007), Hobbs & Stools, (2002).

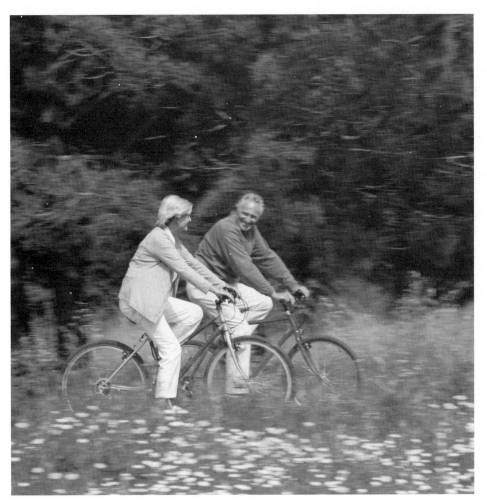

Although many people decrease their physical activity as they age, continuing an active lifestyle is important for helping prevent today's prevalent chronic health conditions.

changes and projected changes in older age groups from 1900 to 2050. All other age groups below age 65 are projected to decline during the first half of the 21st century.

A commonly used statistical indicator of an aging population is the population median age. In 1900 the median age was just under 23. That means that one-half of the population was younger than 23 and one-half was older than 23. In 2000 the median age had risen to over 35. A country with an average age of over 30 can be considered relatively old (Hobbs & Stoop, 2002). The United States is already in the older category, and the average age is expected to increase along with life expectancy.

Because the population is getting older, the pattern of increased prevalence of chronic and degenerative diseases, more common among the elderly, is projected to continue (Institute for the Future, 2000). Not surprisingly, the average level of physical activity is inversely correlated with age groups; that is, the percentage who report no leisure time physical activity increases from about 20% for 18- to 24-year-olds to over 33% in the 65-plus age group (DHHS, 2005). The challenges of keeping the population healthy as

people reach older ages will fall to wellness providers as well as to medical practitioners. Exercise science has an important role in helping to prevent chronic diseases and conditions such as heart disease, cerebrovascular disease, diabetes, obesity, and injuries due to accidents as well as to lessening the severity and minimizing the negative impact of those diseases on the lives of affected individuals.

SOLUTIONS TO HEALTH PROBLEMS

Many factors are responsible for determining the health of an individual. To improve population health, it is essential to consider the various determinants of health. **Health determinants** can be placed in five categories: health behavior, environment, interventions and policies, access to care, and biology (Institute for the Future, 2000).

Of the five categories of health determinants, the Centers for Disease Control estimates health behavior to be responsible for 50% of an individual's health

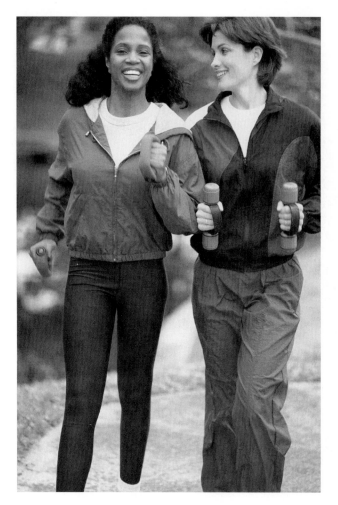

Studies have shown that lifestyle factors such as physical activity are correlated with lower risk of coronary heart disease.

status (Institute for the Future, 2000). This means that health behavior, the category over which individuals have the greatest control, is the most important of the health determinants. One study that strongly demonstrates the impact of health behavior on health status is the Nurses' Health Study (Stampfer, Hu, Manson, Rimm, & Willett, 2000). This comprehensive 14-year study of more than 84,000 women showed the importance of lifestyle factors in coronary heart disease, the number one cause of mortality in the United States. The nurses in the lifestyle low-risk category (including factors such as moderate to vigorous physical activity, nonsmoking, and healthy diet) had a very low risk of coronary heart disease. In addition, each of the lifestyle factors separately predicted low risk. In this study an impressive 82% of the cardiac events in the group were attributable to the lack of lifestyle low-risk factors. Research in exercise science and the work of exercise science professionals will continue to be important in helping people to improve their health, particularly in the health behavior area of health determinants.

The environment, considering both social and physical elements, is a second determinant for population health. Negative physical environment factors such as poor sanitation and housing were addressed nearly a century ago for many Americans; however, for others substandard conditions still exist. Environmental pollutants and toxic substances remain a challenge to population health in many areas, and infectious agents are sometimes a part of the environment. Unsafe conditions where people live or work are also a part of the physical environment. The social environment affects population health through the influence and health habits of coworkers, friends, families, and through institutions such as churches and schools. Violence is also a part of the social environment.

The third category, interventions and policies, refers to government and health or social service groups' programs and campaigns to improve health. Examples would be laws requiring immunizations, seat belt use, and child restraint devices. Health information and health promotion campaigns such as stop smoking campaigns or breast feeding campaigns are also a type of intervention.

Access to care is a fourth category of determinants. Those who are able to both find and afford quality care for treatable or preventable health conditions are likely to have better health than those who are not. Access to care varies widely across the nation, and affordability is related to both income and health insurance availability.

Biology, the fifth category of health determinants, produces or contributes to many health conditions. Genetic makeup is one part of biology that determines health status. A few examples of diseases related to heredity are hemophilia, sickle cell anemia, glaucoma, some types of cancer, and certain congenital conditions such as Down syndrome, spina bifida, autism, and cystic fibrosis. Biology also can alter health through the aging process, producing cataracts or osteoporosis, or through injury, producing conditions such as quadriplegia or traumatic brain injury. Exposure to tobacco, alcohol, or toxic agents can alter biology and cause health problems such as fetal alcohol syndrome and black lung disease.

U.S. Goals for Improving Population Health

By many standards, the health of Americans is good and is improving. In the most recent National Health Interview Survey, nearly 70% of adults 18 and older reported themselves to be in excellent or very good health. Less than 1% of adults considered themselves to be in fair or poor health, and only 2% reported requiring assistance in activities of daily living (Adams & Barnes, 2006). Longevity continues to increase,

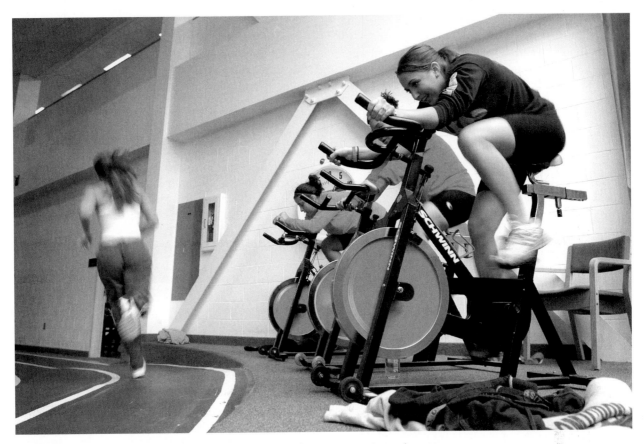

The health benefits from exercise are greatest for those who participate in moderate to vigorous physical activity on a regular basis.

albeit at a slower rate than the dramatic increases in the beginning years of the 20th century. Progress has been made in decreasing the morbidity and mortality caused by a number of conditions, especially communicable diseases; however, major chronic health problems remain as challenges, and health disparities exist between groups of different income levels, racial and ethnic backgrounds, education levels, and geographic locations (DHHS, 2007). An interesting phenomenon, referred to as the "health paradox," is the fact that although the health of the nation has improved, people's satisfaction with their personal health has actually decreased (Barsky, 1988). Possible reasons for this finding are the increased relative prevalence of chronic disorders, greater health consciousness, increased media emphasis on dangers of diseases, and unrealistic expectations for cures of all infirmities (Barsky, 1988).

The U.S. Department of Health and Human Services has been involved in coordinating a national planning process over the past several decades to advance the health of the nation's people and communities. This process has resulted in successive documents outlining a health agenda for the nation. The current document of specific goals and objectives for health improvement is titled *Healthy People* 2010 (DHHS, 2000). The two large, general goals for *Healthy People* 2010 are (1) to increase both the quality and the length of the life and (2) to eliminate disparities in the health status of different subgroups of the population.

Exercise plays an essential role in the plans for health improvement. As a part of the Healthy People project, the Department of Health and Human Services has developed a list of **leading health indicators** to help monitor and evaluate progress toward improving health. The 10 leading health indicators were chosen because they are measurable factors that have a direct connection with important current health issues. Exercise science relates directly to the first two leading health indicators: (1) physical activity and (2) overweight and obesity. Box 10.1 describes the leading health indicators and the goals for percentages of people who will possess the positive indicators by the year 2010.

As the major health problems in the United States have shifted away from communicable diseases and toward chronic and degenerative diseases, personal health decisions and health behaviors have assumed increasing importance in determining health. The first 2 of the 10 *Healthy People* 2010 indicators—physical activity and overweight/obesity—are inextricably linked to exercise. Nearly all of the 10 health indicators relate to individual personal health behavior choices such as being physically active, eating a healthy diet, avoiding tobacco use and substance abuse, practicing responsible sexual behavior, seeking treatment for mental illness, wearing seat belts, receiving immunizations, and receiving prenatal care.

PHYSICAL ACTIVITY AND HEALTH

Physical activity, the first of the *Healthy People* 2010 health indicators, has long been understood to be an important factor for maintaining and improving health.

Physical activity is related to a number of health and disease conditions. Importantly, physical activity correlates negatively with overall mortality, or death from all causes; that is, those with greater levels of physical activity have a lower rate of mortality that those who exhibit sedentary lifestyles (DHHS, 1996). The Harvard Alumni Survey, a study of over 17,000 men from 1962 through 1988, showed a strong inverse relationship between physical activity and mortality: Those who were less physically active had higher mortality rates (Lee, Hsieh, & Paffenbarger, 1995). Numerous studies have found a positive relationship between physical

EXPLORE MORE BOX 10.1

Healthy People 2010 Leading Health Indicators and Goals

1. **Physical activity.** Regular physical activity is correlated with physical health, mental well-being, and lower likelihood of premature death. Increasingly, sedentary lifestyles are the norm among all age groups. The goal is for 80% of adolescents to engage in vigorous, cardiovascular-enhancing physical activity three or more days per week, and for 30% of adults to engage in regular moderate physical activity.

2. **Overweight and obesity.** Overweight and obesity contribute to a number of important preventable causes of death including heart disease and stroke. The *Healthy People* 2010 goal is to reduce the percentage of children and adolescents who are overweight or obese to 5% and the percentage of adults to 15%.

3. **Tobacco use.** Cigarette smoking is the number one preventable cause of morbidity and mortality. It is a risk factor for a long list of conditions including heart disease, stroke, lung cancer, chronic lung diseases, premature births, and sudden infant death syndrome. The *Healthy People* 2010 goal is to reduce the percentage of adolescents who smoke to 16% and the percentage of adults who smoke to 12%.

4. **Substance abuse.** Abuse of drugs and alcohol contribute to violence, accidents, and the spread of HIV/AIDS. The goal is to reduce the percentage of adolescents who use alcohol and drugs to 11% and the percentage of adults who use illicit drugs to 2%.

5. **Responsible sexual behavior.** Sexually transmitted diseases and unintended pregnancies are major health problems that largely can be prevented by responsible sexual behavior. The goal is to increase the proportion of adolescents who abstain from sexual intercourse or use condoms if sexually active to 95% and to increase the percentage of sexually active unmarried women who report condom use by their partners to 50%.

6. **Mental health.** Mental illness is a leading cause of disability, and some types of mental illness are highly correlated with suicides. Among mental illnesses, depression is the most common. The *Healthy People* 2010 goal is to increase, above the baseline level of 23%, the percentage of adults diagnosed with depression who receive treatment.

7. **Injury and violence.** Motor vehicle crashes and homicides are major causes of mortality and morbidity. The number of motor vehicle deaths could be reduced with increased seat belt use and reduced instances of impaired driving. The *Healthy People* 2010 goals are to reduce motor vehicle deaths to 9.2 per 100,000 annually and to reduce homicides to 3.0 per 100,000.

8. **Environmental quality.** Poor environmental quality, especially air pollution and tobacco smoke, is responsible for significant morbidity, most notably from respiratory diseases, cardiovascular diseases, and cancer. The goals are to eliminate exposure to ozone above the EPA standard and to reduce the proportion of nonsmokers exposed to environmental tobacco smoke to 45%.

9. **Immunization.** Immunization can help prevent mortality and morbidity from many infectious diseases. The goals are to increase to 80% the proportion of young children who receive all vaccines recommended for universal administration and to increase the proportion of adults vaccinated against influenza and pneumococcal disease to 90%.

10. **Access to health care.** Access to health care can help prevent or minimize morbidity and mortality. The *Healthy People* 2010 goals are to increase to 100% the persons who have health insurance, to increase to 96% the proportion of people who have a specific source of regular health care, and to increase to 90% the proportion of pregnant women who receive prenatal care in their first trimester of pregnancy.

Source: *Healthy People* 2010 (DHHS, 2000).

activity and prevention of chronic diseases as well as premature death (Arraiz, Wigle, & Mao 1992; Leon & Connett, 1991; Paffenbarger et al., 1993; Paffenbarger, Hyde, Wing, Lee, & Kampert, 1994; Warburton, Nicol, & Bredin, 2006).

The surgeon general's report, *Physical Activity and Health* (DHHS, 1996), provided extensive and important information and recommendations for people wishing to reap the beneficial effects of physical activity. The report indicated that the greatest health benefit from activity will accrue to those who participate on a regular basis at least 5 days per week and that an additional health benefit is available for those who participate in more vigorous activity for longer durations. However, the report emphasized that physical activity need not be at a vigorous level to have significant health benefits. This is a shift in emphasis from earlier years when vigorous physical activity was believed to be necessary for health benefits. In addition to physical activities that build cardiovascular endurance, muscle strengthening activities provide further health benefits such as musculoskeletal health and balance.

The surgeon general's report also described the numerous benefits of physical activity on major causes of morbidity and mortality: helping to prevent or reduce the risk or seriousness of heart disease, high blood pressure, high cholesterol, colon and breast cancer, Type 2 diabetes, arthritis, osteoporosis, depression, and anxiety. The report summarized many studies that have been conducted to show the connection between physical activity and physiological responses. A number of body systems, including cardiovascular, musculoskeletal, respiratory, endocrine, and immune systems, respond to episodes of physical activity with actual physiological changes. Examples are increased cardiac output, increased arterial blood pressure during exercise and decreased arterial blood pressure following exercise, increased blood flow to the coronary arteries, increased pulmonary ventilation, changes in immune function, and changes in levels of hormones including catecholamines, growth hormone, testosterone, estradiol-progesterone, insulin, and glucagon. Long-term physiological changes also occur with exercise. These changes include adaptations in heart rate, heart volume, blood pressure, and respiration rate; and metabolic changes such as oxidative capacity of muscle, capacity of muscle to store glycogen, and ability of muscle to use fat as an energy source (DHHS, 1996).

Lack of physical activity is a contributor to overweight and obesity. Excess weight, in turn, increases the risk and the severity of hypertension, arthritis, and musculoskeletal problems. Among children, obesity also increases the risk of high cholesterol,

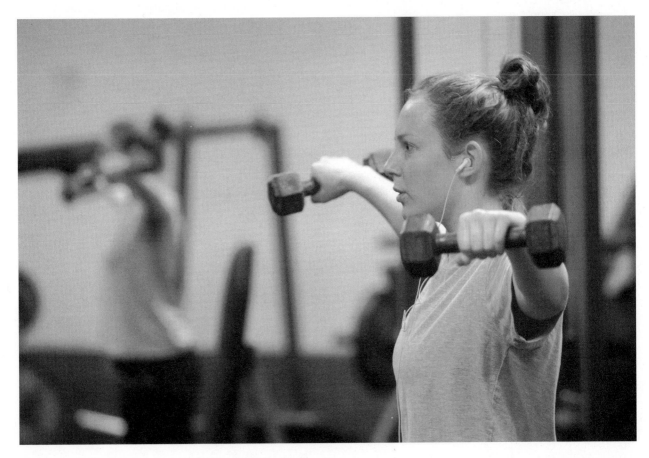

Muscle strengthening activities confer important health benefits.

hypertension, and diabetes (DHHS, 2007). According to National Health and Nutrition Examination Survey data (National Center for Health Statistics, 2004) 65% of U.S. adults are overweight, with 31% falling into the obese category. Among children 6 through 19 years old, 16% are overweight and an additional 15% are at risk for overweight (Hedley et al., 2004).

The level of exercise among Americans is low. Given the potential benefits of physical activity, an increase in physical activity could have a significant impact on population health. Insufficient exercise is a problem for children and adolescents as well as for adults. In 2002 the U.S. Centers for Disease Control conducted a national survey that found that 62% of children ages 9 to 13 participate in no organized physical activity outside of school and that 23% participate in no physical activity in their free time ("Physical Activity," 2003). This means that most activity is occurring during school, and youth may not be developing healthy physical activity leisure time habits. Only 65% of adolescents meet the recommendation for vigorous physical activity a minimum of 20 minutes per day at least 3 days per week. Adults fare less well, with only 15% meeting the recommendation of 30 minutes of moderate physical activity at least 5 days per week. A full 40% of adults do not participate in any type of leisure time physical activity. Certain age, gender, racial, and socioeconomic groups participate in less exercise than the general public (DHHS, 2000).

SUMMARY

Today's major health problems are chronic diseases. Chronic diseases are usually multifactorial, requiring more complex solutions than infectious diseases, which can be solved by destroying a specific microorganism. Comparing today's health problems with those of 100 years ago, a definite shift has occurred away from communicable diseases and toward chronic diseases. Changes in living conditions, in sanitation, in public health, and in effective treatment and prevention therapies for diseases caused by microorganisms have brought the major killers of a century ago under control.

Solutions for today's health problems focus on lifestyle and personal behavior decisions. Critical among the many personal behaviors that can positively affect health today is physical activity. Currently, the majority of adults and many children and adolescents do not meet recommendations for physical activity. Significant progress has been made over the past century in improving the health of the population. The population, facing different health problems in the 21st century, is becoming increasingly older and more diverse. Continued improvement of health status for the nation will almost surely depend on addressing physical activity levels through application of exercise science knowledge.

■ Key Resources

Key Websites

Health, U.S., 2005 (http://www.cdc.gov/nchs/data/hus/hus05.pd)
Healthy People 2010 (http://www.healthypeople.gov/)
Centers for Disease Control and Prevention, U.S. Department of Health and Human Services (http://www.cdc.gov/)

National Center for Health Statistics (http://www.cdc.gov/nchs/)
Physical Activity and Health: Report of the Surgeon General (http://www.cdc.gov/nccdphp/sgr/sgr.htm)

■ Review Questions

1. How was the health of the U.S. population different 100 years ago, and how did the population health relate to differences in the general way of life for people?
2. What statistics describe differences in population health over the past century?
3. Why was exercise not recognized as an important factor for health 100 years ago?
4. What was the nature of the country's first and second health revolutions, and what was the impact of each?
5. How will the increasing racial, ethnic, and cultural diversity in the United States affect the application of exercise science to population health?

6. How will the aging of the population affect the application of exercise science to the country's health?
7. What are the five categories of health determinants? Give examples within each category.
8. What are the 10 leading health indicators in the *Healthy People* 2010 report, and why were the specific 10 chosen?
9. What are the nation's health goals as articulated in *Healthy People* 2010?

■ References

Achievements in public health, 1900–1999: Healthier mothers and babies. (1999). MMWR *Weekly*, 48(38), 849–858.

Adams, P. F., & Barnes, P. M. (2006). Summary health statistics for U.S. adults: National health interview survey 2004. *Vital Health Statistics: 10* (229). Retrieved from http://www.cdc.gov/nchs/data/series/sr_10/sr10_229.pdf

Armstrong, G. L., Conn, L. A., & Pinner R. W. (1999). Trends in infectious disease mortality in the United States during the 20th century. JAMA, 281(1), 61–66.

Arraiz, G. A., Wigle, D. T., & Mao, Y. (1992). Risk assessment of physical activity and physical fitness in the Canada Health Survey mortality follow-up study. *Journal of Clinical Epidemiology*, 45(4), 419–428.

Barsky, A. J. (1988). The paradox of health. *New England Journal of Medicine*, 318(7), 414–418.

Carter, S. B., Gartner, S. S., Haines, M. R., Olmstead, A. L., Sutch, R., & Wright, G. (Eds.). (2006). *Historical statistics of the United States*. New York: Cambridge University Press.

Department of Health and Human Services. (1996). *Physical activity and health: A report of the surgeon general*. Atlanta, GA: Centers for Disease Control and Prevention, National Center for Chronic Disease Prevention and Health Promotion.

Department of Health and Human Services. (2000). *Healthy people 2010: Understanding and improving health* (2nd ed.). Washington, DC: U.S. Government Printing Office.

Department of Health and Human Services. (2005). *U.S. physical activity statistics*. Retrieved from http://apps.nccd.cdc.gov/PASurveillance/DemoCompareResultV.asp#result

Department of Health and Human Services. (2007). *Health, United States, 2007 with chartbook on trends in the health of Americans*. Washington, DC: Centers for Disease Control, National Center for Health Statistics.

Harding, A. S. (2000). *Milestones in health and medicine*. Phoenix, AZ: Oryx Press.

Hedley, A. A., Ogden, C. L., Johnson, C. L., Carroll, M. D., Curtin, L. R., & Flegal, K. M. (2004). Prevalence of overweight and obesity among U.S. children, adolescents, and adults, 1999–2002. JAMA, 291(23), 2847–2850.

Hobbs, F., & Stoops, N. (2002). *Demographic trends in the 20th century*. U.S. Census Bureau, Census 2000 Special Reports, Series CENSR-4. Washington, DC: U.S. Government Printing Office.

Hoyert, D. L., Heron, M. P., Murphy, S. L., & Kung H. (2006). Deaths: Final data for 2003. *National vital statistics reports*, 54(13). [Electronic version] Hyattsville, MD: National Center for Health Statistics.

Institute for the Future. (2000). *Health and health care 2010: The forecast, the challenge*. San Francisco: Jossey-Bass.

Lee, I-M., Hsieh, C. C., & Paffenbarger, R. S., Jr. (1995). Exercise intensity and longevity in men: The Harvard alumni health study. JAMA, 273, 1179–1184.

Leon, A. S., & Connett, J. (1991). Physical activity and 10.5 year mortality in the multiple risk factor intervention trial. *International Journal of Epidemiology*, 20(3), 690–697.

Maddison, A. (2003). *The world economy: Historical statistics*. Paris: Organisation for Economic Co-operation and Development.

National Center for Health Statistics. (2004). NCHS *data on overweight and obesity*. Retrieved from http://www.cdc.gov/nchs/data/factsheets/overweightobesity.pdf

National Office of Vital Statistics. (1947). *Deaths and death rates for leading causes of death: Death registration states, 1900–1940*. Retrieved from http://www.cdc.gov/nchs/data/dvs/lead1900_98.pdf

Paffenbarger, R. S., Jr, Hyde, R. T., Wing, A. L., Lee, I-M., Jung, D. L., & Kampert, J. B. (1993). The association of changes in physical activity level and other lifestyle characteristics with mortality among men. *New England Journal of Medicine*, 328(8), 538–545.

Paffenbarger, R. S., Jr, Hyde, R. T., Wing, A. L., Lee, I-M., & Kampert. J. B. (1994). Some interrelations of physical activity, physiological fitness, health, and longevity. In C. Bouchard, R. J. Shephard, & T. Stephens (Eds.), *Physical activity, fitness, and healh: International proceedings and concensus statement* (pp. 119–133). Champaign, IL: Human Kinetics.

Physical activity levels among children aged 9–13 years—United States, 2002. (2003). MMWR *Weekly*, 52(33), 785–788.

Porter, R. (Ed.). (1996). *Cambridge illustrated history of medicine*. Cambridge, UK: Cambridge University Press.

Stampfer, M. J., Hu, F. B., Manson, J. E., Rimm, E. B., & Willett, W. C. (2000). Primary prevention of coronary heart disease in women through diet and lifestyle. *New England Journal of Medicine*, 343(1), 16–22.

U.S. Census Bureau. (2002). *American housing survey for the United States: 2001*. Current Housing Reports, Series H150/01. Washington, DC: U.S. Government Printing Office.

U.S. Census Bureau. (2004). U.S. *interim projections by age, sex, race, and Hispanic origin*. Retrieved from http://www.census.gov/ipc/www/usinterimproj/

Warburton, D. E. R., Nicol, C. W., & Bredin, S. S. D. (2006). Health benefits of physical activity: The evidence. CMAJ, 174(6), 801–809.

World Health Organization. (2006). *Monitoring and evaluation: Reproductive health indicators database*. Retrieved from http://www9.who.int/familyhealth/reproductiveindicators/countrydata.asp?page=227

CHAPTER 11

Physical Activity Epidemiology

Gregory W. Heath, DHSc, MPH, University of Tennessee at Chattanooga

■ Chapter Objectives

After reading this chapter, you should be able to:

1. Describe the background, importance, and history of physical activity epidemiology.
2. Understand the epidemiologic basis of the *Healthy People* 2010 physical activity and fitness objectives.
3. Identify the epidemiologic methods of rates and proportions and disease and injury occurrence.
4. List the measures of physical activity and fitness used in epidemiologic studies.
5. Describe how common study designs are used in physical activity epidemiology, including cross-sectional, case-control, cohort, and randomized designs.
6. Describe the criteria and assessment for causality in light of epidemiologic, experimental, and clinical findings.

■ Key Terms

agent
association
case-control study
cohort
cross-sectional study
cumulative incidence
diary
direct measurement

environment
epidemiology
host
incidence
longitudinal
observation
prevalence
proportion

prospective cohort study
questionnaire
random assignment
randomized clinical trial
rate
web of causation

Epidemiology is the study of health events in a population (Last, 2000). Epidemiology and biostatistics are the fundamental quantitative sciences of public health. Functionally, epidemiology seeks to address three applications: (1) describe the distribution of a disease/condition/health event; that is, the who, what, where, and when (person, place, and time) of a disease or health event; (2) analyze descriptive information by identifying potential risk factors associated with the increased probability of a health event or disease/condition occurrence; and (3) use this information for the prevention of a health-related occurrence by developing and implementing strategies (i.e., interventions) that address the identified risk factors specific to these health-related events.

Physical activity epidemiology is concerned with the systematic examination of factors related to participation in the health behavior of physical activity and how this behavior relates to the likelihood of improved health or function or disease occurrence. Examples of this investigative effort include descriptive information about the dose or level of physical activity in a population, comparisons across populations regarding the dose of physical activity, identification of factors that are related to varying levels of participation in physical activity, and establishing associations between physical activity and the risk for such chronic diseases as coronary heart disease, stroke, Type 2 diabetes mellitus, osteoporosis, cancer, and obesity.

A BRIEF HISTORY OF PHYSICAL ACTIVITY EPIDEMIOLOGY

The scientific understanding of physical activity, physical fitness, and public health began to come into focus with the early work of Dr. Jeremy Morris and his colleagues as they studied coronary heart disease (CHD) in the late 1940s. As a result of this early work, Morris and Heady (1953) proposed the following hypothesis:

> Deaths from this condition [coronary heart disease] In middle age may be less common among men engaged in physically active work than those in "sedentary" jobs. (p. 145)

This hypothesis was further developed when Morris found that the conductors on London's double-decker buses, who were constantly moving up and down and through the buses, were at lower risk of CHD than the drivers who primarily sat most of their work shift while driving the buses (Morris, Heady, Raffle, Roberts, & Parks, 1953). Those conductors who

did develop CHD had less severe disease, and its onset occurred at later ages. The London bus driver study began a series of investigations that would constitute the beginnings of physical activity epidemiology. Investigations among other occupational groups were carried out that included postmen (Morris, 1957), Finnish lumberjacks (Karvonen, 1962), U.S. railroad workers (Taylor, Blackburn, Puchner, Parlin, & Keys, 1969), and the Seven Countries Study (Keys, 1967). Also, cohort studies of entire communities such as the Framingham Heart Study, begun in 1948 in Framingham, Massachusetts (Dawber, Meadors, & Moore, 1951; Kannel, 1967), and the Tecumseh Community Health Study, begun in Tecumseh, Michigan, in 1957 (Montoye, 1975), added measures of fitness and physical activity.

The San Francisco Longshoremen Study and the College Health Study (Harvard College and the University of Pennsylvania), begun in the 1960s and 1970s (Paffenbarger, Wolfe, Notkin, & Thovne, 1966; Paffenbarger, Lauglin, Gima, & Black, 1970; Paffenbarger, Hyde, & Wing, 1978), have contributed significant information about the relationship of physical activity to selected health outcomes, including CHD, Type 2 diabetes mellitus, hypertension, cancers, obesity, and other chronic conditions/diseases. A premier **longitudinal** study examining the role of both measured cardiorespiratory fitness and physical activity behaviors on longevity and cardiovascular disease risk is the Aerobics Center Longitudinal Study (Blair, et al., 1989). These studies have confirmed the role for physical activity and cardiorespiratory fitness in promoting the longevity and health of the public in both economically developed and developing countries (Haskell et al., 2007; McGinnis, 1992; Pate et al., 1995).

HEALTH GOALS FOR THE NATION

As the link between physical activity and the prevention of CHD and other chronic diseases was confirmed through studies in the 1960s and 1970s, behavioral epidemiologists and public health scientists in the United States acknowledged the importance of shaping public health policy for the purpose of promoting participation in physical activity among all citizens. Such public health policy needed to include ongoing and monitored physical activity data collection as well as the development of specific physical activity and fitness goals for the nation's population subgroups. Each decade since 1980, the U.S. Department of Health and Human Services (DHHS) has published a set of "Objectives for the Nation," which are policy goals for improving the nation's health. Objectives for increasing physical

TABLE 11.1 *Healthy People 2010* Physical Activity and Fitness Objectives

Number Objective

Physical Activity in Adults

22-1   Reduce the proportion of adults who engage in no leisure time physical activity.

22-2   Increase the proportion of adults who engage regularly, preferably daily, in moderate physical activity for at least 30 minutes per day.

22-3   Increase the proportion of adults who engage in vigorous physical activity that promotes the development and maintenance of cardiorespiratory fitness 3 or more days per week for 20 or more minutes per occasion.

Muscular Strength/Endurance and Flexibility

22-4   Increase the proportion of adults who perform physical activities that enhance and maintain muscular strength and endurance.

22-5   Increase the proportion of adults who perform physical activities that enhance and maintain flexibility.

Physical Activity in Children and Adolescents

22-6   Increase the proportion of adolescents who engaged in moderate physical activity for at least 30 minutes on 5 or more of the previous 7 days.

22-7   Increase the proportion of adolescents who engage in vigorous physical activity that promotes cardiorespiratory fitness 3 or more days per week for 20 or more minutes per occasion.

22-8   Increase the proportion of the nation's public and private schools that require daily physical education for all students.

22-9   Increase the proportion of adolescents who participate in daily school physical education.

22-10   Increase the proportion of adolescents who spend at least 50% of school physical education class time being physically active.

22-11   Increase the proportion of adolescents who view television 2 or fewer hours on a school day.

Access

22-12   Increase the proportion of the nation's public and private schools that provide access to their physical activity spaces and facilities for all persons outside of normal school hours (that is, before and after the school day, on weekends, and during summer and other vacations).*

22-13   Increase the proportion of worksites offering employer-sponsored physical activity and fitness programs.

22-14   Increase the proportion of trips made by walking.

22-15   Increase the proportion of trips made by bicycling.

*Developmental objective (i.e., no data source, no baseline data).
Source: DHHS (2000), chap. 22.

activity and physical fitness have figured prominently in these objectives. The main objectives for physical activity pertaining to health status and risk reduction for the year 2010 are listed in Table 11.1 To set realistic national objectives, surveillance systems are necessary to monitor progress. Such systems have only been available since the mid-1980s. These systems (Table 11.2) are best represented by the state-based Behavioral Risk Factor Surveillance System (BRFSS) (CDC, 1998; Marks et al., 1985), the Youth Risk Behavioral Surveiuance System (YRBSS) (CDC, 2008), the School Health Policies and Program Study (SHPPS) (Kann et al. 2007), the National Health Interview Surveys (NHIS) and their supplements on Health Promotion and Disease Prevention (CDC, 2003), as well as the series of National Health and Nutrition Examination Surveys (NHANES I, II, III, IV) and their important follow-up substudies (CDC/NCHS, 2005), and the National Household Travel Surveys (National Household Travel Survey Data, 2001).

EPIDEMIOLOGICAL METHODS

Rates and Proportions

Epidemiologists apply the scientific method to problems of the health sciences. The application of epidemiology requires knowledge of causal factors as they relate to the occurrence of specific health events. This knowledge is often revealed through measures of association that declare suspected causal factors and specific health events.

TABLE 11.2 Summary of U.S. Physical Activity Surveillance Data Sources

Survey	Mode of Data Collection	Target Population	Frequency of Data Collection	Physical Activity Domain(s)
BRFSS	Telephone interview	Adults (>18 years of age) in U.S. states, territories, and the District of Columbia ~240,000 respondents in 2005	Ongoing, annual	Leisure time domestic transportation
NHIS	Personal interview	Adults and children in U.S. states and the District of Columbia ~120,000 respondents in 2004	Ongoing, annual	Leisure time
NHANES	Interview/ examination	Children and adults in the United States ~10,000 respondents in 1999–2000	Ongoing, annual	Leisure time domestic transportation
YRBS	School-based survey	High-school students in the United States >15,000 respondents in 2005	Every 2 years	Leisure time domestic transportation
NHTS	Household survey	U.S. households >25,000 respondents	Every 5 to 7 years	transportation
SHPPS	Mail survey	U.S. school districts, state education organizations, and classrooms	Periodic	Physical activity policies and curricula

The concept of the **web of causation** is an important principle in epidemiology (Last, 2000). The effect of this web may be the result of a complex interaction of causes rather than the result of a single cause (Caspersen, 1989). An important tenet of epidemiology is that effective public health interventions can be carried out without a complete knowledge of the web of causation. Fundamental to understanding the complex nature of a web of causation is assessment of the critical classes of causal factors, which include agent, host, and environment. The **agent** may be one of any number of factors including, but not limited to, genetic or physical (e.g., sunlight, fire, radiation, seat belts), nutritive (excess, deficiency), exogenous chemical (e.g., inhalation, ingestion, skin contact), and physiological or psychological factors, as well as invasive organisms. Personal attributes of the **host** include age, sex, immune status, behavioral attributes (e.g., smoking status, physical activity), race/ethnicity, social class, and genetic predisposition. The **environment** is critical to both the host and agent. Characteristics of the external environment that may influence host-agent interaction include physical (e.g., climate, altitude, urban, rural), biological (e.g., food supply, other animals), and social (e.g., popula-

tion distribution, culture, access to recreation, access to health care) factors.

Disease/Injury Occurrence

Several measures are used to quantify disease, injury, and event occurrence in the population. The **incidence,** or incidence rate, is the number of new cases of disease or injury during a defined period of time, divided by the product of the number of persons monitored during the time period (Savitz, Harris, & Brownson, 1998). Incidence is usually expressed as the number of new cases occurring in a year among a specified population (Kelsey, Whittmore, Evans, & Thompson, 1994). **Cumulative incidence** is the risk of developing a disease over a defined time period, such as 1 year. **Prevalence,** another proportional measure, is expressed as the number of existing cases of disease or injury divided by the total population, with the occurrence of the disease or injury measured at a specific point in time rather than over a certain time period (Savitz, et al., 1998). The prevalence of a disease or injury is influenced both by its incidence and persistence (Kelsey et al., 1994).

If the incidence or prevalence of a condition is known, incidence rates and prevalence rates can be calculated. A **rate** is simply the frequency or number of events that occur over some defined time period, divided by the average size of the population at risk. The usual estimate of the average number of people at risk is the population at the midpoint of the time interval under study. The general formula for a calculating a rate is:

$$\text{Rate} = \frac{\text{Numerator}}{\text{Denominator}} \times \text{Constant}$$

Because rates are usually less than 1, they are generally multiplied by a constant (100, 1,000, or 10,000) for ease of discussion. Therefore, if the death rate in the United States was calculated to be .0090 deaths per year, this could be multiplied by 1,000 and expressed as 9 deaths per 1,000 individuals in the population per year. More simply, when a constant of 100 is used, the rate is a **proportion.**

Prevalence rates are useful for planning purposes. For example, a survey of a city might find that the prevalence of people with coronary heart disease is particularly high; therefore, it may be economically feasible for a local hospital to consider opening a cardiac rehabilitation program. Prevalence data are not useful, however, when trying to determine which factors may be related to an increased probability of disease. High prevalence does not necessarily indicate high risk but could be reflective of increased survival. The high prevalence of coronary heart disease in a city survey may not necessarily indicate that people in that city are at an increased risk of getting coronary heat disease but could be reflective of high-quality emergency services and medical care that increase the rate of survival. In contrast, low prevalence may simply reflect rapid death or rapid cure, not high incidence. When you only have prevalence data, you don't know which of these possibilities is true.

It is particularly important to be sure that the information that you use to make comparisons between groups are actually rates. This may seem obvious, but a number of examples are available in which this fact was overlooked. For example, a sports medicine physician reports that he has seen 100 cases of a torn medial meniscus of the knee in distance runners over the past year. Does this indicate that running is the cause of this problem and that, indeed, it is a large problem that needs to be dealt with? With information only on the number of cases (numerator) and no information regarding the number of people at risk (the denominator) it is impossible to tell. To make these assessments, we need to know how many runners visited the clinic over the course of the year. If 100 runners were seen and 100 cases of torn medial meniscus

were diagnosed, then the incidence would be 100%—a potentially serious problem! On the other hand, if 1,000 runners were seen, the rate would be reduced to 10%—a completely different interpretation. The use of numerator data without considering the size of the population at risk should be avoided; however, numerator data of this nature often can be found in the sports medicine and exercise science literature.

MEASUREMENT OF PHYSICAL ACTIVITY AND FITNESS IN EPIDEMIOLOGICAL STUDIES

Generally, physical activity has been measured in epidemiological studies using three approaches: questionnaires, activity diaries, or direct measurement through either observation or movement technology. Physical activity **questionnaires** ask a respondent to recall and report participation in physical activities, usually over a set period of time. **Diary** assessment of physical activity involves an individual recording all activity for a defined period of time (usually a week or several days). Methods of **observation** include watching and recording playground, park, or facility use during a specified time (e.g., recess, physical education class, set time of day/night) (McKenzie, Marshall, Sallis, & Conway, 2000). **Direct measurement** includes the use of electronic technology (e.g., pedometers, motion detectors, heart rate monitors) designed to record an individual's movements or physiological responses to movement (Chen & Basset, 2005). Once data from each of these assessment methods are gathered, estimates or indicators of energy expenditure can be calculated. U.S. national health surveys typically include a short set of physical activity questions along with many other health-related questions. No national surveys currently use a longer, more detailed physical activity questionnaire, such as those typically used in research studies. In addition to cardiovascular-related physical activities, some national health surveys also query muscle strengthening and flexibility activities (CDC, 1998). Travel and transportation surveys, designed to track individual transportation and movement habits, rely on diaries for information on daily walking and bicycling habits. Measures of physical fitness, in particular measures of cardiorespiratory fitness and aerobic capacity have been used in epidemiological studies examining the relationship between fitness and health outcomes (Blair et al., 1989). Generally, these studies employ the use of either treadmill testing or cycle ergometry, using either maximal or submaximal testing protocols (Blair et al., 1989; Hamalainen et al., 1989).

STUDY DESIGNS IN EPIDEMIOLOGY

Cross-Sectional Study

When attempting to argue an association between a factor and a disease or injury, the least convincing design is **cross-sectional,** in which physical activity or fitness is measured simultaneously with a measure of the frequency of disease, injury, or death. Other risk factors may be measured at the same time. Because this approach is analogous to the "snapshot" in photography (Paffenbarger, 1988), proper temporal sequence is not provided. An example of a physical activity study that uses a cross-sectional approach is the Iowa Farmers Study (Pomrehn, Wallace, & Burneister, 1982), which examined the association of physical activity with mortality. Sixty-two thousand all-cause deaths occurring from 1962 to 1978 in male residents of Iowa aged 20 to 64 years were examined. A randomly selected group of 95 farmers was compared with a group of 158 nonfarmers who lived in a city. Farmers had a 10% lower rate of death due to coronary heart disease, and they were twice as likely to participate in strenuous physical activity compared with the nonfarmers. The farmers also were more fit, as determined by a lower exercise heart rate and longer endurance time on a treadmill test. Because the farmers had higher cholesterol and a higher body mass index, the apparently protective effect attributed to their high activity and fitness could not be explained by lower cholesterol and body mass. In other words, when these known risk factors for CHD were controlled for, the farmers still appeared to benefit directly from their higher fitness levels (i.e., some evidence for independence of the effects of physical activity and fitness was present). However, the farmers had lower estimated body fat, as estimated by skinfold thickness, and their rates of smoking and alcohol consumption were half that of the city dwellers. Therefore, the apparently protective effect of physical activity was not fully independent; it could just as likely be explained by the marked reduction among the farmers in the known risk of smoking and drinking alcohol. Thus, a conclusion that the active lifestyle of the farmers protected against CHD deaths must be accepted with an element of caution.

Another application of the cross-sectional study is in determining the prevalence of selected conditions and health behaviors for the purpose of public health planning and surveillance. For example, through the BRFSS, which is maintained by the Centers for Disease Control and Prevention (CDC), physical activity and other health behaviors are routinely assessed in each of the states (Marks et al., 1985). This information is useful in establishing the current activity patterns among demographic groups and geographic regions. The BRFSS has recently shown that on average about 26% of U.S. adults are inactive during their leisure time (Figure 11.1), failing to meet the recommendations of the U.S. surgeon general (U.S. DHHS, 1996). A wide variation in the prevalence of recommended levels of physical activity among adults across the United States is shown in Figure 11.2, with states in the West most active and states in the Southeast least active (CDC, 2007).

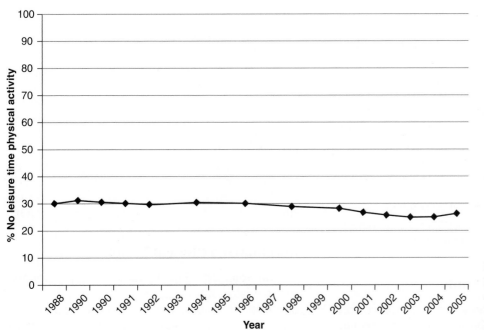

Figure 11.1 Trends in Prevalence of Inactivity Among U.S. Adults 18 Years and Older, 1988–2005. Source: CDC (2007).

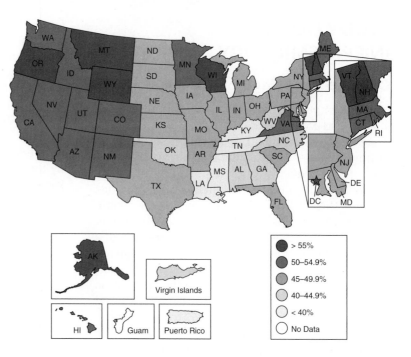

Figure 11.2 Prevalence of Recommended Levels of Physical Activity Among Adults 18 Years and Older, by State, 2005. Source: CDC (2007).

Case-Control Study

When there are no clear suspected causes of a disease, an epidemiologist operates very much like a detective, attempting to piece together causes after the fact. In this situation, the most common design is the retrospective **case-control study.** This approach can be likened to a flashback in cinematography (Paffenbarger, 1988). An example of a retrospective case-control study is the Seattle Heart Watch Study (Siscovick, Weiss, Hallstrom, Inui, & Peterson, 1982), which examined 1,250 cases of sudden cardiac death among men and women, aged 25 to 75 years, living in the Seattle area to determine the association of physical activity habits with risk of sudden cardiac death. Of these cases, 163 were chosen in which the individuals had appeared risk-free prior to the time of their fatal heart attack. Spouses were interviewed about the decedent's physical activity at work and during leisure time during the year preceding death. Each case was paired with a randomly selected control who had similar age, smoking habits, and blood pressure. Low activity on the job and low or moderate activity during leisure were unrelated to death rate. However, people in the top 50% of participants in vigorous leisure physical activities (jogging, climbing stairs, chopping wood, swimming, singles tennis) had just 40% of the risk for sudden cardiac death when compared with individuals who spent no leisure time in those vigorous physical activities (Siscovick et al., 1982).

Prospective Cohort Study

A **prospective cohort study** permits observation of the characteristics and behaviors of a group, or **cohort,**

of people across time. It permits a natural history of physical activity, fitness, and health-related events to be chronicled as they occur, much like a motion picture. Because it is longitudinal, a prospective cohort design enables an investigator to measure physical activity and health-related events at multiple points in time and consequently to test whether an association between physical activity and a low rate of disease is persistent.

The Aerobics Center Longitudinal Study (ACLS) measured physical fitness defined as endurance time on a treadmill test in over 10,000 men and 3,000 women at the time they participated in a preventive medical examination (Blair et al., 1989). The men and women were reexamined about 8 years later. During the period of observation, 240 deaths among men and 43 deaths among women occurred. Age-adjusted death rates from all causes were lower with each successive level of fitness in men from the least fit (64 deaths) to the most fit (19 deaths), and similarly in women from the least fit (40 deaths) to the most fit (9 deaths) (Figure 11.3). The effects of higher fitness were not affected by other factors such as age, smoking, cholesterol concentration, systolic blood pressure, blood sugar, and parental history of coronary heart disease. Much of the decreased total number of deaths was explainable by reduced rates of cardiovascular disease and all-site cancers (Blair et al., 1989).

Randomized Clinical Trials

The **randomized clinical trial** is used to determine whether associations uncovered in epidemiologic observations represent cause-and-effect relations. The validity of the trial depends on having a representative

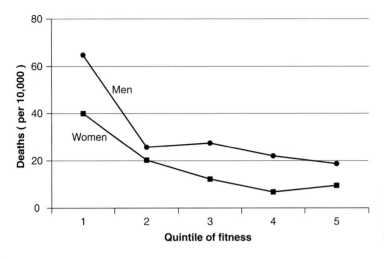

Figure 11.3 Physical Fitness and All-Cause Mortality Among Men and Women: The Aerobics Research Center Longitudinal Study. Source: Adapted from Blair et al. (1989).

population sample and matching treatment and control groups with respect to characteristics thought to affect outcome. The **random assignment** of subjects to the treatment or control group is essential to equally distribute known and unknown confounding variables between groups.

Examples of a randomized study design in exercise science are the secondary prevention trials among heart attack survivors to determine whether exercise training reduces recurrence rates of myocardial infarction and death.

In one study from Finland, 375 men and women who had survived a heart attack at the time of hospitalization were randomized into a multiple risk factor intervention group, which included exercise, or a control group. The intervention group had a significant reduction in total cardiovascular disease mortality and cardiac sudden death but not in repeat heart attacks. However, because there was no evidence of improved physical fitness on bicycle ergometer testing in the intervention group, the independent effect of exercise was not clearly shown (Hamalainen et al., 1989).

In the United States, the National Exercise and Heart Disease Project was carried out in the mid-1970s (LaRosa, cleary, muesing, Gorman, & Hellerstein, 1982). About 651 men aged 30 to 64 years from five medical centers who had suffered a heart attack from 1976 to 1979 were randomly assigned to a control group or to a supervised exercise program. The program consisted of 15 minutes of jogging, cycling, or swimming followed by 25 minutes of aerobic games at an intensity of 85% of maximal exercise heart rate. The men were retested after 9 weeks, after 6 months, and at the end of each year.

The risk of dying of cardiovascular disease during the 4 years following initiation of the study was significantly less likely for the exercise group than for the control group. These reduced risks were not affected by smoking, blood lipids, hypertension, and parental history of CHD (LaRosa et al., 1982).

ASSESSMENT OF CAUSALITY

Community or clinic interventions are based on the presumption that the associations found in epidemiological studies are causal rather than occurring by chance or through some bias. However, in most instances in which epidemiological methods are used to observe health events in the population, the circumstances do not permit the investigator to absolutely prove that an association is causal. Certain criteria have been used in epidemiological research for judging the strength of inference drawn from studies about the cause-and-effect relationship between a factor such as physical inactivity and a disease or injury. These criteria were initially defined by Sir Bradford Hill (1965) and are often cited as a checklist for causality in epidemiological studies.

Strength of Association

The first criterion is that studies show a statistically meaningful **association** (i.e., not likely to be explainable by random or chance observation) between physical activity and lowered prevalence or incidence of disease. The stronger these associations, the less likely it is that they are the result of confounding or bias.

Consistency of Association

Consistency is achieved when the association of increased physical activity or fitness with lower rates of disease is similar for different types of people, in different geographical regions, and when different measures or components of physical activity or fitness are used. Consistency of association makes a particular bias an unlikely explanation for such a series of observations.

Specificity of Association

Even though a study may show a dose-response pattern between increasing levels of physical activity and decreased risk for disease, the pattern of reduced risk seen with increasing levels of physical activity must remain in the presence and in the absence of other potential causes of the disease. An illustration of this criterion, taken from the physical activity and CHD literature, is the Harvard Alumni Study carried out by Dr. Ralph Paffenbarger (Paffenbarger et al., 1978), in which he showed that the health benefits of regular physical activity were persistent among these male alumni even considering the effects of other risk factors such as smoking, obesity, hypertension, and elevated blood lipids.

Temporality

For a lower rate of disease or death associated with higher levels of physical activity or fitness to be interpreted as being possibly caused by activity or fitness, sedentary or unfit participants must be just as health at the onset of the study as are participants judged to be more active or fit. Also, the measurement of activity or fitness must precede the measurement of subsequent events of disease or death.

Biological Gradient

If physical activity exerts a protective effect for reducing disease, injury, or death (or conversely, causing some kinds of injury), it should be possible to determine some pattern of relationship between increasing levels of physical activity and change in the rates of disease, injury, or death. If the rates of events vary randomly across levels of activity or across differing changes in physical activity, an argument that physical activity was causally responsible for such variation would not be convincing. The most convincing pattern is a linear dose-response of activity to decreased occurrence of an outcome (i.e., disease, injury, death) that was proportional to each increment of increased physical activity or physical fitness. It is also possible that the dose-response relationship could be curvilinear, such that each successive increment in physical activity or fitness corresponds with an accelerating change in the rate of disease, injury, or death. A negatively accelerating dose-response would indicate a reduced modification of the benefit. Finally, there may be some minimal level of physical activity or physical fitness that explains all or nearly all of the altered outcome rates. Thus, once the minimal threshold was exceeded, no further change in disease, injury, or death would be observed.

Plausibility

Even when the preceding criteria have been met, the overall case established for cause and effect will remain weak if the association between increased physical activity and decreased disease or death cannot be explained. A convincing explanation requires evidence that physical activity or physical fitness induces biological changes that are consistent with current understanding of the causes and course of development of a disease or condition and the process by which the function of cells and systems deteriorate because of a disease or condition.

Coherence

Once the proper temporal sequence has been established, it is important to determine whether an association seen between physical activity or fitness and disease rates holds as time passes and that the evidence is not contradictory to the known biology and natural history of the disease.

Experimental Evidence

The most compelling evidence that increased physical activity reduces rates of disease or death would come from an experiment conducted in a large group of initially healthy people drawn randomly from a total population, in which the participants would be randomly assigned to at least three levels of physical activity of differing intensity or amount, or to a control group that remained sedentary for several years.

In the absence of a population experiment, confirmation must come from studies of lower animals. Studies using rats, dogs, and nonhuman primates have shown favorable changes in the cardiovascular system after exercise training. In addition, many clinical studies with small groups of humans have shown that physical activity can reduce mild hypertension and alter blood lipids, blood sugar, clotting factors, and white blood cells in positive ways; stimulate bone mineral density; and reduce depression, to name a few benefits. Such clinical experiments are important for demonstrating the health benefits of physical activity. Nonetheless, they cannot demonstrate that the benefits observed for small select groups of people are generalizable to the population as a whole.

Analogy

When many studies find associations between physical activity or fitness and reduced risks of disease or death, it is more likely that each study estimated the same true effect of physical activity. The number of studies finding results that agree determines the confidence with which it can be concluded that physical activity or fitness improves health or longevity. As is the case for the other criteria, the number of studies that agree differs widely according to the disease or health outcome studied. An example of the application of the Hill criterion is the review by Powell and coworkers (Powell, Thompson, Caspersen, & Kendrick, 1987) examining the relationship between physical activity and the incidence of coronary heart disease (CHD). These authors set forth a compelling case for the cause and effect relationship between increasing levels of physical activity and the prevention of CHD (Powell et al., 1987).

CAREERS IN PHYSICAL ACTIVITY AND EXERCISE EPIDEMIOLOGY

Those interested in pursuing physical activity and exercise epidemiology as a career should have undergraduate training in exercise science, kinesiology, social sciences, or life sciences with good quantitative skills and an inquisitive mind.

Most entry-level positions require a master's degree, preferably the Master of Public Health (MPH) in epidemiology, biostatistics, or health promotion. A Master of Science degree in epidemiology, population science, or clinical research is also an acceptable graduate degree for entry-level positions in epidemiology.

Positions for physical activity and exercise epidemiologists with master's or doctoral level training can be found within the following agencies and institutions:

Federal, state, and local public health agencies

Universities and colleges

Nongovernmental health agencies (e.g., American Heart Association, American Cancer Society)

Private and community foundations

Regional and local health care service institutions (e.g., hospitals, clinics, professional organizations)

National, regional, and local foundations and agencies

National, regional, and local park and recreation organizations

SUMMARY

We have observed that the principles of epidemiology can be an important scientific foundation within exercise science, kinesiology, and physical education. Because epidemiology is an eclectic scientific enterprise, it is based on the scientific method and an understanding of potentially causal factors relative to the occurrence of specific health events. The epidemiological measures of rates and proportions, variation in occurrence of disease or injury, and the application of risk all provide the exercise scientist with useful tools in understanding the relationship between physical activity, health outcomes, and other correlates. The methods of study employed by epidemiologists include cross-sectional study designs, case-control studies, prospective cohort designs, and randomized controlled trials, providing the exercise scientist which an array of sources of evidence linking physical activity and exercise to specific health and performance outcomes, all with their inherent strengths and weaknesses. The exercise scientist, thus, has the task of assessing the array of evidence from such studies based on a specific set of criteria to determine the causal link between physical activity, exercise, fitness, and health, and in establishing appropriate and meaningful health policies regarding the role of exercise, fitness, physical activity, and health.

■ Key Resources

Key Journals
American Journal of Epidemiology
American Journal of Health Promotion
American Journal of Preventive Medicine
American Journal of Public Health
British Journal of Sports Medicine
Journal of Physical Activity and Health

Medicine & Science in Sports & Exercise
Preventing Chronic Disease
Preventive Medicine: An International Journal Devoted to Practice and Theory
Research Quarterly for Exercise and Sport

■ Review Questions

1. What is the web of causation?
2. When examining the effects of physical activity interventions among children and youth, what would be considered the strongest study design and why?
3. What is an example of informational bias?
4. What is an example of confounding in research data?
5. What is the definition of the prevalence rate of a condition or behavior in the population?

6. Researchers identify 10 competitive cyclists who suffer severe muscle cramping following a 90-minute ride at 75% of maximal oxygen uptake. Each cyclist is given an experimental sports drink prior to their next 90-minute ride. The researchers identify that following the second 90-minute ride, 80% of the cyclists experience no muscle cramping, while 20% of the cyclists had no improvement with their post-ride muscle cramping. What type of study design does this represent?

7. Researchers are interested in assessing a possible association between living in the space station for 6 months and a reduction of bone mineral density. What is the best study design to assess this possible association?

8. What is an advantage of conducting case-control studies rather than randomized controlled trials?

9. When assessing causality, what are the nine criteria outlined by Sir Bradford Hill?

■ References

Blair, S. N., Kohl, H. W., Paffenbarger, R. S., Jr., Clark, D. G., Cooper, K. H., & Gibbons, L. W. (1989). Physical fitness and all-cause mortality: A prospective study of health men and women. *JAMA* 262, 2395–2401.

Caspersen, C. J. (1989). Physical activity epidemiology: Concepts, methods, and applications to exercise science. *Exercise and Sport Sciences Reviews*, 17, 423–474.

Centers for Disease Control and Prevention. (1998). *Behavioral risk factor surveillance system user's guide*. Atlanta, GA: Author.

Centers for Disease Control and Prevention. (2007). Prevalence of regular physical activity among adults—United States, 2001 and 2005. *Morbidity and Mortality weekly Report*, 56(46), 1209–1212.

Centers for Disease Control and Prevention. (2008). *Youth risk behavior surveillance—United States, 2007*. Surveillance Summaries. MMWR 2008; 57 (No. SS-4). Washington, DC; Author.

Centers for Disease Control and Prevention and National Center for Health Statistics. (2005). *National health and nutrition examination survey questionnaire*. Hyattsville, MD: U.S. Department of Health and Human Services, Centers for Disease Control and Prevention. Retrieved from http://www.cdc.gov/nchs/about/major/nhanes/nhanes99_00.htm

Centers for Disease Control and Prevention and U.S. Department.of Health and Human Services. (2003). NHIS *survey description*. Hyattsville, MD: Division of Health Interview Statistics, National Center for Health Statistics.

Chen, K. Y., & Bassett, D. R., Jr. (2005). The technology of accelerometry-based activity monitors: Current and future. *Medicine & Science in Sports & Exercise*, 37(11 Suppl), S490–500.

Dawber, T. R., Meadors, G. F., Moore, F. E. J. (1951). Epidemiological approaches to heart disease: The Framingham Study. *American Journal of Public Health*, 41, 279–286.

Hamalainen, H., Luurila, O. J., Kallio, V., Knuts, L. F., Arstila, M., & Hakkila, J. (1989). Long-term reduction in sudden deaths after a multifactorial intervention programme in patients with myocardial infarction: 10-year results of a controlled investigation. *European Heart Journal*, 10, 55–62.

Haskell, W. L., Lee, I. M., Pate, R. R., Powell, K. E., Blair, S. N., Franklin, B. A., Macera, C. A., et al. (2007). Physical activity and public health: Updated recommendation for adults from the American College of Sports Medicine and the American Heart Association. *Circulation*, 116, 1–13.

Hill, A. B. (1965). The environment and disease: Association or causation? *Proceedings of the Royal Society of Medicine*, 58, 295–300.

Kann, L., Brener, N. D., & Wechsler, H. (2007). Overview and summary: School health policies and programs study 2006. *Journal of School Health*, 77, 385–397.

Kannel, W. B. (1967). Habitual level of physical activity and risk of coronary heart disease: The Framingham Study. *Canadian Medical Association Journal*, 96, 811–812.

Karvonen, M. J. (1962). Areriosclerosis: Clincial surveys in Finland. *Proceedings, Royal Society of Medicine*, 55, 271–274.

Kelsey, J. L., Whittemore, A. S., Evans, A. S., & Thompson, W. D. (1994). *Methods in observational epidemiology* (2nd ed.). New York: Oxford University Press.

Keys, A. (1967). Epidemiological studies related to coronary heart disease: Characteristics of men aged 40–59 in seven countries. *Acta Medica Scandinavica*, 460(Suppl), 1–392.

LaRosa, J. C., Cleary, P., Muesing, R. A., Gorman, P., Hellerstein, H. K. (1982). Effect of long-term moderate physical exercise on plasma lipoproteins. The National Exercise and Heart Disease Project. *Archives of Internal Medicine*, 142, 2269–2274.

Last, J. M. (2000). *A dictionary of epidemiology* (3rd ed.). New York: Oxford University Press.

Marks, J. S., Hogelin, G. C., Gentry E. M., et al. (1985). The Behavioral Risk Factor Surveys: State-specific prevalence estimates of behavioral risk factors. *American Journal of Medicine*, 1, 1–8.

McGinnis, J. M. (1992). The public health burden of a sedentary lifestyle. *Medicine and Science in Sports and Exercise*, 24(6 Suppl), S196–200.

McKenzie, T. L., Marshall, S. J., Sallis, J. F., & Conway, T. L. (2000). Leisure-time physical activity in school environments: An observational study using SOPLAY. *Preventive Medicine*, 30(1), 70–7.

Montoye, H. J. (1975). *Physical activity and health: An epidemiologic study of an entire community*. Englewood Cliffs, NJ: Prentice-Hall.

Morris, J. N. (1957). *Uses of epidemiology*. London: Churchill Livingstone.

Morris, J. N., & Heady, J. A. (1953). Mortality in relation to the physical activity of work: A preliminary note on experience in middle age British. *Journal of Industrial Medicine*, 10, 245–255.

Morris, J. N., Heady, J. A., Raffle, R. A. B., Roberts, C. G., & Parks, S. W. (1953). Coronary heart disease and physical activity of work. *Lancet*, 2, 1111–1120.

National Household Travel Survey Data, 2001. (2001). Washington, DC: U.S. Department of Transportation, Federal Highway Administration. Retrieved December 18, 2006, from http://nhts.ornl.gov/download.shtml#2001

Paffenbarger, R. S., Jr. (1988). Contributions of epidemiology to exercise science and cardiovascular health. *Medicine and Science in Sports & Exercise*, 20, 426–438.

Paffenbarger, R. S., Jr., Hyde, R. T., & Wing, A. L. (1978). Physical activity as an index of heart attack risk in college alumni. *American Journal of Epidemiology*, 108, 161–175.

Paffenbarger, R. S., Jr., Lauglin, M. E., Gima, A. S., & Black, R. A. (1970). Work activity of longshoremen as related to death from coronary heart disease and stroke. *New England Journal of Medicine*, 282, 1109–1114.

Paffenbarger, R. S., Jr., Wolf, P. A., Notkin, J., & Thorne, M. C. (1966). Chronic disease in former college students: I. Early.precursors of fatal coronary heart disease. *American Journal of Epidemiology*, 83, 314–328.

Pate, R. R., Pratt, M., Blair, S. N., Haskell, W. L., Macera, C. A., Bouchard, C., Buchner, D., et al. (1995). Physical activity and public health: A recommendation from the Centers for Disease Control and Prevention and the American College of Sports Medicine. *Journal of the American Medical Association*, 273, 402–407.

Pomrehn, P. R., Wallace, R. B., & Burneister, L. F. (1982). Ischemic heart disease mortality in Iowa farmers. The influence of lifestyle. JAMA, 248, 1073–1076.

Powell, K. E., Thompson, P. D., Caspersen, C. J., & Kendrick, J. S. (1987). Physical activity and the incidence of coronary heart disease. Annual Review of Public Health, 8, 253–287.

Savitz, D. A., Harris, R. P., & Brownson, R. C. (1998). Methods in chronic disease epidemiology. In R. C. Brownson, P. L. Remington, & J. R. Davis (Eds.). Chronic disease epidemiology and control (pp. 27–54). Washington DC: American Public Health Association.

Siscovick, D. S., Weiss, N. S., Hallstrom, A. P., Inui, T. S., & Peterson, D. R. (1982). Physical activity and primary cardiac arrest. JAMA, 248, 3113–3117.

Taylor, H. L., Blackburn, H., Puchner, V., Parlin, R. W., & Keys, A. (1969). Coronary heart disease in selected occupations of American railroads in relation to physical activity. Circulation, 40(Suppl 3), 202.

U.S. Department.of Health and Human Services. (1996). Physical activity and health: A report of the surgeon general. Atlanta, GA: U.S. Department.of Health and Human Services, Centers for Disease Control and Prevention, National Center for Chronic Disease Prevention and Health Promotion.

U.S. Department of Health and Human Services. (2000). Healthy people 2010: Understanding and improving health (2nd ed.). Washington, DC: U.S. Government Printing Office.

CHAPTER 12

Laws That Affect Exercise Science

Dan Connaughton, PhD, University of Florida
Thomas Baker, JD, PhD, University of Georgia

■ Chapter Objectives

After reading this chapter, you should be able to:

1. Understand how certain areas of the law affect exercise science professionals.
2. Understand the basics of civil law and the steps in a civil lawsuit.
3. Understand the basics concepts of negligence, defenses of negligence, and risk management.
4. Understand the importance of being aware of, and operating within, the law as it applies to the field of exercise science.
5. Recognize some of the journals and professional literature that publish legal information and research regarding exercise science.
6. Identify professional organizations that involve law and exercise science.

■ Key Terms

civil law
contract
intentional

negligence
risk management
standard of care

strict liability
waiver

This chapter briefly introduces major areas of law that affect the exercise science field. In today's litigious society, exercise science professionals can benefit from understanding and operating within the law; however, few academic programs require a legal aspects course. Research has revealed that the majority of academic programs (84% of undergraduate and 68% of graduate) in exercise science or related areas that prepare students for employment in the health/fitness field, do not offer, or require their students to take, a legal aspects course (Eickhoff-Shemek & Evans, 2000).

In addition to the law, it is important for the exercise science professional to know where to obtain legal and risk management information. Professional associations publish standards and guidelines that can be used to demonstrate the standard of care owed to clients, athletes, and health/fitness club members. The general information presented in this chapter in not intended as a substitute for legal advice. Specific legal advice should be obtained from a competent attorney in your jurisdiction. However, acquiring the knowledge in this chapter will help you to communicate better with legal counsel and may assist you in reducing liability.

OVERVIEW OF THE UNITED STATES LEGAL SYSTEM

In the United States, three levels of government exist: local, state and federal. Each level is comprised of three branches that create laws: executive, legislative, and judicial. Within the judicial system, criminal and civil matters are litigated.

Criminal and Civil Law

Both criminal and civil law attempt to encourage people to act for the benefit of society. However, they differ in their means of accomplishing this.

CRIMINAL LAW The body of state and federal law that declares what conduct is criminal and prescribes penalties for violating the law is known as criminal law. In criminal courts, which hear cases concerning the alleged commission of misdemeanors and felonies, the people (society) are represented by the government (district attorney). To convict a criminal, it must be shown that the person committed the crime beyond a reasonable doubt. A convicted criminal may be punished by community service, fines, imprisonment, or, in some cases, death. For all practical purposes, the victim of a crime will leave the courtroom empty-handed.

CIVIL LAW Civil law, in contrast, is the body of state and federal law that pertains to civil, or private,

rights that are enforced by civil actions. The vast majority of lawsuits involving exercise science involve civil law. Civil courts hear noncriminal matters between individuals, businesses, organizations, and governmental units and agencies; however, it is possible for a person to face both a criminal trial and a civil trial for the same wrongful action. The two parties involved in a civil lawsuit are the plaintiff (e.g., the participants injured in a sport event who are bringing the lawsuit) and the defendant the plaintiff is suing (e.g., the coaches and athletic director). Often several defendants are named in a civil suit. A plaintiff suing in civil court only has to show by a preponderance (a greater amount) of evidence that the defendant is guilty (liable). The criminal law standard requires that a jury finds the criminal 100% guilty whereas the civil standard only requires the jury to find the defendant 51% guilty (responsible) (Fried, 2007). As opposed to in a criminal trial, the victim (plaintiff) may leave the courtroom with a verdict that will require the defendant to provide financial compensation to the plaintiff or to right (correct) the alleged wrong.

Anatomy of a Civil Lawsuit

A civil lawsuit starts with filing a complaint. This document, which initiates a lawsuit, provides the facts the plaintiffs believe justify their claim and requests damages, or other relief, that they are seeking from the defendant. Typically, the complaint is served via a summons, often delivered by a court officer, which informs the defendant that a lawsuit has been filed against him or her and gives the defendant a certain time period to respond to the complaint.

Upon receipt of the complaint, a defendant will often retain the services of an attorney who will represent his or her interests. The defendant's attorney normally files an answer, which typically denies some or all of the allegations in the complaint. The complaint and answer combined are termed pleadings.

After these initial pleadings, the case proceeds to what is commonly known as the discovery phase. The period of discovery encompasses the time period from filing the answer to the beginning of the actual trial. This pretrial procedure is when the parties acquire facts and information regarding the case, including from the other parties, to assist in preparing for trial. Common discovery techniques are requests to produce physical evidence, interrogatories, and depositions. A request to produce evidence is a request by one party to another to produce, and allow for the inspection of, any designated physical evidence that the party currently controls or possesses, and that is believed to be pertinent to the case. For example, it is not uncommon for attorneys to request to examine equipment (e.g., a treadmill, swimming pool, gymnasium) that was used by a plaintiff at the time of an injury or death. Documents such as preparticipation questionnaires, medical records, health history questionnaires, parental permission forms, accident/incident reports, facility and equipment inspection/maintenance records, informed consents, and waivers may also be requested. An interrogatory is a set of written questions sent by an attorney from one party in the lawsuit to another party named in the suit. The questions must be answered within a specified time period, and the answers may be used as evidence in a later trial. A deposition is an out-of-court, pretrial questioning of a witness. Attorneys representing both parties are usually present at depositions, and the witness answers questions, under oath, that are recorded by a court stenographer. Similar to interrogatories, deposition transcripts also may be used as evidence at a trial.

If there are no disputes over the facts of the case that need to be resolved, the case may be decided without having to go to trial. In a motion for summary judgment, the moving party (the one making the request) argues that there is no question of material fact and therefore the party is entitled to judgment as a matter of law. This motion may be requested at any time, but it is typically brought after discovery, when a party believes discovery has shown that there are no real disputes as to the facts. If the motion is granted, a trial will not occur.

Usually, any party or the court can request a pretrial conference or hearing, which typically takes place after the discovery process is complete. The primary purpose of these informal conferences is to identify the matters in dispute and to plan the course of the trial. At a pretrial hearing, a judge can encourage the parties to attempt an out-of-court settlement. If a settlement cannot be reached, the case typically proceeds to trial.

In a civil trial, the plaintiff typically can choose whether the case will be heard by a jury or not. The plaintiff provides the opening statement, which may be followed by the defendant's opening statement, and is designed to inform the triers of fact (the judge or the jury) about the case and what types of evidence will be presented during the trial. After opening statements, the plaintiff presents his or her case first. The plaintiff calls witnesses and examines them. Typically, the witnesses are then cross-examined by the defendant, redirected by the plaintiff, and then recrossed by the defendant. The defendant then repeats the process previously described with his or her witnesses.

During a trial, two types of witnesses are often called. Fact witnesses are utilized because they had specific facts (maybe something they saw or heard) regarding the lawsuit. Expert witnesses are called to educate the judge or jury by sharing their expertise and knowledge. Expert witnesses are often asked to testify regarding the professional standards that apply to the incident in question and to the degree that the defendant met those standards. For example,

an exercise science expert could be called to testify on the legal standards imposed on fitness club directors in a case concerning a fitness club injury.

Once both sides have finished their questioning, final closing statements are made with the defendant proceeding first. Following these final statements, the judge, in a jury trial, gives the jury instructions regarding the options they have in reaching a decision based on the applicable laws. After deliberating, the jury renders a verdict. In a trial without a jury, the judge may either recess the court while making a decision or render a decision directly after closing statements.

Verdicts rendered by lower level courts can be appealed. The party that lost the case can make a request to have the initial proceedings reviewed by a higher court in hope that the lower court's decision will be reversed. The appellate court may agree with (affirm) the lower court's decision, disagree with (reverse) it, send it back to the lower court (remand) for a new trial, or modify the lower court's judgment in some manner (Fried, 2007; Wong, 2002).

TORT LAW

Tort law, an area of civil law, involves an infringement (a civil wrong) by one person of the legally recognized rights of another. The infringement (conduct that is an error or omission of certain conduct) can be categorized according to three levels of fault (Keeton, Dobbs, Keeton, & Owen, 1984). First, **intentional** requires the legal "intent" to harm. Second, **negligence** requires the plaintiff's harm to have occurred by an unintentional act or unintentional inaction. Third, **strict liability** does not require any level of fault; it is liability without fault. Intentional torts and strict liability are each briefly discussed; negligence is given more attention because liability associated with negligence is generally more of a concern for the exercise science professional than liability due to intentional conduct or strict liability.

Intentional Torts

Intentional torts can be classified as follows: (a) disturbances of intangible interests, such as invasion of privacy and defamation (libel and slander); (b) interference with property, such as trespass to land, trespass to chattels (property other than land); and (c) interference with person, such as assault, battery, and false imprisonment (van der Smissen, 1990). Intentional torts require the legal "intent" to harm, which means that it was the purpose of the wrongdoer to bring about a certain harm or that the wrongdoer knew that harm was substantially certain to happen (Keeton et al., 1984). Though it is beyond the scope of this chapter to discuss intentional torts in detail, it is important to note that a victim of an intentional tort could file a civil lawsuit against the person who committed the act (the defendant). Furthermore, the government could also prosecute the defendant in criminal court if the conduct also violated a state or federal statute. For example, a personal trainer who assaults his client could face a civil lawsuit (e.g., a battery claim made by the client) as well as criminal charges.

It is also important to note that the doctrine of *respondeat superior* (in which an employer could be held liable for the "negligent" actions of his or her employees) only applies to intentional acts committed during the scope of employment. For instance, in most cases the employer could not be held liable for an intentional tort such as battery committed by one of its employees. However, if the battery took place within the parameters of the employee's job duties, the employer could be sued and held liable. Furthermore, if the employer had knowledge that such conduct was occurring and chose to do nothing about it, or if the employer negligently hired the employee, the employer also could be held liable.

Negligence

The vast majority of lawsuits brought against exercise science professionals allege negligence on the part of the exercise science facility owner, administration, or staff. Allegations have included, but are not limited to, the failure to provide reasonable (1) exercise instruction, (2) exercise progression, (3) supervision, (4) inspection and/or maintenance of exercise equipment, (5) warnings regarding the risks associated with physical activity, (6) screening of participants prior to engaging in physical activity programs, and (7) emergency medical planning and care.

According to Dougherty, Goldberger, and Carpenter (2007), "negligence is essentially failing to do something that a reasonable, prudent and up-to-date person would have done under the same or similar circumstances or doing something that a reasonable, prudent and up-to-date person would not have done. Negligence may therefore arise from an act of omission or commission" (p. 187). To hold a defendant liable for negligence, all four elements of negligence must be shown by the plaintiff. These include a legal duty, the act, causation, and damage or harm (van der Smissen, 2007).

Duty arises from a special relationship between the exercise science professional and the participant that requires the exercise science professional to protect the participant from exposure to unreasonable risk that may cause injury (van der Smissen, 2007). Although a special relationship may exist, it also must be shown that the defendant should have been able to predict the possibility of an injury under the circumstances in question. In other words, the

exercise science professional (fitness director, aerobics instructor, personal trainer, etc.) should have realized that an exercise science participant might suffer some type of harm. This is known as *foreseeability* (Dougherty et al., 2007). One is not typically liable for injuries that were not foreseeable.

The act (also known as the breach of duty) is the error, or omission (failure to act), that injured the participant. The major issue is essentially whether the defendant failed to act reasonably under the specific circumstances at the time of the incident. In reaching its decision, the court will apply the "reasonable person" test to determine if the **standard of care** was met under the circumstances. Determination of negligent conduct is made by comparing the defendant's behavior against the conduct of a hypothetical, ordinary, reasonable, and prudent person under like or similar circumstances. In other words, the court will consider what a typical, reasonable person would have done in the same circumstances. How that hypothetical person would have acted will be considered in a negligence case. However, in the case of a professional, he or she will not be judged as a typical individual but rather as a member of a specified class. When acting in a professional capacity, the exercise science professional (program director, fitness instructor, personal trainer, etc.) will be judged by the standards of the profession that were in existence at the time of the incident.

In general terms, standards describe the level of care that is owed to participants that reasonably protect their health and safety (Napolitano, 1997). The standard of care may be determined by legislation, by organizations and associations, or by the profession. When published standards do not exist, the practices of the profession are often considered the norm. Typically, expert witnesses will attest to the accepted, desirable practices and standards. Therefore, the standard of care provided by exercise science professionals should be that of the best professional practices (van der Smissen, 1990). In an attempt to provide this, it is necessary for exercise science professionals to stay abreast of the developments and modifications to the ever-changing standard of care. It is important to be well versed and current regarding the newest and best practices. Several professional associations in the exercise science field have published position statements, standards, and guidelines that are frequently referenced in court to attack or defend a defendant's conduct. For example, the National Athletic Trainers' Association (2006) has published several position statements including for (a) emergency planning in athletics, (b) lightning safety for athletics and recreation, and (c) exertional heat illnesses.

Of particular relevance to health/fitness professionals is the ACSM's *Health/Fitness Facility Standards and Guidelines* (Tharrett, McInnis, & Peterson, 2007), which includes 21 standards and 36 guidelines. It states that standards "are base performance criteria or minimum requirements that ACSM believes each health/fitness facility must meet to satisfy a facility's obligation to provide a relatively safe environment in which every physical activity or program is conducted in an appropriate manner" (p. xi). Furthermore, guidelines "are recommendations that ACSM believes health and fitness operators should consider using to improve the quality of service they provide to users. Such guidelines are not standards, nor are they applicable in every situation or circumstance; rather, they are illustrative tools that ACSM believes should be considered by health and fitness operators" (p. xi).

In addition, the following statements, standards, and guidelines regarding exercise science could be utilized in court to help establish the standard of care in exercise science lawsuits:

> *American College of Sports Medicine Guidelines for Exercise Testing and Prescription* (American College of Sports Medicine, 2006)
>
> "Recommendations for Cardiovascular Screening, Staffing, and Emergency Policies at Health/Fitness Facilities" (American College of Sports Medicine and American Heart Association Joint Position Statement, 1998)
>
> "Automated External Defibrillators in Health/Fitness Facilities" (American College of Sports Medicine and American Heart Association Joint Position Statement, 2002)
>
> NSCA *Strength & Conditioning Professional Standards & Guidelines* (National Strength and Conditioning Association, 2001)
>
> "IHRSA Club Membership Standards" (International Health, Racquet and Sportsclub Association, 2005)
>
> *Canadian Fitness Safety Standards & Recommended Guidelines* (Ontario Association of Sport and Exercise Sciences, 2004)
>
> *The Medical Fitness Model: Facility Standards and Guidelines* (Medical Fitness Association, 2006)
>
> *Exercise Standards & Guidelines Reference Manual* (Aerobics and Fitness Association of America, 2005).
>
> *Medical Advisory Committee Recommendations: A Resource Guide for YMCAs* (YMCA of the USA, 2007)

Compliance with such position statements, standards, and guidelines will not guarantee that exercise science participants won't get injured. However, in a lawsuit, standards published by professional associations can be introduced as evidence to establish the standard of care, as is often done in other professions

such as medicine. In an effort to support or attack a defendant's conduct, which allegedly caused the injury, an expert witness will often compare the defendant's conduct to published professional standards. Proof of adherence to such standards could be extremely helpful in defending a negligence claim, or even in discouraging or preventing lawsuits from being filed. Exercise science professionals can stay abreast regarding current standards and other important legal-related developments in the field by attending professional conferences and workshops, reading relevant literature, and maintaining appropriate certifications through continuing education (van der Smissen, 2007).

To show negligence, the defendant's act, which did not meet the standard of care that a prudent person should have provided, must have actually caused or aggravated the plaintiff's injury. This is referred to as *causation*. Just because the standard of care was not met does not mean the defendant was negligent. For example, a fitness instructor may have given a health club member improper instructions for performing a certain exercise, but inadequate instruction may not have been the cause of the member's injury.

Finally, the act, or inaction, must have resulted in damages or losses to the plaintiff. Often, in exercise science cases, this is bodily injury or emotional harm. There is no liability if there is no damage. Plaintiffs can be compensated for injuries that resulted in physical impairment, physical pain and suffering, emotional distress, or economic loss (van der Smissen, 2007).

Defenses to Claims of Negligence

The fact that an exercise science business or professional is sued does not necessarily mean he or she will be held liable. Several effective defenses to negligence claims can be utilized by a defendant. Some of these defenses are based on common, statutory, and contract law (Cotten, 2007).

Common law defense examples include proving that one or more of the elements required for negligence does not exist, assumption of risk, and governmental immunity. If any of the elements of negligence, as previously described, do not exist, a court cannot impose liability for negligence. Primary assumption of risk involves the plaintiff assuming known risks that are inherent to participating in the activity. For example, when participants know and understand the inherent risks involved in fitness testing and they voluntarily participate, they assume those inherent risks and the exercise science program and staff are not liable, absent negligence on their parts, for injuries resulting from those inherent risks. The following three elements must exist to successfully utilize the primary assumption of risk defense: (a) the risk was inherent

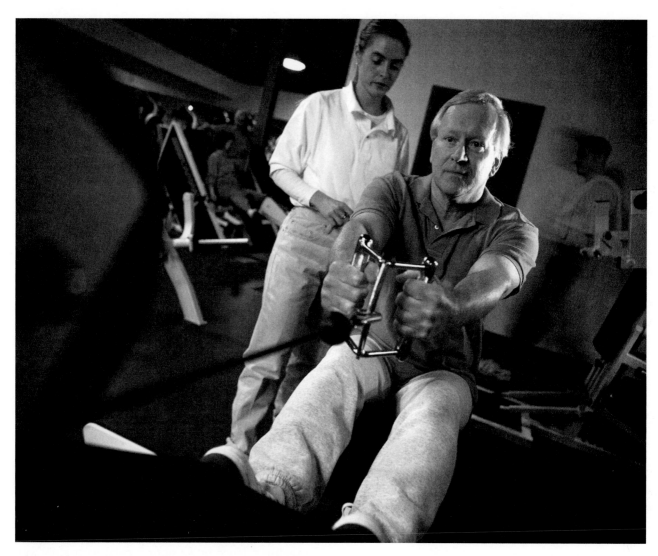

When a client is injured, inadequate instruction or supervision are frequent allegations in lawsuits filed against health/fitness professionals.

to the activity, (b) the participant voluntarily agreed to participate, and (c) the participant knew, understood, and appreciated the inherent risks. An effective method of meeting these requirements is through the use of informed consent and agreement to participate forms (Cotten, 2007).

Governmental immunity originally barred lawsuits against governmental entities, although not, usually, against their employees individually. However, the federal and state governments have approved varying degrees of tort claims legislation that permit injured parties to sue governmental entities under certain circumstances (Dougherty et al., 2007).

Defenses based on statutory law include statute of limitations and comparative fault. The statute of limitations limits the amount of time an injured party has to file suit. The time limitations vary among states and depend on the type of claim. Many states allow 1 to 3 years to file a tort claim (Cotten, 2007).

Although not a true negligence defense, comparative fault is a manner for apportioning damages based on the responsibility (fault) for the injury. A jury will compare the fault of both the defendant and the plaintiff, and then allocate liability by percentage. For example, if a jury award was $100,000 and the fault was apportioned 25% to the plaintiff and 75% to the defendant, the plaintiff would receive $75,000. Comparative negligence schemes vary from state to state, and many states bar recovery if the fault of the plaintiff is 50% or higher (Cotten, 2007).

Contributory fault, previously known as contributory negligence, occurs when the plaintiff's conduct, in any manner, helped to cause or aggravate the plaintiff's own injuries. For states that use this doctrine, it acts as a complete bar to recovery if the plaintiff is negligent and the plaintiff's negligence, no matter how minor, contributed to the harm (Cotten, 2007). Very few states still use contributory fault because its all-or-nothing approach can lead to very harsh results. The vast majority of states instead use a comparative fault system.

Defenses based on contract law include the use of waivers, independent contractors, and facility lease agreements. A waiver, or release of liability, is a contract in which the signer agrees to relinquish the right to sue the exercise science provider in the event that the exercise science provider's ordinary negligence caused an injury to the signer. Validity of waivers varies greatly from state to state. In addition, waivers must be properly written and administered to be legally upheld. The use of independent contractors also may provide an effective defense from negligence claims. Typically, if an injury occurs due to the negligence of an independent contractor, the liability for that injury is shifted from the exercise science program to the independent contractor. For example, many personal trainers are independent contractors rather than employees. Accordingly, health/fitness facilities are generally not liable for the negligent acts committed by personal trainers who are independent contactors. A facility lease agreement may be useful for exercise science facility owners/operators who permit other individuals to use their facilities. For example, a local youth sports team may request to use an exercise science facility (e.g., gymnasium, weight room, exercise testing laboratory) to conduct a practice, workout, or assessment. Waivers and facility lease agreements must be carefully drafted and should always be approved by an attorney prior to use (Cotten, 2007).

Strict Liability

Strict liability is a term given for liability regardless of fault. This means that plaintiffs using strict liability as a basis for their lawsuit, rather than ordinary negligence, need not prove that the defendant acted wrongfully in order to prevail in court. Numerous circumstances exist where strict liability would apply. The following three examples will be briefly discussed: (a) product liability, (b) workers compensation, and (c) *respondeat superior*. There are several theories of strict liability for product-related injuries, but perhaps the most important is strict liability for unsafe products. For example, manufacturers of fitness equipment can be held strictly liable for defective products if they are manufactured with a defect. Strict liability, however, is not available if the defect is found in the design of the product rather than the manufacturing of the product. In design defect cases, plaintiffs must base their claims in negligence. A defect is anything that renders a product unreasonably dangerous (Keeton et al., 1984). It is important to realize that not all fitness equipment-related injuries are due to manufacturer defects. For instance, they also may be caused by the negligence of the exercise science professional for not providing proper instruction, supervision, or maintenance.

Workers' compensation is a form of strict liability that is imposed on the employer without fault. Workers' compensation covers an employee for employment-related injuries that arise out, and in the course, of employment. If an employee of an exercise science program is injured while on the job, the employee receives a fixed amount of compensation (e.g., medical expenses, a part of lost wages). Workers' compensation laws benefit both the employee and the employer. The employee receives some compensation without the time, inconvenience, and risk associated with a negligence lawsuit that he or she might not win, and the employee is not allowed to sue the employer for negligence, thereby protecting the employer from potentially large costs.

Under the doctrine of *respondeat superior*, an employer can be held strictly liable for an employee's negligence that occurred within the scope of employment. Because of this, it is important that managers and owners of exercise science facilities develop operating procedures that reflect the legal duties that exercise science programs have, and then provide proper training and supervision of employees to help ensure that they are effectively carrying out those procedures.

CONTRACT LAW

Contract law is another area of civil law that is an integral part of the exercise science field. For example, exercise science professionals need to comply with contract law when making equipment purchases, obtaining insurance coverage, utilizing waivers, and negotiating employee contracts. Other common exercise science-related contract examples may include facility rental agreements, personal training packages, and event contracts.

What Is a Contract?

Simply put, a **contract** is an agreement that can be enforced in court. Typically, a contract is formed when two (or more) parties exchange binding promises. When making a promise, a party states that he or she will, or will not, take a specified action in the future. If that promise is not performed, the contract has been breached and the party that did not keep the promise must compensate the party to whom the promise was made. The nonperforming party is often required to pay financial damages for the failure to perform the promise. In some situations a court instead may require actual performance of the promised act. However, in many cases when a contract is breached, the parties agree to some acceptable alternative without litigation and the payment of damages (Carper, Mietus, & West, 2000).

Contract law varies between states and among major types of businesses. Contracts are often based on common law (court decisions) and specialized statutes for certain types of contracts (e.g., real estate transactions, insurance policies, employment contracts). Many contracts involve the sale or purchase of goods, which are governed by the *Uniform Commercial Code* (American Law Institute, 1987). All states have adopted, at least in part, the UCC as an element of their statutory law. Since the UCC does not attempt to answer every contract question, common law rules provide answers to most contract questions. Additionally, although the *Restatement of the Law of Contracts* (American Law Institute, 1981) does not have the force of law, it is a highly persuasive summary that provides guidance and clarity for the U.S. common law of contracts.

Four Elements of a Valid Contract

The following four elements must be met for a contract to be considered valid. If any of these elements are absent, a contract will not have been legally formed.

Agreement. An agreement to form a contract includes an offer and an acceptance. One party must offer into a legal agreement and another party must accept the terms of the offer.

Consideration. Any promises made by the parties to the contract must be supported by legally sufficient and bargained-for consideration (something of value received or promised, such as money, to convince a person to make a deal).

Contractual capacity. Both parties entering into the contract must have contractual capacity to do so; the law must recognize them as possessing characteristics that qualify them as competent parties.

Legality. The contract's purpose must be to accomplish some goal that is legal and not against public policy. (Clarkson, Miller, Jentz, & Cross, 2001, p. 199)

Types/Classifications of Contracts

In the majority of contracts, both parties exchange promises. These types of agreements are known as bilateral contracts: a promise made in exchange for another promise. For example, a personal trainer promises to provide several private training sessions to a client in exchange for the client's promise to pay the trainer a set amount of money. Bilateral contracts are the most common type of contract utilized in the exercise science field. In comparison, a unilateral contract involves a promise in exchange of an act. This occurs when one party makes a promise to induce some completed act by another party. For example, a health club offers members a free, 2-week membership extension for every new member they refer to the club. No member is legally obliged to refer members, nor is the facility obliged to extend memberships by 2 weeks unless the requested act is performed.

VOID, VOIDABLE, AND UNENFORCEABLE CONTRACTS A contract must comply with certain essential elements for it to be legally valid. If the effort to create a contract is totally ineffective, there is no contract, but rather a void agreement. An example would be the agreement to commit a theft or other crime.

If an essential element of a valid contract is absent, the contract is considered to be *voidable* and either party may withdraw without liability. For example, a minor (less than 18 years old) can typically void a contract even if freely and intentionally made.

A contract will be considered unenforceable if it violates a statute or is contrary to public policy. For example, agreements that contemplate violating statutory laws such as antitrust or tax laws, or the commission of torts such as fraud or defamation, may be declared illegal and unenforceable (Sharp, 2007).

A legally valid contract must be made with mutual assent. Assent can be negated if either party acted under duress or because of undue influence. Assent will also be negated if it resulted from fraud or certain mistakes. Duress can occur when one party is unfairly persuaded or coerced by a wrongful act or threat from the other party. The threats to rescind an employee contract or to physically harm are examples. A victim of duress can typically choose to carry out the contract or cancel the contract.

Undue influence, although often more peaceful and subtler than duress, can have the same effect. Wrongful persuasion and persistent pressure may deprive a party from exercising sound judgment and free will. This can occur when one party is in a position of authority over the other (e.g., a health club owner and a fitness instructor) and unfairly exploits the victim's trust and confidence when entering a contract.

Misrepresentation is a false assertion of fact that induces a party to enter into a contract. The misrepresentation may be intentional and fraudulent or unintentional and a mistake. If the misrepresentation is fraudulent, the victim has the option of canceling the contract without liability. If the misrepresentation was innocent, the party that relied on the misrepresentation may cancel the contract with no penalty; however, this must be done promptly upon discovering the true facts (Sharp, 2007).

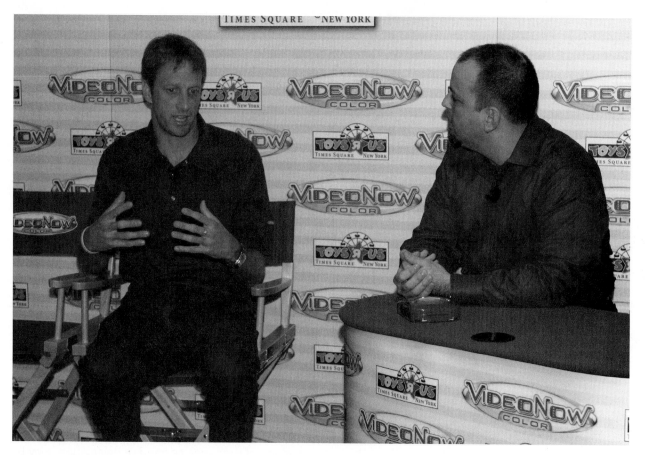

Professional athletes frequently enter into contractual agreements to endorse products and make public appearances.

When both parties have a false understanding about a fact that is an important element to the contract, there is a bilateral mistake that typically makes the contract voidable by either party. In other words, when both parties are mistaken about an important fact, either party may cancel the contract without penalty. A unilateral mistake occurs when just one party is mistaken about a vital fact. In these situations, the contract may not be voided if the mistaken party assumed the risk of mistake. For example, if the mistake should have been detected and was not, then the party that is mistaken may still be bound by the mistake.

Breach of Contract

Except in unusual cases, a breach of contract is not a crime or a tort. If litigation becomes necessary, the breaching party can be required by a court to pay compensatory damages. These compensatory (monetary) damages are designed to put the victim in essentially the same economic position that would have resulted from the performance of the contract. A damaged party's ability to recover damages for such a breach is limited by his or her duty to mitigate. The party may not collect for damages that he or she allowed to accumulate or those that may have reasonably been avoided (Sharp, 2007).

If financial damages are inadequate, a court may require a party to fulfill the specific performance of the contract. This is sometimes granted when the interest involves land or the sale of goods that are very rare or unique (e.g., limited sports memorabilia). On the other hand, courts will not usually require a contract for personal services such as personal training to be specifically performed (Sharp, 2007).

Specific Applications of Contract Law in the Exercise Science Field

There are many specific examples in which contract law applies to the exercise science field. Three of these are discussed briefly here: waivers, independent contractors, and purchasing/leasing equipment.

WAIVERS Prior to participation, many exercise science programs require their participants to sign a **waiver.** When someone signs a waiver, he or she agrees to release the exercise science program for any liability associated with negligence on the part of the exercise science program or its employees. The exculpatory clause within the waiver contains specific language that releases the exercise science program from its own negligence.

The four requirements of a legal contract are applied to waivers as follows:

Agreement. The exercise science program offers to enter into a legal agreement and the participant accepts.

Consideration. The participant receives all the services included in the program (the promises) in exchange for giving up (waiving) his or her right to file a negligence claim against the exercise science programs.

Contractual capacity. Minors, mentally incompetent, or intoxicated individuals do not have contractual capacity and therefore should not be allowed to sign waivers.

Legality. The waiver must be lawful and not against public policy.

Contractual capacity and legality are issues that often arise in waiver cases.

Regarding contractual capacity, some states allow minors to waive their rights if their signature is accompanied by the signature(s) of their adult parent(s) or legal guardians. In many jurisdictions, minors cannot be bound by a waiver they sign, even if there is also parental or guardian authorization. In these jurisdictions, a minor upon reaching the age of majority (18 years old) can disaffirm (or void) the waiver (Cotten & Cotten, 2000). Therefore, it is recommended that minors (and their parents) sign a participation agreement, which is a document that specifies the types of inherent injuries that can occur by participating in sports or physical activity. This document can assist with an assumption of risk defense for an exercise science program if a child or parent claims he or she was unaware of the inherent risks and should have been informed of them. It does not, however, protect an exercise science program from its own negligence.

In many waiver cases, courts have ruled the exculpatory clause unenforceable because it did meet the requirements of a legal contract. Courts carefully examine the words utilized in the exculpatory clause. For a waiver to be upheld, it must clearly and unequivocally express the intention of the exercise science program to absolve itself from its own negligence. It is recommended that the word *negligence* be included in the exculpatory clause to minimize any ambiguity. However, state laws vary regarding how explicit the exculpatory clause needs to be in order to be enforceable. In addition to a waiver's specific wording, courts will also determine whether or not the exculpatory clause was conspicuous. Courts have ruled exculpatory clauses embedded within lengthy membership contracts, or other contracts, unenforceable because they were not conspicuous to the reader. It is therefore recommended that waivers be separate, stand-alone documents. They should be very conspicuous in

a large font and bold lettering, and titled something like "WAIVER—READ BEFORE SIGNING."

In addition to claims that an exculpatory clause was ambiguous or inconspicuous, plaintiffs also have alleged that a waiver did not meet the legality requirement of a contract because it was against public policy. Public policy refers to something that is in the best interest of the public as a whole or is an essential service to the public as a whole (Cotten & Cotten, 2000). Courts rely on many different factors to determine whether a waiver is against public policy (*Tunkl v. Regents of University of California*, 1963). One of such factor (the party seeking exculpation is performing a service of great importance) often arises in waiver cases involving health/fitness clubs. When examining this factor, courts typically have ruled that the services provided by health/fitness club facilities are not against public policy because they do not provide an essential service to the public as a whole.

INDEPENDENT CONTRACTORS Many fitness facilities utilize independent contractors to carry out various programs and services. For example, independent contractors often teach group exercise classes, serve as personal trainers, and maintain or clean facilities. As previously discussed, under *respondeat superior*, employers can be held liable for the negligent acts of their employees. Because independent contractors are not employees, *respondeat superior* would not apply. However, if a court determines that an independent contractor was indeed an employee, the employer could be liable for the negligent acts of the independent contractor. Courts often consider the following questions when determining whether a worker was an employee or independent contractor (Clarkson et al., 2001, pp. 573–574):

1. How much control can the employer exercise over the details of the work? If an employer can exercise considerable control over the details of the work and the day-to-day activities of the worker, this often indicates employee status. This is perhaps the most important factor weighed by the courts in determining employee status.
2. Is the worker engaged in an occupation or business distinct from that of the employer? If so, this points to independent contractor status, not employee.
3. Is the work usually done under the employer's direction or by a specialist without supervision? If the work is usually done under the employer's direction, this typically indicates employee status.
4. Does the employer supply the tools at the place of work? If so, this may indicate employee status.

5. For how long is the person employed? If the person is employed for a long period of time, this often indicates employee status.
6. What is the method of payment—a set time period or at the completion of the job? Payment by time period, such as once every 2 weeks or once a month, typically indicates employee status.
7. What degree of skill is required of the worker? If a great degree of skill is required, this may indicate that the person is an independent contractor hired for a specialized job and not an employee.

Another way that exercise or fitness programs could be held liable for the negligent acts of their independent contractors is through agency by estoppel. Estoppel is a legal doctrine designed to protect individuals from false expectations. For example, this can occur if the exercise program's actions have created the appearance that an independent contractor is an employee. If a health/fitness club allowed their independent contractors to wear an employee uniform or T-shirt, it may have appeared to members that the independent contractors were actual employees of the facility. In such a situation, the health/fitness club could be liable for the negligent acts of those independent contractors. A plaintiff in this type of negligence lawsuit would have to prove in court that he or she reasonably believed that the independent contractor was an employee of the health/fitness club (Clarkson et al., 2001). To minimize this type of liability, exercise programs should take the necessary steps so that their participants will not perceive their independent contractors to be employees. It is suggested that exercise programs post notices to inform participants that independent contractors carry out certain services, and also inform them orally and in writing of such (Herbert, 1994). To minimize liability associated with independent contractors, exercise programs should contract only with competent professionals, have a written contract with all independent contractors, require independent contractors to purchase their own liability insurance, and do not attempt to control the means or methods the independent contractor uses to accomplish his or her work.

PURCHASING OR LEASING EQUIPMENT As a sound business practice, contracts should be in writing because a written contract will provide evidence of what was agreed to by the two parties should a dispute arise. All states have statutes (collectively termed the Statute of Frauds) that require certain types of contracts to be in writing in order to be enforceable. For instance, contracts involving the sale of goods for a price of $500 or more or lease contracts requiring payments of $1,000 or more must be in writing. Article 2 of the Uniform Commercial Code (UCC) governs contracts for the sale of goods, and Article 2A addresses contracts for the lease of goods. A good is an item of property that is tangible (has physical existence and can be touched or seen) and movable (can be carried from place to place). Many types of equipment (e.g., fitness and office equipment) purchased or leased by exercise science programs would be defined as goods according to the UCC. To satisfy the Statute of Frauds when purchasing equipment, the UCC only requires a writing or memorandum indicating the intention of the parties to form a contract as long as it is signed by the party against whom enforcement is sought. When leasing equipment, the writing must identify and describe the equipment leased and the lease terms (Clarkson et al., 2001).

Although verbal contracts can be enforced in court, as a matter of good business practice, contracts should be written because they will provide documentation of what the parties agreed to should a contractual dispute arise. While exercise science professionals can draft contracts, it is recommended that a lawyer, knowledgeable of contract law in the relevant state, review all contracts prior to being used.

AMERICANS WITH DISABILITIES ACT

The Americans with Disabilities Act (ADA) is a federal statue that prohibits discrimination against otherwise qualified individuals with disabilities in situations involving employment (Title I), public services (Title II), public accommodations and services operated by private entities (Title III), and telecommunications and common carriers (Epstein, 2003). Exercise programs often fall within the ambits of the ADA as they tend to provide services that are deemed public accommodations. For example, exercise programs provide public accommodations if they provide (a) food or drink service, (b) exhibition or entertainment services, (c) sale or rental establishment services, (d) recreational services, or (e) exercise services.

Whether an exercise program provides employment opportunities, spectator opportunities, or even participatory opportunities, the ADA requires such programs to provide reasonable accommodations to those with disabilities. First, it is important to note that the term *disability* is broadly defined by the ADA to include any physical or mental impairment that substantially limits one or more of the major life activities of an individual, a record of such impairment, or being regarded as having such an impairment (42 U.S.C.A. § 12102).

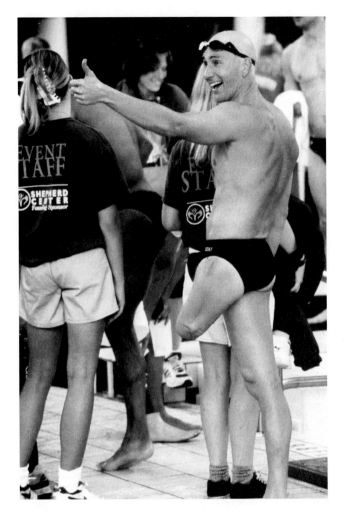

The Americans with Disabilities Act gives civil rights protections to individuals with disabilities.

Second, when a person has a disability, it is important that exercise science programs make reasonable accommodations, when possible, which allow the person with the disability to participate in whatever services the program provides. The ADA does not require programs to make accommodations that result in undue hardship. *Undue hardship* is defined as those accommodations that are significantly difficult or unreasonably expensive (Epstein, 2003). Thus an exercise program must be mindful in accommodating individuals with disabilities. This includes making reasonable accommodations for current or potential employees in the workplace and adapting services and facilities to accommodate the needs of those with disabilities who may wish to participate in exercise programs. Examples of reasonable service accommodations in an exercise program may include ensuring wheelchair access to the facility via ramps and proper equipment spacing, allowing people in wheelchairs equal access to tennis and basketball courts, and using tactile end of lane markers to assist those who are visually impaired and wish to swim.

RISK MANAGEMENT

Risk management (RM) can be defined as controlling the financial and personal injury losses from sudden, unforeseen, atypical accidents and intentional torts (Ammon & Brown, 2007). RM is the process by which businesses utilize operational policies and practices to decrease their exposure to risk (van der Smissen, 1990). An effective RM plan will assist in controlling the risks that today's exercise science professionals face. A comprehensive RM plan should address risks related to public liability caused by negligence (e.g., injuries and deaths caused by negligence), public liability excluding negligence (e.g., product liability, sexual harassment, intentional torts, employment practices), business operations (e.g., financial risks resulting from employee accidents and injuries, theft, business interruption), and property exposures (e.g., risks due to floods, hurricanes, fire) (van der Smissen, 1990).

Establishing an effective RM program consists of developing an RM plan, implementing the RM plan, and managing the RM plan. The development stage consists of three distinct steps: (a) identifying risks, (b) classifying risks, and (c) choosing methods to treat the risks. Every program and activity is different and has it own unique risks, so identifying risk should be an ongoing process. Risks should be identified and classified into the categories of risk previously described. Methods used to assist in identifying risks include surveys and discussions with frontline staff members, reading literature and standards or guidelines published by professional organizations, consulting with colleagues, and utilizing various professionals such as insurance agents and RM consultants (Ammon & Brown, 2007).

After potential risks have been identified, the next step is to classify the risk. The purpose of this step is to determine how frequent the risk may occur and the severity of the potential loss arising from the risk. Frequency may be categorized as low, medium, or high. Severity may be categorized as low, moderate, critical, or catastrophic. To aid in consistency, a matrix may be created to aid in the classification process (Ammon & Brown, 2007).

The last step in developing an RM plan is to select a treatment for the identified and classified risks. Four general treatments are typically available. First, a risk may be eliminated or avoided (e.g., the removal of a diving board in a health club swimming pool or the decision not to offer a certain fitness program). Second, a risk may be transferred to another party (e.g., the use of waivers, obtaining appropriate insurance coverage, utilizing independent contractors). Third, a risk may be retained by an organization (also termed *self-insurance*). This method is typically used for minor or insignificant risks and may be less expensive than purchasing insurance to cover such risks. Fourth, risks may be reduced by an organization. This proactive approach is most important to reduce the chances that loss will occur and reduce the severity if a loss does occur. It is important to realize that all risks cannot be eliminated from activities, but risk reduction strategies can be employed. These would include establishing an ongoing, systematic inspection program; developing a regular maintenance program for facilities and equipment; training staff members; and designing a filing system for RM-related documents (e.g., waivers, parental permission forms, participation agreements, facility contracts, accident report forms, inspection checklists, facility use agreements). Such forms should be easily retrievable and retained for the length of the state's statute of limitations (Ammon & Brown, 2007).

Once a risk management plan is developed, it must be implemented and managed. Effective implementation requires proper communication. All staff members must not only understand the overall RM plan but must also understand their roles in the plan. In addition to oral communication, written guidelines should be utilized. These guidelines can be incorporated in employee manuals. A sound training program (including both initial orientation and regular in-service training) with two-way communication between staff and management is encouraged and will assist with the implementation of the RM plan (Ammon & Brown, 2007).

Managing the RM plan involves designating a risk manager and selecting a risk management committee. These individuals should monitor the RM plan, assist with RM training, review accidents, evaluate the RM plan, and implement changes. Another step in managing the plan is to encourage employee input regarding the RM plan. This will assist in fostering an overall pro RM attitude. Finally, because risks are constantly changing, RM plans must also evolve. Risk management is a constant, fluctuating process (Ammon & Brown, 2007).

PROFESSIONAL ORGANIZATIONS

Several professional organizations related to sport law exist. Membership benefits typically include a subscription to journals and other related publications, discounted conference fees, and the opportunity to network with others who have similar professional interests. The Sport and Recreation Law Association's (SRLA) purpose is to further the study and dissemination of information regarding legal aspects of sport and recreation. The association addresses legal aspects of sport, fitness, and recreation within both the public and private sectors. Student and profes-

sional memberships are available. Further information regarding SRLA can be obtained from their Web site.

Other professional organizations, although primarily geared toward law students and attorneys, include the Sport Lawyers Association, Black Entertainment and Sport Lawyers Association, and Marquette University's National Sports Law Institute. The American Bar Association and many state bar associations also have forums and organizations specific to sports law.

PROFESSIONAL OPPORTUNITIES

The vast majority of professional opportunities in exercise science as it relates to the law are for those who obtain a law degree (Juris Doctorate) or complete advanced academic studies in law. Those with a law degree may practice law in the many areas that pertain to the exercise science industry. Others who obtain appropriate legal knowledge may have opportunities as a risk manager, consultant, or expert witness as it pertains to exercise science.

SUMMARY

Exercise science professionals are challenged to identify and understand potential legal problems, to effectively manage such problems, and to reduce the probability of legal problems occurring. An exercise science professional can better manage legal issues by understanding key aspects of the law. By being familiar with legal issues, one can eliminate, or reduce, many types of problems. For instance, a well-developed and implemented risk management plan can assist an exercise science professional in avoiding or reducing legal liability (Wong & Masteralexis, 2005). This chapter focused on the two areas most likely to affect the field of exercise science, tort and contract law, but many other areas of the law may affect the field of exercise science including, but not limited to, employment law, disability law, constitutional law, and trademark/patent law. These subjects are typically discussed in legal issues courses but may be introduced in other management/administration courses in many academic programs.

Knowledge and understanding of key aspects of the law has become increasingly important for the exercise science professional in today's litigious environment. Likewise, it is important to realize when to seek legal assistance. The law is constantly evolving, and a wise professional will continue to stay abreast in this area by attending conferences, reading the professional literature, and seeking advice from legal professionals.

Key Journals

Athletic Business
Club Industry
Exercise Standards and Malpractice Reporter

Fitness Management
Journal of Legal Aspects of Sport

Key Websites

Club Industry (http://fitnessbusinesspro.com/)
FindLaw (http://www.findlaw.com/)
Fitness Management (http://www.fitnessmanagement. com/)
Legal dictionaries (http://www.legal-dictionary.org/) (http:// legal-dictionary.thefreedictionary.com/)
Legal Information Institute from Cornell Law School (http:// www.law.cornell.edu/)
Link to U.S. federal courts (http://www.uscourts.gov/)

National Center for State Courts (http://www.ncsconline. org/D_KIS/info_court_web_sites.html)
PRC Publishing (http://www.prcpublishingcorp.com/)
Source for legal blogs (http://www.blawg.com/)
Sport and Recreation Law Association (www.srlaweb.org)
Sports law-related blogs (http://sports-law.blogspot.com/) (http://www.blawgrepublic.com/cat/Sports-Law/)
WashLaw from Washburn University School of Law (http:// www.washlaw.edu/)

■ **Review Questions**

1. Identify the three branches of government that create law. Provide an example of a type of law each branch creates that potentially affects the exercise science field.
2. Explain the primary differences between criminal and civil law.
3. Identify the steps in a civil trial.
4. Provide an exercise science-related hypothetical example of negligence. Identify the four elements of negligence in your example.
5. Describe the essential elements of a valid exercise science-related contract.

6. What do the courts consider when determining if a worker was an employee or an independent contractor?
7. Identify and provide examples of the three steps in developing a risk management plan.
8. Discuss the four options available for treating risks. Provide examples for each that could be utilized in a typical health club setting.
9. Research the Americans With Disabilities Act and identify how it may apply to an exercise science program.

■ **References**

Aerobics and Fitness Association of America. (2005). *Exercise standards & guidelines reference manual* (4th ed.). Sherman Oaks, CA: Author.

American College of Sports Medicine. (2006). *American College of Sports Medicine guidelines for exercise testing and prescription* (7th ed.). Philadelphia, PA: Lippincott Williams & Wilkins.

American College of Sports Medicine and American Heart Association Joint Position Statement. (1998). Recommendations for cardiovascular screening, staffing, and emergency policies at health/fitness facilities. *Medicine and Science in Sports and Exercise*, 30, 1009–1018.

American College of Sports Medicine and American Heart Association Joint Position Statement. (2002). Automated external defibrillators in health/fitness facilities. *Medicine and Science in Sports and Exercise*, 34, 561–564.

American Law Institute. (1981). *Restatement of the law of contracts* (2nd ed.). St. Paul, MN: Author.

American Law Institute. (1987). *Uniform commercial code* (UCC). 2-206(1)(a). St. Paul, MN: Author.

Ammon, R., & Brown, M. T. (2007). Risk management process. In D. J., Cotten & J. T. Wolohan (Eds.), *Law for recreation and sport managers* (4th ed., pp. 288–300). Dubuque, IA: Kendall/Hunt.

Carper, D. L., Mietus, N. J., & West, B. W. (2000). *Understanding the law* (3rd ed.). Cincinnati, OH: West.

Clarkson, K. W., Miller, R. L., Jentz, G. A., & Cross, F. B. (2001). *West's business law* (8th ed.). St Paul, MN: West.

Cotten, D. J. (2007). Defenses against negligence. In D. J. Cotten & J. T. Wolohan (Eds.), *Law for recreation and sport managers* (4th ed., pp. 58–70). Dubuque, IA: Kendall/ Hunt.

Cotten, D. J., & Cotten, M. B. (2000). *Waivers & releases for the health & fitness club industry* (2nd ed.). Boston, MA: IHRSA.

Dougherty, N. J., Goldberger, A. S., & Carpenter, L. J. (2007). *Sport, physical activity and the law* (3rd ed.). Champaign, IL: Sagamore.

Eickhoff-Shemek, J. M., & Evans, J. A. (2000). An investigation of law and legal liability content in master academic programs in sports medicine and exercise science. *Journal of Legal Aspects of Sport*, 10(3), 172–179.

Epstein, A. (2003). *Sports law*. New York: Thompson.

Fried, G. B. (2007). The legal system. In D. J. Cotten & J. T. Wolohan (Eds.), *Law for recreation and sport managers* (4th ed., pp. 2–11). Dubuque, IA: Kendall/Hunt.

Herbert, D. (1994). Avoiding liability for independent contractors. *The Exercise Standards and Malpractice Reporter*, 8(3), 33, 36–37.

International Health, Racquet & Sportsclub Association. (2005). IHRSA club membership standards. In IHRSA's *guide to club membership & conduct* (3rd ed.). Boston, MA: Author.

Keeton, W. P., Dobbs, D. B., Keeton R. E., & Owen, D. O. (1984). *Prosser and Keeton on torts* (5th ed.). St Paul, MN: West.

Medical Fitness Association. (2006). *The medical fitness model: Facility standards and guidelines*. Richmond, VA: Author.

Napolitano, F. (1997). What do lawn mower safety and Par-Q have in common? ACSM's *Health & Fitness Journal, 1*(1), 38–39.

National Athletic Trainers' Association. (2006). NATA *statements*. Retrieved October 3, 2007, from http://www.nata.org/statements/index.htm

National Strength and Conditioning Association. (2001). NSCA *strength & conditioning professional standards & guidelines*. Colorado Springs, CO: Author. Retrieved October 2, 2007, from http://www.nscalift.org/Publications/standards.shtml

Ontario Association of Sport and Exercise Sciences. (2004). *Canadian fitness safety standards & recommended guidelines* (3rd ed). Ontario, Canada: Author. Retrieved.October 2, 2007, from http://www.oases.on.ca/safety/safetyStdsCurrent.htm

Sharp, L. A. (2007). Contract essentials. In D. J. Cotten, & J. T. Wolohan (Eds.), *Law for recreation and sport managers* (4th ed., pp. 364–374). Dubuque, IA: Kendall/Hunt.

Tharrett, S. J., McInnis, K. J., & Peterson, J. A. (Eds.). (2007). ACSM's *health/fitness facility standards and guidelines* (3rd ed.). Champaign, IL: Human Kinetics.

Tunkl v. Regents.of University of California, 383 P.2d 441 (1963).

van der Smissen, B. (1990). *Legal liability and risk management for public and private entities*. Cincinnati, OH: W. H. Anderson.

van der Smissen, B. (2007). Elements of negligence. In D. J. Cotten & J. T. Wolohan (Eds.) *Law for recreation and sport managers* (4th ed., pp. 36–45). Dubuque, IA: Kendall/Hunt.

Wong, G. M. (2002). *Essentials of amateur sports law* (3rd ed.). Westport, CT: Greenwood.

Wong, G. M., & Pike Masteralexis, L. (2005). Legal principles applied to sport management. In L. Pike Masteralexis, C. A. Barr, & M. A. Hums (Eds.), *Principles and practice of sport management* (2nd ed.). Sudbury, MA: Jones and Bartlett.

YMCA of the USA. (2007). *Medical advisory committee recommendations: A resource guide for YMCAs*. Chicago, IL: Author.

CHAPTER 13

Ethical Considerations in Exercise Science

Matthew J. Robinson, PhD, University of Delaware

■ Chapter Objectives

After reading this chapter, you should be able to:

1. Understand the critical role ethics play in a career in exercise science.
2. Appreciate the importance of values and principles in acting ethically within the exercise science profession.
3. Comprehend the major ethical theories that are applicable to a career in exercise science.
4. Appreciate the importance of morality in conducting oneself professionally in a career in exercise science.

5. Recognize what is considered ethical behavior as defined by professional codes and standards established for the field.
6. Assess your level of moral development as it applies to a career in exercise science.
7. Understand which ethical theory to which you adhere.
8. Appreciate the different professional situations that will arise that can potentially lead to an ethical dilemma.

■ Key Terms

applied ethics
Belmont Report
codes of ethics
conflict of interest
deontological theories
egoism
ethics

Institutional Review Boards
morality
Nuremberg Code
personal ethics
principles
professional ethics
situational ethics

social responsibility
stages of moral development
teleological theories
utilitarian
values

The majority of this text focuses on the technical areas of the exercise sciences and the skills and training necessary for a person who wants a career in the exercise science field. This chapter's focus is not on what a person does as a professional but rather on how a person conducts him- or herself in the exercise science field. The Greek Philosopher Heraclitus said, "Day by day what you chose, what you think, and what you do is who you become. Your integrity is your destiny" (as cited in Goree, Pyle, Baker, & Hopkins, 2004, p. v). As a professional, a person will be judged as much on his or her professional ethics as on his or her professional competence. That integrity comes from the daily practice of moral and ethical behavior.

Coming to terms with one's ethics, values, and morals is an important step in becoming a professional. Whether a student wants to be an athletic trainer, an academic researcher, a strength and conditioning coach, or a sport psychologist, one unethical act can ruin his or her professional reputation, which may have taken many years to develop. The purpose of this chapter is to present a theoretical framework for the aspiring professional to determine which ethical theories and beliefs to adhere to and to challenge you to consider the degree of rightness and wrongness with situations you may face in the various exercise science fields.

A BRIEF HISTORY OF ETHICAL CONSIDERTATIONS IN EXERCISE SCIENCE

Exercise science as a discipline was created to systematically inquire and empirically examine the physiological and psychological aspects of those who participate in these activities. Exercise science encompasses biomechanics, athletic medicine, exercise physiology, physical therapy, cardiac rehabilitation, motor control, sport nutrition, sport psychology, and athletic training (Hall, 2007). Academic inquiry in these areas has led to research that has advanced the performance and abilities of athletes through better training methods in the areas of strength and conditioning, improved technical instruction by coaches for athletes, development of more effective ways to address injury reduction and rehabilitation, and better understanding of the individual and team psychological aspects of athletic competition. Some of this research has led to unethical behaviors by professionals who have utilized methods or substances that can create an unfair ad-vantage for an unethical athlete, coach, or team over those playing by the rules. Recently, major league baseball's image has been tarnished by accusations and allegations that some of the game's biggest stars used performance enhancing drugs and human growth hormones to enhance their performance. Scientists developed these drugs, and trainers and strength and conditioning coaches supplied and in many cases injected the athletes with the chemicals and hormones. Although baseball did not have any rules against the use of such enhancers nor did it drug test, the actions by the exercise science professionals were as wrong as the athletes were who utilized these methods.

The origins of Western ethical theory can be traced to Ancient Greece and the teachings of Socrates, Plato, and Aristotle (Goree, 2004). Human beings face ethical dilemmas on a daily basis in their personal and professional lives. Exercise science is not immune to this ethical discourse. Ethical questions over the treatment of subjects, falsifying results to ensure publications or to secure grant funding, and development of training methods or performance enhancing drugs detrimental to the health and well-being of the participants while also creating an unfair advantage in competition are prevalent and will arise in any environment in which a professional practices: an academic position, a university or high school athletic department, a professional sport franchise, the Olympic movement, or a physical therapy clinic. In these scenarios and within these environments, individuals utilize theoretical ethics and morality in an attempt to gain an understanding of the intent behind the actions. Specific ethical issues are open for debate, and different interpretations may be made as to the degree of rightness or wrongness of an act.

BASIC ETHICS CONCEPTS IN EXERCISE SCIENCE

Goree (2004) defined ethical issues as those questions, problems, situations, or actions that contact legitimate questions of right or wrong. When a personal trainer, who is compensated handsomely, is asked by a client if he or she can secure performance-enhancing drugs for the athlete and utilize a method to prevent detection of the use, the personal trainer must make a choice. To address this situation, an individual refers to his or her own code of ethics. DeSensi and Rosenberg (2003) described **ethics** as the objective basis upon which judgments are rendered regarding right or wrong, good or bad, authentic or inauthentic behavior.

Values

A person's ethics are based on values. A **value** is anything an individual assesses to be worthwhile, interesting, excellent, desirable, or important (DeSensi & Rosenberg, 2003). These values can come in the form of virtues or moral values such as loyalty, integrity, honesty, compassion, courage, and perseverance. Values may also come in the form of tangible outcomes such as money and material objects or intangible outcomes such as fame, prestige, or reputation. Values are derived from a variety of sources such as family, friends, teachers, life experiences, or religion.

Principles

Principles are universal guides that tell what actions, intentions, or motives are prohibited. Principles enable values to be translated into action. For example, if a person values honesty, he or she will develop a principle not to falsify the results of a study. If another person values compassion, he or she will not disregard the well-being of an athlete and rush the athlete back from an injury rehabilitation for the sake of winning a contest.

Action

The action of an individual is the ultimate statement of ethics. An exercise scientist can value honesty and develop a principle that he or she would not be dishonest in training athletes, but when placed in the situation of being asked to provide an illegal performance-enhancing drug, whether he or she does or does not do so defines that person's ethics.

Morality

DeSensi and Rosenberg (2003) defined **morality** as the principles and theories of that ethics derived from or that explain the way of life, beliefs, attitudes, intentions, and motives that are judged to possess moral qualities. Morality is the debate over the rightness and wrongness of the action. A person may report findings in a study to secure grant money or to ensure tenure at an institution. The exercise scientist who falsifies the results can justify his or her action based on loyalty and or self-interest in that he or she needs to stay employed to continue with his or her research career. If discovered, others would view that action as being wrong and would make a moral judgment on the actions of their peer.

Morality is learned and inherited, not inherent. Most of us begin to understand morality early in life through parental and other influences, and our ideas evolve throughout life. Thus it has been argued that acquiring moral reasoning skills is a development process.

Moral Development

Kohlberg (1987) quantified this process of developing morality by the presentation of a theory on moral development. Kohlberg presented six **stages of moral development.** Kohlberg proposed that children and adolescents move through distinct moral stages in which different levels of moral judgment can be identified. Kohlberg's model consists of three levels: preconventional, conventional, and postconventional. Each level includes two moral stages, one being more advanced than the other.

At Stage 1 of the preconventional level, rules are obeyed in order to avoid punishment. A strength and conditioning coach does not supply performance-enhancing drugs to athletes for fear of being discredited professionally or dismissed from his position if it is discovered. At Stage 2, rules are obeyed in order to obtain rewards and have favors returned. The strength and conditioning coach does not supply performance-enhancing drugs because he wants to continue in his career and the benefits that go along with practicing his profession the right way. In both of these stages, there is a self-interest orientation on the part of the person.

At Stage 3 in the conventional level, rules are obeyed to avoid disapproval by others; meeting the expectations of others is the most important element. The strength and conditioning coach does not supply the drugs because he does not want to be viewed as a cheat by his family, his close friends, and his mentors. At Stage 4, the coach does what is deemed right to avoid guilt as well as to recognize that he is a member of society. Here the coach does the right thing because he does not want to be discredited and viewed as a dishonest professional by his peers and society as a whole. In these stages the incentive to do the right thing is based more on the person's desire to meet the approvals of others.

At Stage 5 in the post conventional level, rules are obeyed for the sake of social and community welfare. In this case the coach does not provide the performance enhancing drugs because if he does others may do so as well and there will be a total breakdown of the integrity of competition as it is known. By being honest he is working within the social order and meeting his responsibility to society and to the profession. At Stage 6, rules are obeyed in order to abide by universal ethical principles. At this stage, the scientist does not fabricate results for it is not the right thing to do. There is no benefit or punishment, no judgments of others—it is just the right thing to do. Kohlberg proposed that transition from stage to stage is driven primarily by social interaction, especially interaction with others at those higher levels of development.

Social Responsibility

Social responsibility involves an entity's obligation, whether it is a state, government, corporation, organization, or individual, to act in a manner that recognizes and accepts the consequences of each action and decision it undertakes (DeSensi & Rosenberg, 2003). Social responsibility is an integral component in the exercise scientist's career and decisions. Upholding this conviction can be a challenge based on pressures that may range from securing tenure for a faculty member, training a world champion, prescribing an exercise program for an individual, or treating or rehabilitating a high school athlete.

Exercise scientists interact with varied populations and in most cases conduct their research and work with human subjects; therefore, it is important to consider issues such as gender, race, special needs, and varying mental and physical capabilities whether doing research or training athletes. It is important to take these social issues into account and treat all with dignity and respect and in a morally appropriate way that meets established codes and standards.

ETHICAL THEORIES

After laying the foundation for the discussion of ethics and morality, individuals must choose which ethical theories they will adhere to. For some this process is a matter of classifying themselves based on the beliefs, values, and principles they practice. For others it may be a process of self-discovery in terms of which ethical theory meets how they should, desire to, or will act professionally.

Ethical theories can be broken down into two broad categories: those that focus on the consequences of actions (teleological theories) and those that do not consider the consequences when action is taken (deontological theories).

Teleological Theories

Teleological theories are characterized by a focus on the consequences or the end to which an action is directed. Decisions are dependent on an understanding of what will result from a person's choices. Actions that lead to good and valuable consequences are right; actions that lead away from them are wrong. Teleology is the "science of ends." Two teleo-

logical theories are egoism and utilitarianism; both focus on the consequences of action but differ in intent. A third teleological theory involves situational ethics.

EGOISM **Egoism** is the belief that all actions are motivated by selfish interest (DeSensi & Rosenberg, 2003). A person may act on behalf of another, but ultimately each person is concerned about him- or herself and never sacrifices on behalf of others. An egoist strength and conditioning coach will prescribe a training program to create a world champion not for the benefit of the athlete but for his or her own benefit or values (e.g., monetary reward, enhanced reputation, personal glory).

UTILITARIANISM **Utilitarianism** contends that the only moral duty one has is to promote the greatest amount of happiness, and pleasure and happiness are the only goods worth pursuing. From a utilitarian perspective, the end justifies the means, and behavior must be practical and useful, or have "utility." A behavior is right if the consequences lead toward a positive outcome.

A utilitarian can justify doing an experiment on a person that may cause that individual personal harm because the results of that study could lead to a treatment that will cure many in the future. On a more positive note, a sport trainer may not prescribe a training method that may lead to a championship for one athlete because it may cause long-term ill effects on all that use it. In both cases it is the greatest good for the greatest number that drives the action.

SITUATIONAL ETHICS **Situational ethics,** a third type of teleological theory, does not take into account particular rules when faced with a moral problem. Every moral situation begins with a blank slate, and each case must be viewed independently (DeSensi & Rosenberg, 2003). This trait is often viewed as a weakness of teleological theory because it leads to inconsistency and begs the question: Can an individual ignore values and principles and truly look at each situation differently?

Deontological Theories

Deontological theories maintain that one has a moral obligation to do right without considering the outcome or the consequences of a decision. The sport trainer will not practice blood doping because it is wrong. Doing the right thing supersedes the consequences associated with the ethical action. Other athletes may do it and perform better and win the competition, but the sport trainer did the right thing by not cheating.

PERSONAL VERSUS PROFESSIONAL ETHICS

Each person has his or her own **personal ethics**, which are distinct, and people may not always agree with one another. There is room for variation and different styles even within the framework of values and principles. For example, to receive a promotion, one person may spend 60 to 70 hours on a project that only requires 40 hours a week, and another person may spend only 40 hours of work in order to have more time for family. Morally speaking, neither person is better.

Developing good **professional ethics** starts with having a solid personal ethical framework. It is impossible to separate personal and professional ethics. An individual's ethics must act as a guide from both the personal and professional level. Professional ethics involve taking on an additional burden or ethical responsibility.

It is extremely important for exercise scientists to have a strong personal ethical framework so they can confront the ethical shortcomings they may encounter. By making bold and solid decisions in their professional life, exercise scientists can uphold the values and virtues of scientific inquiry in their treatment of other human beings, whether they be world class athletes or sedentary individuals looking for a workout program. Morals should not be sacrificed for prestige, positions, or funding. Rather, both objectives can be pursued simultaneously.

Those in the exercise science field must also recognize that their actions are highly scrutinized. Whether it is a refereed paper or prescribing an exercise program for a person looking to become more fit, it is extremely important for the exercise scientist to be cautious and to avoid unethical behavior.

PROFESSIONAL CODES OF ETHICS

Appropriate or ethical behavior in a given profession or organization is defined in a code of ethics. Goree (2004) characterized a **code of ethics** as a written set of principles and rules that serve as a guideline for what is considered ethical behavior for those under its authority. It is often the middle ground between professional etiquette and what is required by law.

An exercise scientist may be under the authority of multiple codes of ethics, and one of the limitations of a code of ethics is that these codes may conflict. For example, an exercise science professor at a university falls under the purview of the professional codes of ethics for the American Association of University Professors (AAUP) as well as those for the American College of Sport Medicine (ACSM). Along with those, the particular university may have established its own code of ethics, and finally, the individual may have created his or her own code.

Kultgen (1988) believed that professional codes of ethics are instruments for persuasion both of members of a profession and the public. They enhance the sense of community among members, of belonging to a group with common values and a common mission.

Goree (2004) argues that an effective code maintains a sense of professionalism, offers guidance to individuals facing ethical dilemmas in a given profession, and gives the public a standard to which it can hold those in a given profession. Goree identified seven characteristics of effective professional codes of ethics:

- The content and quality of professional codes cover the important ethical issues in the field clearly, thoroughly, and adequately.
- Effective professional codes are protective of the public interest and the interests of the individuals who are served by that profession.
- The members of the profession must be familiar with the code of ethics and its contents.
- Quality professional codes are specific and honest.
- Professional codes must be enforceable and policed.
- Professional codes must be revised periodically.
- Professional codes must be regulative to be effective.

Elements of a Code of Ethics

Kultgen (1988) identified four basic elements that comprise a code of ethics.

An ethical code. This component brings legitimacy to the field by creating standards for a profession.

Model laws. This component regulates the action of the professional by stating minimum standards to be viewed as professional and discipline for those who do not follow the laws.

Basic ideals. This component express the values of the profession and what is viewed as moral behavior.

Rationale. This component allows for the interpretation of the code.

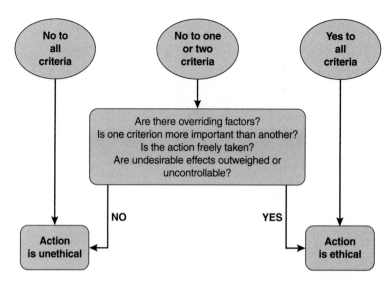

Figure 13.1 Ethical Decision-Making Model.
Source: Cavanaugh, G. F. (1990). *American Business Values*, 3rd ed. American Management Association. p. 195.

The American College of Sports Medicine's Code of Ethics was established for those who are interested in researching, teaching, or practicing sport medicine. The Web site is listed at the end of the chapter. For those with an interest in other fields, visit the professional organization for that field and review its code of ethics.

ETHICAL DECISION MAKING

Decisions are based on judgments and involve choice. When making a decision that would be morally appropriate within exercise science, it is useful to develop a decision-making strategy. As stated previously, action is the ultimate statement of one's ethics. The following sections discuss concepts that will assist you in moving in the direction of making an ethical decision.

Ethical Decision-Making Model

Cavanaugh (1990) proposed a model in which the exercise scientist asks whether an action is acceptable based on principles of utility, rights, and justice: Does it optimize benefits? Does it respect the rights of those involved? Is the action fair? If the answer is "no" to all three, the action is unethical. If the answer is "yes" to all three, the action is ethical. If two of the three are "yes" or "no," then overriding factors must be considered. For example, is one criterion more important than the other? Is the action freely taken? Are the undesirable effects outweighed or uncontrollable? This will enable a person to determine whether the action is ethical or unethical (see Figure 13.1).

As discussed earlier in the chapter, the individual's values and principles will determine his or her views of utility, rights, and justice and will ultimately dictate whether the action is ethical or unethical.

Right Versus Right Decision Making

Often making a decision is not a choice between right and wrong but between two rights. Kidder (1995) proposed that resolution is based on selecting the action that is nearest right for the circumstance and offers an ends-based resolution, which is the greatest good for the greatest number; a care-based resolution, which follows the golden rule; and a rule-based resolution, which states we should act in a manner that we hope the rest of the world would choose if placed in the same situation.

Practical Application

Kidder (1995) provides a rather simplistic method in determining the rightness of an action. Before acting, a person first should consider how he or she would feel if this action would be reported on the front page of a newspaper. Second, how would the person feel if his or her grandmother discovered this act? In both cases Kidder appeals to the moral development of the individual: If the person does not want to be held up to public scorn or let down a significant other, the person should not do the act. If the trainers for major league baseball players had utilized this approach, perhaps they would not have supplied the human growth hormones or performance-enhancing drugs and would not have been held up for public scorn for their actions.

CAREERS IN APPLIED ETHICS IN EXERCISE SCIENCE

Having established a theoretical framework for ethics for the exercise scientist, we turn our attention to **applied ethics** in a professional context. Regardless of the professional setting, ethics will play an important part in the careers of those in the exercise sciences. Exercise scientists will be challenged to act on the values, principles, and codes they possess or develop and are expected to follow. No professional, whether an academic researcher, an athletic trainer in the high school setting, or a coach working with a world class athlete, will be able to avoid situations with moral and ethical ramifications.

Academic Research

At the heart of exercise science is the research process. Research implies a careful approach to solving problems and has the enduring traits of being systematic, logical, empirical, reductive, and replicable (Tuckman, 1978). Ethics play an important role in research, for research endeavors are grounded in values such as integrity, honesty, trust, curiosity, and respect for intellectual achievement (National Academies Press, 1992). Scientists trust that the results reported by others are in fact valid, and society as a whole trusts that the study was conducted and the results reported in a manner that is fair, unbiased, and truthful. This trust will endure only so long as the scientific community devotes itself to exemplifying and transmitting the values associated with ethical scientific conduct (National Academies Press, 1992).

Along with reporting results, ethical issues arise with regard to the research process. The Tuskegee Study of Untreated Syphilis in the Negro Male is considered one of the most infamous experiments in the history of the United States (Loue, 2000). The study involved African American males being left untreated for syphilis in the name of science (Jones, 1981). Ethical transgressions were also found in the treatment of prisoners in the Holmsburg Prison Experiments, in which prisoners were enticed into participating in various studies that exposed them to untested materials or infected them with diseases. Although in these cases a utilitarian could claim that the results of the studies were for the greater good and the egoist could view the findings as a way to advance his or her career, those practicing deontological ethics would view the studies as being wrong or immoral based on the deplorable treatment of the participants.

Immoral, unethical, dishonest, or untrustworthy researchers become known to their colleagues through various mechanisms, including discovery of the research methods and treatment of human subjects that led to the results, word of mouth, and the inability of other scientists to confirm or replicate the work in question. Such irreproducible work is recognized and discredited through the processes of peer review and evaluation, which are critical to making professional appointments, accepting work for publication, and awarding research support (National Academies Press, 1992). Therefore, it is not wise from many ethical perspectives to develop an unethical reputation whether it be in the conduct, reporting, or acquiring funding for research. The ethical transgressions could haunt a professional for the rest of his or her career.

CONDUCT OF RESEARCH The classic model of scientific inquiry entails defining the problem, formulating the hypothesis, gathering data, and analyzing, interpreting, and reporting the results. Each of these steps has the potential for ethical dilemmas for the researcher. The majority of research conducted in exercise science involves humans and, in many instances, children. With this in mind, the well-being of the human subject must be of the utmost concern. "In the United States, regulations protecting human subjects first became effective on May 30, 1974. Promulgated by the Department of Health, Education and Welfare (DHEW), those regulations were raised to regulatory status in the National Institute for Health's (NIH) Policies for the Protection of Human Subjects, which were first issued in 1966. The regulations established the **Institutional Review Boards** (IRB) as one mechanism which would offer protection to human subjects through the evaluation and approval of the research methods" (Protecting Human Research Subjects, n.d.).

In 1978, the National Commission for the Protection of Human Subjects of Biomedical and Behavioral Research produced *The Belmont Report: Ethical Principles and Guidelines for the Protection of Human Subjects of Research.* The **Belmont Report** identified the underlying principles researchers must adhere to. The principles of respect for persons, beneficence, and justice are now accepted as the three quintessential requirements for the ethical conduct of research involving human subjects in the United States (U.S. Department of Health and Human Services, 2006).

University IRBs assume an important responsibility in the process of protecting the rights of human research subjects. The IRB's role ultimately is to make sure researchers at the institution are living up to their moral and ethical obligations in working with human subjects. In addition to these U.S. standards, international standards were established in the form of the **Nuremberg Code** (Box 13.1) and the Declaration of Helsinki.

EXPLORE MORE BOX 13.1

The Nuremburg Code

The impetus for the Nuremburg Code was the treatment of human subjects by the Nazis during World War II. The Nuremburg Code presents 10 basic principles that are viewed as being universally applicable to research involving human subjects.

1. The prospective participant's voluntary consent is essential.

2. The results to be obtained from the experiment must be beneficial to society, and those results cannot be obtained through other means.

3. The study must have as its foundation the result of animal experiments and a knowledge of the natural history of the disease so that the anticipated results justify the conduct of the experiment.

4. All unnecessary physical and mental injury or suffering must be avoided during the course of the experiment.

5. No experiment should be conducted if it is believed that death or disabling injury will occur except where the research physician also serves as a research participant.

6. The degree of risk should not exceed the humanitarian importance of the problem being addressed.

7. Adequate facilities and preparation should be used to protect the participant against death or injury.

8. Only scientifically qualified persons should contact the experiment.

9. The participant has a right to end his or her participation at any time if he or she reaches a point where continuation seems impossible.

10. The scientist in charge must be prepared to end the experiment if there is probable cause to believe that continuing the experiment will likely result in the injury, disability, or death of the research participant.

Source: World Medical Association (1964).

The Declaration of Helsinki addresses issues related to a surrogate giving permission to a potential subject who is incapable of consenting and distinguishes between clinical research combined with professional care and nontherapeutic clinical research (Loue, 2000). At the heart of both codes is the ethical and humane treatment of the participants in the study.

In applying an ethical perspective in the conduct of research, an egoist may put aside the well-being of the subject if it advances his or her research, and a utilitarian may view the mistreatment of a subject as being justified based on the results from the study that will bring a greater good to society in the form of a new treatment. But it also could be argued that an egoist would not do the study for fear of the mistreatment being discovered and harming the egoist's professional reputation. Those who practice the deontological theories would not do the research because it is morally wrong. It is important to consider the moral development of the researcher in trying to understand the intent behind the action as well as the action itself.

REPORTING RESEARCH The final stage of the research process is reporting the results in published form. Drowatzky (1996) stated that the two purposes of publishing research are to make new knowledge available and to allow for replication and reproduction of the study. A researcher has the moral obligation to report the actual results of a study as opposed to falsifying results to report conclusions that may benefit the researcher or the funding agency. As stated earlier, a published article is held up for scrutiny. If multiple researchers replicate the study and come to different conclusions, the original researcher may be viewed as being unethical.

Another ethical issue in reporting research is tied to how the research was conducted. If the results were obtained using a research protocol that is viewed as immoral or unethical or does not meet either United States or international codes, the data are termed *morally tainted* (Greene 1992; Luna 1997). Pozos (1992) presented the ethical arguments for and against the use of data gathered from morally tainted experiments.

For

Use of the data will advance knowledge.

The data gathered are independent of the questions over the ethics of the collection method.

There is no relationship between the characteristics of the researcher and the validity of the data.

Referencing the data does not constitute or condone the unethical behavior that was used to acquire it.

Against

Nothing good can come from evil.

Referencing the data will encourage similar studies to be conducted.

Referencing the data acknowledges the unethical researcher.

Referencing the data casts doubt on scientific research in general.

Referencing the data condones dehumanization of the subjects.

THE CASE OF ERIC POEHLMAN Dr. Eric Poehlman was a leading researcher in the area of obesity and metabolic changes during aging. In 2005 Poehlman admitted to fabricating data on 17 applications for federal grants to make his work seem more promising, helping him win nearly $3 million in government funding. His actions also led to his papers being more publishable, helping Poehlman to be viewed as a leading expert in the study of obesity. Poehlman's unethical and illegal behavior was discovered by a research assistant who noticed that data were changed to exaggerate the findings of a study.

Poehlman benefited both in a material sense (he received millions of dollars in grant money) and by advancing his career as a university professor and scholar. But his unethical behavior compromised the research process, fooled his peers, and filled the literature with inaccurate findings. Poehlman has admitted his wrongdoing and faces criminal charges. Also, all of his work over his two-decade career has been called into question, and his professional reputation is damaged.

On the surface it appears that Poehlman valued material gains and prestige over his obligation to science and the public to conduct and report his research in a manner consistent with the appropriate ethical code established for scientists. Poehlman's story is a cautionary tale for aspiring researchers who value prestige, fame, and fortune over acting within the appropriate ethical norms.

CONFLICTS OF INTEREST Beauchamp (1991) defined **conflict of interest** as being whenever a personal interest or a role obligation conflicts with an obligation to uphold another party's interest, thus compromising objectivity in regard to the other party. In exercise science there are several potential sources of conflict of interest including financial reward, desire for personal recognition, and altruism. An athletic trainer is pressured by a head coach to clear an athlete to compete in an important contest. The coach has control over hiring and firing the athletic trainer. In conflict is the self-interest of the trainer in keeping the position and the well-being of the athlete.

Conflicts of interest also arise for those who seek careers in the field of academic study. Loue (2000) stated that maintaining objectivity in research while maintaining an economic interest in the outcome is universally viewed as being difficult. The Council on Scientific Affairs and the Council on Ethical and Judicial Affairs (1990) of the American Medical Association noted that economic incentives may introduce subtle biases in the research process that may escape detection by even careful peer review.

Although ethical concerns about conflicts of interest in regard to financial incentives have been documented, the reality is that corporations provide a significant source of research funding. This increased pool of available research funding can create temptations for ethical digressions on the part of the researcher. The sport scientist must decide what the ethical behavior is based on his or her own ethical and moral beliefs.

Loue (2000) observed that a person's desire to make a significant mark in the exercise sciences, advance his or her career, increase power, or enhance prestige may lead to actions that are in the researcher's self-interest instead of in the interest of science, thus creating a conflict of interest. One only has to recall the Poehlman cased mentioned earlier in this chapter to see what lies down that slipping slope.

Finally, a conflict of interest may arise based on a exercise scientist's desire to do the right thing. In the hope of using an experimental treatment on a person he or she knows is suffering, the exercise scientist may disregard standard random selection for participation in the group that would get the treatment as opposed to the control group. Although the intent may be good, the researcher's interest in the well-being of that person compromises the research process.

Exercise scientists must be aware of potential conflicts of interest and take action that will ensure that their actions are not biased based on the conflicts mentioned here and that their actions meet the ethical standards of their profession.

Professional Careers

A number of career opportunities are presented to professionals in the exercise and sport field. These opportunities range from athletic trainers, to coaches, to fitness instructors, to judges and officials. For each of these areas, acceptable ethical behavior is codified, and individuals who do not adhere to these codes are not viewed favorably by their peers. Practitioners must determine their ethical views on a variety of specific ethical issues. Their views will reflect their values and principles and should be consistent with the ethical theory to which they adhere.

Olympic Movement

The International Olympic Committee serves as the umbrella organization for the Olympic movement. Under it auspices are international federations, national Olympic committees, national governing bodies, and the organizing committees of the Olympic Games as well as the athletes, coaches, judges, and officials. It can be argued that the IOC touches all aspects and participants in sport in the world. The goals of the Olympic movement are to promote a peaceful and better world through sport and without discrimination.

Over the course of the rise of the modern Olympics, a variety of ethical situations have arisen. These include amateur athletes accepting endorsement money, thus nullifying their amateur status; athletes who have used performance-enhancing drugs; IOC members being bribed to vote for a particular city to be the host city for an Olympic Games; officials being bribed to vote a certain way in a subjective competition like figure skating or boxing; officials voting in line with their political beliefs; and countries using the games to promote a political agenda. For all of the goodness that the Olympic movement wants to promote, the movement's reputation has been soiled by the ethical transgressions of those who are a part of the movement.

In each of the cases just mentioned, the entity or individual who committed the act may be able to justify the action based on the ethical theory to which he or she adheres. For example, when the leaders of the bid for Salt Lake City to host the 2002 Winter Games bribed IOC members to vote for the city, they could justify the action based on the economic benefits brought to the city and its population. In their minds, the end justified the means, but the public judged the behavior unethical and immoral. The officials viewed it as doing what needed to be done to secure the bid. Amateur athletes justified their decision to take endorsement money on egoist principles, asserting that they had earned it, but again the public viewed them with scorn for compromising the purity of the Olympic Games. American athlete Jim Thorpe was stripped of his medals at the 1912 Stockholm Games for accepting money to play minor league baseball prior to the games. The Olympics of today allow professional athletes to compete, and Thorpe's performance was reinstated and his medals given to his daughter in 1982.

Finally, judges in Olympic competition have not practiced moral behavior, sometimes voting as part of a bribe or voting in the national interest. In the 1988 Seoul Summer Games, United States boxer Roy Jones Jr. appeared to have won a Gold Medal in his weight class. At the conclusion of the bout, the Gold Medal was given to a South Korean boxer who was clearly defeated. It was determined later that the fight was fixed against Jones. In this case, a hard-fought victory was denied based on the unethical behavior of a sport judge.

If these types of ethical transgressions continue, the integrity of the Olympic movement and games will be weakened. All performances will be called into question, and the intent and actions of those who make up the Olympic movement will be questioned.

With the potential problems associated with these types of ethical transgressions, the IOC developed a code of ethics for those involved in the Olympic movement. Along with a preamble, the IOC Code of Ethics addresses dignity, integrity, resources, candidature, relations with state, confidentiality, and implementation. The code addresses the ethical digressions of members of the movement both in competition on the field and in the governance of the Olympic movement. The IOC also has established an Ethics Commission to oversee implementation of the code of ethics.

Performance Enhancement and Doping

Some exercise scientists will work in the area of international world class, professional, or major intercollegiate sport. Within these environments, highly competitive athletes and coaches search for ways to gain an edge over the competition. This has led to unethical practices by sport scientists to develop means to provide that competitive edge. Those means include the use of performance-enhancing drugs, blood doping, and questionable training methods. Wilson and Derse (2001) stated that there is a deeply held belief that athletes' use of banned substances threatens the very essence of sport, and it is the sport scientist who has the knowledge and the means to partake in the practice of developing and or using banned substances or doping blood. These actions lead to one competitor gaining an advantage over another who is following the prescribed rules.

There is potential for great financial reward to the exercise scientist who is able to develop and perfect a drug or a doping method that can go undetected and enhance the performance of an athlete. Recent scandals in professional sport in the United States (e.g., steroid use in professional baseball) and at the international level (e.g., Olympic track athletes, Tour de France bike race) have soiled the reputation of many famous athletes and have disgraced exercise scientists who developed and administered these performance-enhancement techniques. In the process they cheated other competitors, the public who believed these athletes were playing by the rules, the sport itself, and finally the field of exercise science.

Governing bodies at the national, international, intercollegiate, and professional levels have established drug testing mechanisms and policies to combat the use of these practices. The fact that they have been established is a statement in itself that their use by athletes and their development by sport scientists is ethically wrong.

Doping refers to the use of performance-enhancing drugs such as anabolic steroids. Historians recognize that as early as the 8th century athletes were using these kinds drugs: Ancient Greek Olympians ate sheep testicles, which have now been recognized as a form of testosterone. Athletes have much more complex means to enhance performance today. These progressions in pharmacology always surpass the ability of sports federations to implement the necessary testing to catch athletes.

In 1998, a doping scandal of unprecedented scale occurred during the world's premier cycling event, the Tour de France. Willy Voet, a masseur for the French Festina team, was arrested after being found with large quanitities of doping products. As a result, police raids also found drugs in the rooms of team members of the Dutch team. The athletes were enraged by the controversial treatment and staged a sit-down protest. After being urged by the ONCE team, the Spanish teams also pulled out of the race. This scandal was one of the sport's biggest wakeup calls. The controversy resulted in the creation of the World Anti-Doping Agency (WADA) in 1999. The battle against doping woud no longer be handled sport by sport, but instead would be a worldwide effort.

In recent years many ethical questions have surrounded doping and antidoping practices. The ethical considerations of the war on doping exist on the foundation of fairness in sports and the concept of a level playing field. The invasion of privacy some claim results from drug testing is considered acceptable because an athlete's health is being protected and because the athlete's sport achievements should reflect his or her natural abilities. In *Doping in Elite Sport*, Schneider and Butcher (2001) write that an intervention can be justified in two ways. First, intervention can be justified by an overwhelming need to pursue other moral values: The moral value of privacy is superseded by some other moral value, such as harm to others. Second, intervention can be justified by permission. Therefore, if consent is gained for an intervention, then that individual has waived his or her right to privacy.

In recent times, athletes and athletic personnel have become extremely sophisticated in their attempts to gain an advantage, often without consideration of possibly severe health consequences. One of the most common justifications for the bans on doping are those from harm. Misuse of substances has led to cardiovascular disorders, liver and kidney disease, psychological or physical dependence, and even death.

In addition to harm to users, harm to society is another argument stemming from this justification. Paul Weiss argues that sport is one of the very first arenas young people experience and in which they gain excellence: the excellence of their heroes. From a societal perspective, if this hero is morally despicable, this will be a negative influence because young people will not separate the athletic abilities of their heroes from the quality of their personal lives, especially when fame and glamour surround the hero (as cited in Schneider & Butcher, 2001). In addition, the benefits from sport surpass the playing field. Sports are an important learning tool, draw people together,

REFLECTION QUESTIONS

1. List five values and the principles that you have created from those values.

2. What have been the sources of your values?

3. At what stage of moral development are you? In expressing your view also state why you are not at the other stages.

4. To which theory of distributive justice do you adhere and why?

5. Visit a professional organization's Web site and review its code of ethics. What values and principles are being promoted? What behavior is encouraged? What behavior is not condoned?

6. To what ethical theory do you adhere and why?

7. Which ethical theory do you not adhere to and why?

8. Discuss how the Belmont Report findings would influence how you would conduct a research experiment.

9. Your mentor asks you to lie to his supervisor about his use of institutional funds. Your mentor has made your career possible and you owe him loyalty, but you know for a fact that he/she spent funds for personal use and created a false expense report that is being called into question. What do you do in this right versus right conflict? What resolution strategy would you use?

10. A private corporation asks you to conduct a test on a new exercise machine it has developed. If the results of the test you do show that the machine will improve performance, you will receive royalties on the sale of every machine. Your results are indicating the machine does not do what it claims to do. What do you do and why?

11. If you were told there was a 100% guarantee that you would not be caught, would you fabricate data in the manner that Dr. Poelhman did? Why or why not? Are there any ethical theories that would defend his actions? Explain.

12. Does the Olympic movement live up to its lofty ideals, or have the ethical digressions of members of the movement irreparably damaged its image and legacy?

13. Make an argument for and against doping using the deontological and teleological theories of ethics.

and are a powerful vehicle for peace. From an ethical perspective, doping has the potential to undercut these benefits.

Another argument stemming from this justification is harm to other athletes (other referring to the "clean" athletes). At the elite level of play, athletes are willing to do whatever it takes to get a step ahead. Clean athletes are harmed, so the argument goes, because the dopers "up the ante." If some competitors are using steroids, then all who wish to compete at that level will need to take steroids or other substances to keep up. (Schneider & Butcher, 2001) Doping harms other athletes in that it coerces them into accepting risks that are not essential to practicing their sport.

Doping and antidoping practices are receiving an increasing amount of coverage, and ethical concerns continue to surround the issue. Recently, the World Anti-Doping Association held a 2-day meeting with United Kingdom Sports. During the meeting, ways other than collecting urine and blood samples were discussed in order to continue the fight against doping. One new measure that has been considered is to target large-scale manufacturers and distributors of illegal anabolic steroids. This will require the cooperation of governments and law enforcement agencies. The world will continue to watch, condemn, and applaud these actions as long as anabolic steroids exist within sport.

SUMMARY

Exercise scientists have the opportunity to make significant contributions to society and the discipline through both theory and practice. How people conduct themselves professionally is as important if not more important than what they do professionally. Aspiring exercise scientists should come to terms with their ethical beliefs, be aware of what is considered ethical and unethical in their field, and conduct themselves in a manner that meets the accepted practices in the field. By doing so, exercise scientists may have long and productive careers where they will be respected by their peers while making valuable contributions to sport and society as a whole.

■ Key Resources

Key Web Sites

ACSM Code of Ethics (http://www.acsm.org/Content/NavigationMenu/MemberServices/MemberResources/CodeofEthics/Code_of_Ethics.htm)

International Olympic Committee Code of Ethics (http://multimedia.olympic.org/pdf/en_report_17.pdf)

■ Review Questions

1. What are examples of moral values?
2. What are principles, and what is their purpose?
3. What are the four distinguishing points of morality?
4. What are the six stages of moral development?
5. What is the fundamental difference between deontological and teleological ethical theories?
6. What is the basic tenet of a person who practices egoism?
7. What are the seven characteristics of an effective code of ethics?
8. What are the four elements of a code of ethics proposed by Kultgen?
9. What are three underlying principles presented in the Belmont Report?
10. What are the arguments for and against the use of morally tainted data?
11. What are four strategies to prevent conflict of interest in research?

■ References

Beauchamp, T. L. (1991). *Philosophical ethics: An introduction to moral philosophy* (2nd ed.). New York: McGraw-Hill.

Cavanaugh, G. F. (1990). *American business values* (3rd ed.). American Management Association. Englewood, NJ: Prentice Hall.

Council on Scientific Affairs and Council on Ethical and Judicial Affairs. (1990). Conflicts of interest in medical/industry research relationships. *Journal of the American Medical Association, 263,* 2790–2793.

DeSensi, J. T., & Rosenberg, D. (2003). *Ethics and morality in sport management.* Morgantown, WV: Fitness Information Technology, Inc.

Drowatzky, J. N. (1996). *Ethical decision making in physical activity research.* Champaign, IL: Human Kinetics.

Goree, K., Pyle, M. D., Baker, E., & Hopkins, J. V. (2004). *Ethics applied* (4th ed.). Boston, MA: Pearson Education.

Greene, V. W. (1992). Can scientists use information derived from concentration camps? Ancient answers to new questions. In A. L. Caplan (Ed.), *When medicine went mad: Bioethics and the Holocaust* (pp. 155–170). Totowa, NJ: Humana Press.

Hall, S. J. (2007). *Basic biomechanics* (5th ed.). New York: McGraw-Hill.

Jones, J. (1981). *Bad blood: The Tuskegee syphillis experiment: A tragedy of race and medicine.* New York: Free Press.

Kidder, R (1995). *How good people make tough choices.* New York: Harper.

Kohlberg, L. (1987). *Child psychology and childhood education: A cognitive-development view.* New York: Longman.

Kultgen, J. (1988). *Ethics and professionalism.* Philadelphia, PA: University of Pennsylvania Press.

Loue, S. (2000). *Textbook of research ethics: Theory and practice.* New York: Kluwer Academic/Plenum.

Luna, F. (1997). Vulnerable populations and morally tainted experiments. *Bioethics, 11,* 256–264.

National Academies Press. (1992). *Panel on scientific responsibility and the conduct of research. National Academy of*

Sciences, National Academy of Engineering, Institute of Medicine. Washington, DC: Author.

National Commission for the Protection of Human Subjects of Biomedical and Behavioral Research. (1978). *The Belmont report: Ethical principles and guidelines for the protection of human subjects of research*. Washington, DC: Author.

Pozos, R. S. (1992). Scientific inquiry and ethics: The Dachau data. In A. L. Caplan (Ed.), *When medicine went mad: Bioethics and the Holocaust* (pp. 95–108). Totowa: NJ: Humana Press.

Protecting human research subjects: Institutional Review Board Guidebook. (n.d). Retrieved from http://www.hhs.gov/ohrp/irb/irb-introduction.htm

Schneider, A J., & Butcher, R. B. (2001). An ethical analysis of drug testing. In W. Wilson & E. Derse (Eds.), *Doping in elite sport: The politics of drugs in the Olympic movement* (pp. 129–152). Champaign, IL: Human Kinetics.

Tuckman, B. W. (1978). *Conducting educational research*. New York: Harcourt Brace Jovanovich.

U.S. Department of Health and Human Services. (2006). IRB *guidebook*. Washington, DC: Author.

Wilson, W., & Derse, E. (2001). *Doping in elite sport: The politics of drugs in the Olympic movement*. Champaign, IL: Human Kinetics.

World Medical Association. (1964). *Declaration of Helsinki: Ethical principles for medical research involving human subjects*. Adopted by the 18th WMA General Assembly Helsinki, Finland, June 1964 and amended by the 29th WMA General Assembly, Tokyo, Japan, October 1975; 35th WMA General Assembly, Venice, Italy, October 1983; 41st WMA General Assembly, Hong Kong, September 1989; 48th WMA General Assembly, Somerset West, Republic of South Africa, October 1996; 52nd WMA General Assembly, Edinburgh, Scotland, October 2000.

CHAPTER 14

The Future of Exercise Science: Transdisciplinary Approaches to Research and Applied Intervention Strategies

Beverly Warren, PhD, EdD, FACSM, Virginia Commonwealth University

■ Chapter Objectives

After reading this chapter, you should be able to:

1. Identify the approved special interest groups within ACSM.
2. Define unidisciplinary, multidisciplinary, interdisciplinary, and transdisciplinary approaches to exercise science research and interventions.
3. Describe the transition of exercise science research from the organ level of observation to cellular and subcellular reactions.
4. Define and describe the impact of genomics, proteomics, and nanotechnology on recent scientific advances.
5. Describe new frontiers and career options in the exercise sciences.
6. List career options and appropriate preparation for 21st century careers in the exercise sciences.

■ Key Terms

genomics
interdisciplinary approach
multidisciplinary approach

nanotechnology
proteomics
transdiscipslinary approach

unidisciplinary approach

Within the last 50 years, exercise science has transitioned from a relatively new scientific discipline devoted to the science of human movement to a field of study that encompasses a number of subdisciplines. This text has focused on nine of the major subdisciplines within exercise science. The heightened interest in preventive medicine and a focus on public health initiatives have resulted in the vast expansion of knowledge and the evolution of a multitude of subdisciplines within the field. For example, the subdiscipline of exercise physiology is now comprised of specialty areas including the biochemistry of exercise, neuromuscular physiology, cardiovascular physiology, clinical exercise physiology, environmental physiology, and the physiology of aging, to name a few. As a result of the growth in subdisciplines within exercise science, the American College of Sports Medicine (ACSM) has formed a number of special interest groups. Table 14.1 provides a description of these special interest groups. As can be seen from this listing, this national organization presents a broad-based approach to the exercise sciences.

This increased specialization has produced a knowledge explosion that has resulted in a multitude of new discoveries in the basic and applied sciences. In addition, a number of applied intervention strategies have been developed from these subgroups targeted at improving the quality of human performance or the human condition. In addition to the subdisciplines mentioned in the table, ACSM works in a wide range of medical specialties, allied health professions, and scientific disciplines to improve the diagnosis, treatment, and prevention of sports-related injuries and the advancement of the science of exercise. Individuals who are interested in the science of exercise may find employment not only as exercise scientists but also as physical therapists, physicians, athletic trainers, nutritionists, sport psychologists, and a whole host of positions ranging from medical/therapeutic opportunities to the more health-related/preventive medicine careers often associated with exercise science professionals.

Although the increased specialization within the exercise sciences has advanced our knowledge of health and human performance, it can also lead to unidimensional research outcomes. This unidimensional approach to intervention occurs when multiple research or performance-enhancement teams work in isolation, often largely unaware of the findings of other research groups. In recent years, however, there appears to be a paradigm shift toward the expansion of interdisciplinary research. This type of intervention incorporates the physiological and neuromuscular sciences with social and behavioral sciences to explore new approaches to still unanswered questions in the area of human movement studies (Reis, 2000).

UNIDISCIPLINARY TO TRANSDISCIPLINARY APPROACHES

Research or intervention strategies can be classified on a continuum from unidisciplinary to transdisciplinary approaches to the study of human movement. **Unidisciplinary approaches** include the pursuit of a research question or intervention strategy from one unique subdiscipline perspective. Results are typically presented in journals that are read predominantly by those with a specific interest within the discipline, and there is very little crossover into other fields of study (Baldwin, 2000).

Multidisciplinary approaches incorporate more than one subdiscipline in the research or intervention team. In a multidisciplinary team, specialists from a number of subdisciplines contribute to the investigation of a common problem. However, each subdiscipline works independently within the boundaries of its own discipline (Abernathy, Harahan, Kippers, McKinnon, & Pansy, 2005). For example, a world-class cyclist works with a number of specialists to improve his performance. The exercise physiologist strives to improve the cyclist's VO_2max; the biomechanist investigates methods to improve the force and velocity of the pedaling technique; the sport psychologist works to improve focus and mental imagery; and the sports nutritionist develops a high-performance dietary regimen. Although much information is being provided to the cyclist, this multidisciplinary approach to training leaves the synergy and combined training strategy in the hands of the cyclist or coach. An **interdisciplinary approach** to intervention or to basic science research involves representatives from a number of subdisciplines who identify a common problem and explore discipline-specific contributions toward comprehensive solutions. Interdisciplinary pursuits are best thought of as bringing together distinctive components of two or more disciplines to produce a more comprehensive solution to the identified problem.

The most current research/intervention model is the **transdisciplinary approach,** which brings together specialists from two or more distinct specialties who work together on a problem with the intent of integrating their views to develop new and unique solutions. It is thought to be a blurring or blending of the specialties to develop new knowledge and unique interventions. Researchers or practitioners on transdisciplinary teams attempt to understand the others' perspective so that a new consolidated solution can be formulated (Rosenman, 1992).

TABLE 14.1 American College of Sports Medicine Approved Interest Groups

Interest Group	Mission
Aging	To support and promote basic, applied, and clinical research in exercise science as it relates to aging
Biomechanics	To promote biomechanics research
Biostatistics	To promote use of research design and statistical analysis in exercise science and sports medicine
Bone and Osteoporosis Network Exchange	To develop collaborative research groups facilitating approaches to the study of bone health and to develop recommendations for the prevention of osteoporosis
Cancer	To promote the study of physical activity/exercise and cancer
Cardiorespiratory Interests	To support scientific research in the areas of cardiovascular and respiratory physiology
Combative Sports	To provide a forum for the discussion and dissemination of the relevant sport science research as it pertains to the health, safety, and performance of athletes participating in combative sports, including the Olympic combative sports of wrestling, judo, tae-kwon-do, and boxing, as well as other martial arts competitions
Clinical Exercise Physiology	To provide opportunities for discussion of clinical issues and to improve training of exercise laboratory operation
Endurance Athlete Medicine and Science	To provide a multidisciplinary forum to develop standardized care for endurance athletes
Environmental Physiology	To provide a forum for exchange of research on the demands, challenges, and consequences of performing exercise in environmental extremes
Exercise Sciences Education	To develop and promote methods to enhance the lecture and laboratory exercise sciences pedagogy
Health Education and Promotion	To promote networking and interaction involved in health promotion and to provide a forum for discussion of contemporary health promotion issues
Health, Fitness, and Wellness Coaching	To network to share coaching experiences and practice new coaching skills to assist clients in taking responsibility to discover their own answers and solutions
Military Sports Medicine	To provide a forum to assemble and discuss issues regarding sports medicine in the military
Minority Health and Research	To provide a multidisciplinary forum for discussion and collaboration on minority health issues
Molecular and Cellular Regulatory Mechanisms	To provide a forum for focused discussion and debate among ACSM members with this interest
Motor Control	To provide a forum for individuals with interest in neurological aspects of movement to formulate, discuss, and refine ideas related to current topics
Noninvasive Investigation of the Neuromuscular System	To support and promote the use of noninvasive techniques in exercise sciences with particular reference to the neuromuscular system
Nutrition	To promote the science of nutrition within ACSM
Occupational Physiology	To promote and facilitate applied research and communication among ACSM members with interest in the relation of physical performance occupations with environmental or occupational demands

(continues)

(continued)	
Oxidative Stress	To foster exchange of information and research in the area of oxidative stress interventions that may influence and improve health and performance
Pediatric Exercise Science	To provide a forum for scientific and clinical communication regarding the acute and chronic exercise in the healthy and diseased child
Psychobiology and Behavior	To promote research and the advancement of sport psychology with particular emphasis on psychobiology and health
The Science in Winter Sports	To foster, enhance, and promote interdisciplinary scientific inquiry in Winter Sports activities
Strength and Conditioning Specialties	To support and promote an interdisciplinary forum for the exchange of interests with a focus on research and the development of a cooperative relationship between strength and conditioning professionals and the medical and applied sciences
Worksite Health Promotion	To promote networking and interaction with ACSM members involved in health promotion and to provide a forum for discussion of contemporary health promotion issues

EXAMPLES OF TRANSDISCIPLINARY MODELS

Research on the promotion of physical activity in youth and adults has evolved over time. In the 1970s, the focus was on the physiological variables targeted at defining the amount of vigorous activity needed to improve fitness. A second phase developed in the late 1970s and early 1980s in which a number of epidemiological studies linked physical activity and fitness with a multitude of important physiological and psychological health outcomes. By the 1990s, these studies led to the recognition of physical activity as a major public health priority, and new recommendations focused on increasing the amount of moderate physical activity in one's daily life. A third phase developed in the late 1990s and was characterized by an emphasis on behavioral/psychological theories to inform the most effective health promotion strategies. Despite these efforts and the development of new knowledge in areas of physiology, psychology, and health promotion, a significant proportion of the U.S. population remained irregularly active or sedentary (Powell, Bricker, & Blair, 2002).

In the early 2000s, a fourth phase of physical activity research has emerged and is characterized by a focus on a broader and more global range of influence. It involves blending physiological and behavioral research with environmental strategies and public policy mandates. The Robert Wood Johnson Foundation has supported this new approach to research in its target on "Active Living." Dr. James Sallis (Sallis, Linton, & Kraft, 2005) reported that this concept of encouraging physical activity through an increased emphasis on environmental and policy-driven factors has brought together individuals who have not previously partnered to enhance the promotion of physical activity in the U.S. population. King, Stokols, Talen, Brassington, and Killingsworth (2002) proposed a continuum to explain the conceptual approaches to physical activity and to propose a transdisciplinary paradigm to explore physical activity behaviors. Figure 14.1 provides a synopsis of this transdisciplinary approach involving a spectrum of choice-driven (physiological and behavioral parameters) and choice-enabling factors (environmental and public policy parameters).

By exploring physical activity from both an environmental and health behavior perspective, new ideas are formulated through cross-fertilization of two very different fields of study. The Active Living research initiative is directed at identifying environmental factors and policies that influence physical activity behavior. The Active Living research teams are transdisciplinary groups that are forging new concepts and designs that would not be possible in a single research field or even within an interdisciplinary research team. Stokols, Harvey, Gress, Fuqua, and Phillips (2005) reported that these efforts in transdisciplinary research on active living will facilitate scientific advances and improved public health outcomes in the 21st century.

As a result of these transdisciplinary efforts, a growing interest has developed in understanding how features of city design can facilitate or impede physical activity. Transdisciplinary models have fostered a "new urbanism" that seeks to promote a pedestrian-oriented environment. New design principles include walkable urban areas (more dense urban designs versus suburban sprawl), ample well-designed public spaces, and the provision for nonautomotive modes

Conceptual Approaches to Physical Activity		
Choice-Driven ←		→ **Choice-Enabling**
Intrapersonal	Behavior Micro-environment	Macro-environment
Health locus of control	Operant condition	Neighborhood disorder
Reasoned action/ Planned behavior	Social learning/ Social cognitive	Urban imageability
Relapse prevention	Behavioral economics	Environmental psychology & the Internet
Expectancy-value	Meso-environment	Urban design
Transtheoretical model	Environmental stresses	Transportation planning
Self-determination	Restorative environments	Land use

Figure 14.1 Transdisciplinary Approach to the Study of Physical Activity.

Source: King et at. (2002).

of travel such as bike lanes and public transit (King et al., 2002). A number of studies have been conducted that indicate a higher prevalence of obesity and overweight exists in locales where segregated land use makes walking to destinations difficult (Brown, Khattak, & Rodriguez, 2008). Through this impetus to examine the relationship between environmental conditions and level of physical activity, there is an emerging understanding of the shortcomings associated with treatment strategies targeted solely at individual interventions. Many treatment strategies are now targeted at social and environmental determinants of health as well as stressing individual responsibility for health behavior change (Heinrich et al., 2008). The combined efforts of physiological and behavioral scientists with public policymakers and urban developers provide a ray of hope in creating a larger impact on the fight against the increasing levels of inactivity in the American culture.

NEW FRONTIERS IN THE EXERCISE SCIENCES

Specialty Groups and Innovative Practices

The new millennium in exercise science will be defined, in large part, by new technologies and innovative practices to address the need to encourage a physically active lifestyle for individuals of all ages. Much of the success of exercise science professionals in the 21st century will be determined by their understanding of the health needs of target populations and their use of new and innovative strategies to encourage a healthy lifestyle.

Two unique populations that have received recent attention from exercise science professionals are children/youth and older adults. Many children are overweight, physically inactive, and have poor eating habits, resulting in greater risks for the development of major chronic diseases. The number of children who are overweight has doubled over the last 20 years, and the prevalence of obesity continues to increase, especially among Mexican American and African American adolescents. Much of the increase in the number of youth who are obese is attributed to decreased physical activity, particularly in the adolescent years (Ogden, Carrol, Curtin, McDowell, Tabak, & Flegal, 2006). This increase in obesity rates coincides with recent federal education mandates that have resulted in decreased time spent in quality physical education classes in schools. The Centers for Disease Control and Prevention (2008) found that participation in physical education has declined significantly among high school students. As a result, alternative programs have evolved to provide children and youth with safe and effective physical activity programs. Many fitness facilities have begun to offer specialized children's fitness and exercise programs, and many new entrepreneurial franchises have evolved such as My Gym Children's Fitness Centers, Fun Bus, The Little Gym, and Kidokinetics. These franchises offer programs focused on innovative approaches to developmentally appropriate physical activity for children in a for-profit enterprise. In addition, a number of hospital or university-based facilities have been developed to assist in the prevention and treatment of childhood obesity. A strong background in pediatric exercise physiology as well as a general understanding of human growth and development principles is highly recommended for the 21st century exercise scientist.

At the other end of the age spectrum is the growing population of older adults. By the year 2030, Americans age 55 and older will number 107.6 million and will account for 31% of the population. Those over 65 will account for 20% of the total population. This aging of the population will be one of the major health and business issues of the 21st century. It is estimated that the number of jobs in gerontology-related fields will increase by more than 36% by 2012 (Bureau of Labor Statistics, 2008). The trend in this gerontological market will be a focus on ways to assist older adults to lead productive lives and to remain healthy and independent for as long as possible. Senior exercise programs are offered at health clubs, community centers, churches, retirement communities, park and recreation departments, and in colleges and universities. In addition to the general undergraduate preparation in exercise science, additional certifications and training programs are offered to better prepare exercise scientists to meet the needs of these unique age groups.

Sport Performance Enhancement

The training of the elite athlete has led to a reidentification of effective training techniques. At the United States Olympic Training Center, the subdisciplines of sport science have become more tightly integrated to improve performance. The typical boundaries of the sport sciences of physiology, biomechanics, psychology, motor learning and control, nutrition, and sports medicine have been blended for a more focused approach to skill advancement. For example, sport biomechanists and engineering scientists are able to transform athletic performance into two or three dimensional pictures for precise movement analysis. From this information, they can build custom sensing equipment to measure the most subtle aspects of performance such as oar positions for rowing teams, the position and force of the barbell in weightlifting, or the body position of the gymnast in a vaulting maneuver. This information is coupled with sport physiologists and motor learning specialists to determine the most effective training strategy for elite U.S. athletes. The end result is a very effective interdisciplinary team that works to improve performance in all areas of sport science (Sands, 2004).

Medicine and Health

Over the last 30 years, the exercise sciences have moved from research investigations targeted at whole body or organ level observations to research models that explore cellular and subcellular reactions. The 1970s and 1980s have been identified as the "biochemistry of exercise" era, and the 1990s to early 2000s have been linked to the study of "molecular exercise science" (Abernathy et al., 2005). Many of the recent advances have resulted from the introduction of more sophisticated instrumentation that permits cellular and subcellular observations. Just as radioisotope and imaging technologies advanced our understanding of exercise biochemistry, an explosion of molecular biology tools has created new fields of study in the life sciences. The areas of genomics, proteomics, and nanotechnology have the potential to improve our understanding of

chronic diseases and to offer treatment solutions that can improve our success rate in combating these life-threatening conditions (U.S. Department of Heath and Human Services, 2004). **Genomics** is the study of genes and their function. It typically involves the high-speed sequencing of a large number of genes, which will help researchers identify specific genes responsible for specific functions within an organism. **Proteomics,** a related and emerging field, is the study of proteins that are expressed in a cell. This field of study attempts to catalog and characterize proteins derived from genetic coding. **Nanotechnology** researchers work at the molecular level to create and use devices and structures that can be controlled or manipulated on the atomic scale. These new technologies will enable scientists to identify the specific sets of genes that are involved in areas such as behaviors related to adherence to physical activity or the identification of the specific etiology of various disease processes or the effects of aging on human cells (Baldwin, 2000). For example, recently funded work by the National Cancer Institute has developed a nanotechnological tool called PEBBLEs (Probes Encapsulated by Biologically Localized Embedding). These tiny plastic beads hold promising hope of delivering therapeutic drugs with exceptional precision to target only the cancerous cells in the body, thus sparing healthy cells from the debilitating effects of toxic chemotherapy treatments. With the development of PEBBLEs, chemotherapy may work on a microscale to direct medicine exactly where it is needed and avoid the damage to healthy tissues (Buck et al., 2004). These new levels of treatment will have a tremendous impact on the quality of life of the cancer patient and the ability of the patient to improve health through exercise. The amalgamation of biomedical research with health care prevention and treatment is certainly the wave of the future. Preparation for applied health careers will necessarily require a broader level of training that spans molecular biology through integrative systems physiology as well as applied health behavior interventions.

The four main research priorities established by the Federation of American Societies for Experimental Biology support this need for transdisciplinary approaches to improving health and human performance. They include (1) exploiting genomics to determine the origins of diseases, to design new therapies, and to predict responses to environmental influences; (2) revitalizing clinical research through increasing the number of funded General Clinical Research Centers at major research institutions; (3) collaborating with other disciplines such as biology, engineering, environmental science, and medicine to explore new knowledge and treatment regimens; and (4) eliminating health disparities by improving living conditions, access to health, and general health knowledge for all components of our society and for all nations (Baldwin, 2000).

CAREERS IN
EXERCISE SCIENCE

With the focus on preventive medicine and the dramatic increase in adults who are over 50 years of age, careers in the exercise sciences will continue to expand (Kravitz & Rockey, 1999). Just as the focus in research has experienced a shift toward interdisciplinary approaches to new discoveries, the future careers in the exercise sciences will involve a blending of science, health, and technology. Kravitz and Rockey suggest that preparing for careers in the new millennium will involve greater understanding of the health needs of target populations. These authors identified four evolving career tracks: health and fitness, alternative wellness, health rehabilitation, and specialty areas. In the area of health and fitness, the emerging positions are in medical health and fitness facilities that work with high-risk clients in a tightly supervised exercise environment. Alternative wellness therapies are receiving more attention as many individuals seek nonpharmacological and nonsurgical solutions to the health issues arising from chronic disease states. Opportunities exist in private practice clinics, chiropractic offices, nursing homes, and wellness retreats. The field of health rehabilitation has experienced a shift to an interdisciplinary approach, with physicians and physical therapists working hand in hand with cardiac rehabilitation specialists, clinical exercise physiologists, and athletic trainers to improve health. A comprehensive clinical program may include the following treatment team:

- Physicians and physician assistants
- Nurse practitioners
- Nurses
- Physical therapists
- Clinical exercise physiologists
- Cardiac rehabilitation specialists
- Occupational therapists
- Social workers
- Psychologists and mental skills coaches
- Functional capacity clinicians
- Athletic trainers
- Certified exercise specialists
- Preventive and rehabilitative exercise directors

Likewise, many specialty areas are emerging in health, fitness, and sport performance areas. For example, pediatric exercise specialists will be in high demand to counteract the surge of heightened obesity in children and adolescents. Many weight management clinics have surfaced as a result of Medicaid support for the morbidly obese. In addition, with the

aging of the baby boomer population, there are more individuals over the age of 50 than ever before. To take advantage of this market, many health clubs are specializing in the health and fitness needs of seniors. Finally, a new frontier in the area of sport performance involves the emergence of performance-enhancement centers focusing on adolescents who are striving to become elite athletes. These centers are employing strength and conditioning specialists and exercise physiologists who apply the latest sport science research and improved technology to develop the elite athlete of tomorrow.

Table 14.2 lists occupations available to the student prepared in the exercise sciences.

TABLE 14.2 Potential Careers in the Exercise Sciences	
Career Type	**Possible Job Title**
General Wellness	Aerobic Instructor
	Exercise Program Director
	Health Fitness Instructor
	Corporate Fitness Director
	Personal Trainer
	Recreation Fitness Specialist
	Group Exercise Instructor
	Health Promotion Specialist
	Community Center Director
Rehabilitation and Therapy	Athletic Trainer
	Kinesiotherapist
	Recreation Therapist
	Exercise Specialist
	Exercise Test Technologist
	Occupational Physiologist
	Cardiopulmonary Rehabilitation Specialist
	Physical Therapist
	Occupational Therapist
	Physician's Assistant
Sport Performance Enhancement	Biomechanist
	Exercise Physiologist
	Strength and Conditioning Specialist
	Sports Nutritionist
	Sport Psychologist
	Athletic Trainer
Business/Innovative Practices	Pharmaceutical Sales
	Corporate Health Adviser
	Sports Agent
	Fitness Marketing and Sales

Credentialing and Licensure of Exercise Science Professionals

There is a growing interest in the regulation or licensing of the exercise science professions. Although state and national licensure is required for some exercise science professions such as physical therapy, occupational therapy, and athletic training, other fields of study related specifically to exercise physiology remain largely unregulated. Many states have explored the development of state certification examinations for the position of clinical exercise physiologist; however, no broad national accreditation or licensure exists to certify exercise physiologists.

Despite the lack of uniformity in the licensure of exercise science professionals, a number of organizations offer training and certification programs related to career tracks in fitness, health promotion, and rehabilitative/preventive medicine. Table 14.3 lists organizations offering certification for a broad array of exercise and physical activity areas. Some certifications are offered online and do not require that individuals have appropriate academic credentials, but many national organizations have established rigorous criteria for validating the knowledge, skills, and abilities (KSAs) of exercise science professionals. The American College of Sports Medicine certifications have been recognized as the gold standard in the health, fitness, and clinical physiology professions.

Another initiative targeted at enhancing the professionalism of the exercise science fields is the development of an accreditation process for university-based academic programs that prepare candidates for employment in the health, fitness, and clinical physiology areas. The Committee on Accreditation for the Exercise Sciences (CoAES) was established in 2004 as a subset of the Commission on Accreditation of Allied Health Education Programs (CAAHEP). Programmatic accreditation through CAAHEP is intended to provide academic standardization for college and university programs with professional preparation tracks in health wellness, fitness, or clinical exercise science. The importance of the accreditation established by CoAES is that it provides objective third-party evaluation of academic programs and ensures consistency in the preparation of exercise science practitioners.

These 21st century advances in university program accreditation and the enhancement of certifications through requiring appropriate academic preparation will assist in the recognition of exercise science practitioners as equals among colleagues in other professional practices such as physical therapy, nursing, and athletic training.

TABLE 14.3 Organizations Offering Certification Programs Related to Physical Activity

Organization	Areas of Certification
Aerobics and Fitness Association of America (AFAA)	AFP Fitness Practitioner Primary Aerobics Instructor Step Reebok Certification Weight Room/Resistance Training Certification
American College of Sports Medicine (ACSM)	Certified Personal Trainer Exercise Specialist Certified Health Fitness Specialist Registered Clinical Exercise Physiologist
American Council on Exercise (ACE)	Group Fitness Instructor Personal Trainer Lifestyle and Weight Management Consultant Clinical Exercise Specialist
American Fitness Professionals and Associates (AFPA)	Certified Personal Trainer Cardio Kickboxing Instructor Cycle Instructor Nutrition and Wellness Consultant Pilates Fitness Instructor Yoga Fitness Instructor
The Cooper Institute	Coaching Health Behaviors Cooper Fitness Specialist Group Exercise Leader Master Fitness Specialist Personal Trainer
International Sports Sciences Association (ISSA)	Certified Fitness Trainer Endurance Fitness Trainer Fitness Therapy Youth Fitness Trainer
National Strength and Conditioning Association (NSCA)	Certified Personal Trainer Certified Strength and Conditioning Specialist
National Federation of Personal Trainers (NFPT)	Certified Personal Fitness Trainer
YMCA of the USA	Certified Fitness Leader Certified Specialty Leader Trainer of Fitness Leader Trainer of Trainers

Preparing for the 21st Century Workforce

As individuals seek exercise science careers in the 21st century, it is important that their academic preparation matches the expectations of a transdisciplinary, globalized marketplace. In *The World Is Flat*, Thomas Friedman (2007) makes the case that the globalization of the marketplace has leveled the competitive playing fields between modern, industrialized countries and the emerging market countries such as China, Japan, and India. To prepare for this flattened world, Friedman suggests that a new kind of education will be required for individuals to get ahead. Individuals will need to see connections never before visualized and must be able to effectively communicate those complex connections to others. He indicates that the first and foremost trait to develop is a passion for learning. Because much of what is learned becomes quickly outdated, employers are seeking individuals who can think critically and who can learn readily on the job. In *A Whole New Mind*, Daniel Pink (2005) emphasizes the need for these skills as he describes the world changing from an Information Age to what he calls a Conceptual Age. Pink argues that we are leaving behind the Information Age, based on acquired knowledge and logical analysis, and entering a new Conceptual Age, requiring inventive, empathic, big picture capabilities. Pink calls these aptitudes "high concept" and "high touch."

Based on these theories, 21st century exercise science careers will require individuals who can work effectively in teams, who can blend existing ideas into new knowledge, and who can understand the subtleties of human interaction. Therefore, the most effective approaches to learning and preparing for new careers in the exercise sciences will require the motivated student to do the following: (1) nurture a passion for learning new things; (2) seek an academic degree from an accredited program that provides the KSAs needed to be successful; (3) develop an interdisciplinary academic program of study that is well grounded in the humanities and the sciences; (4) acquire appropriate certifications that become validating credentials; and (5) develop experience in working with people through internships and participation on transdisciplinary research teams.

SUMMARY

A tremendous challenge remains to solve the health issues of chronic disease and advance new frontiers in elite athlete performance, and these issues are best resolved with an integrative approach of the many subdisciplines within exercise science. We need to continue to develop specialists with specific technical capabilities who can contribute to solving these complex health and performance issues. However, it is imperative that the future preparation of exercise scientists include a transdisciplinary approach to understanding the complexity of the issues we face in improving the health and well-being of all people. We must reach out to link with professionals from other disciplines where the combined skills and talents can be utilized to improve performance, increase physical activity, and offer effective health promotion access for everyone. The best institutions of the future are those that can reorganize themselves to address scientific and educational questions in an interdisciplinary way. Likewise, the best exercise scientists and practitioners of the future are those who have received a broad-based yet focused education to become key contributors on the transdisciplinary teams of the future.

■ Key Points

- There are more than 20 approved special interest groups within the American College of Sports Medicine.
- Transdisciplinary approaches to research and intervention strategies within exercise science have the potential to produce a more comprehensive solution to identified health and performance issues.
- Over the last 30 years, the exercise sciences have moved from a whole body/organ level of observation to the study of cellular and subcellular reactions.
- Sport performance teams have blurred the boundaries of the sport science specialties to focus on effective, comprehensive performance enhancement.

- Careers in the exercise sciences continue to expand and to focus on interdisciplinary and transdisciplinary approaches to exercise intervention.
- There is growing interest in the credentialing and licensure of exercise science professionals.
- The American College of Sports Medicine offers the gold standard for certifications for exercise science professionals.
- It is imperative that the future preparation of exercise scientists include a transdisciplinary approach to understanding the complexities involved in improving the health and well-being of all individuals.

■ Review Questions

1. List and briefly describe the mission of the special interest groups within ACSM.
2. Define the following: unidisciplinary, multidisciplinary, interdisciplinary, and transdisciplinary.

3. Describe the history of research on the promotion of physical activity and the impact of the Robert Wood Johnson Foundation's Active Living initiative.

4. Define the fields of genomics, proteomics, and nano-technology and their impact on the exercise sciences.
5. List the four main research priorities of the Federation of American Societies for Experimental Biology.
6. List and describe four evolving career tracks in the exercise sciences.
7. What is the main accrediting organization for allied health professions?

8. List five organizations that offer certification for exercise science professionals.
9. List possible career opportunities in each of the evolving tracks in the exercise sciences.
10. Describe a current unresolved issue in health or sport performance and outline a transdisciplinary approach to its resolution.

■ References

Abernethy, B., Harahan, S., Kippers, V., Mackinnon, L. T., & Pansy, M. O. (2005). *The biophysical foundations of human movement*. Champaign, IL: Human Kinetics.

Baldwin, K. M. (2000). Research in the exercise sciences: Where do we go from here? *Journal of Applied Physiology*, 88, 322–336.

Brown, A. L., Khattak, A. J., & Rodriguez, D. A. (2008). Neighbourhood types, travel and body mass: A study of the new urbanist and suburban neighbourhoods in the US. *Urban Studies*, 45, 963–988.

Buck, S. M., Lee Koo, Y. E. Park, E., Hao, X., Philbert, M. A., Brasuel, M. A., & Kopelman, R. (2004). Optochemical nanosensor PEBBLEs: Photonic explorers for bioanalysis with biologically localized embedding. *Current Opinion in Chemical Biology*, 8, 540–546.

Bureau of Labor Statistics, U.S. Department of Labor. (2008). *Occupational outlook handbook*, 2008–09 Edition. Retrieved from http://www.bls.gov/oco/ocos054.htm

Centers for Disease Control and Prevention. (2008). Retrieved from http://www.cdc.gov/needphp/publications2008

Friedman, T. L. (2007). *The world is flat: A brief history of the twenty-first century*. New York: Picador.

Heinrich, K. M., Lee, R.E., Regan, G. R., Reese-Smith, J. Y., Howard, H. H., Haddock, C. K., Poston, W. S., & Ahluwalia, J. S. (2008). How does the built environment relate to body mass index and obesity prevalence among public housing residents? *American Journal of Health Promotion*, 22, 187–194.

King, A. C., Stokols, D., Talen, E., Brassington, O. S., & Killingsworth, R. (2002). Theoretical approaches to the promotion of physical activity: Forging a transdisciplinary paradigm. *American Journal of Preventive Medicine*, 23, 15–25.

Kravitz, L., & Rockey, M. S. (1999). Career growth tips for the 21st century: A resource guide to career opportunities. *American College of Sports Medicine Health and Fitness Journal*, 3, 15–18.

Ogden, C. L., Carrol, M. D., Curtin, L. R., McDowell, M. A., Tabak, C. J., & Flegal K. M. (2006). Prevalence of overweight and obesity in the United States, 1999–2004. *Journal of the American Medical Association*, 295, 1549–1555.

Pink, D. H. (2005). *A whole new mind: Moving from the Information Age to the Conceptual Age*. New York: Penguin Group (Riverhead).

Powell, K. E., Bricker, S. K., & Blair, S. N. (2002). Treating inactivity. *American Journal of Preventive Medicine*, 23, 1–2.

Reis, R. M. (2000, September 29). Interdisciplinary research and your scientific career. *The Chronicle of Higher Education*. Retrieved from http://chronicle.com/jobs/news/2000/09/2000092903.htm

Rosenman, P. L. (1992). The potential of transdisciplinary research for sustaining and extending linkages between the health and social sciences. *Social Science and Medicine*, 35, 1343–1357.

Sallis, J. F., Linton, L., & Kraft, M. K. (2005). The first active living research conference: Growth of a transdisciplinary field. *American Journal of Preventive Medicine*, 28, 93–95.

Sands, W. A. (2004). Sport biomechanics and engineering. *Olympic Coach*, 16, 4–5.

Stokols, D., Harvey, R., Gress, J., Fuqua, J., & Phillips, K. (2005). In vivo studies of transdisciplinary scientific collaboration: Lessons learned and implications for active living research. *American Journal of Preventive Medicine*, 28, 202–213.

U.S. Department.of Health and Human Services. (2004). Cancer nanotechnology. NIH Publication No 04-5489. Washington, DC: National Cancer Institute.

Credits

Photo Credits

pp. 1, 11, 57, 95, 113, 127 © Thomas Northcutt/PhotoDisc/Getty Images; p. 4, © Hulton-Deutsch Collection/Corbis; pp. 17, 21, Courtesy Dr. David L. Costill, Human Performance Laboratory, Ball State University; p. 31, Photo by Ian Soper; p. 32, Courtesy of Fitness Institute of Texas; pp. 35, 37, 40, Photo by author; p. 42, Courtesy of Fitness Institute of Texas; p. 43T, Courtesy William E. Prentice; p. 43B, Courtesy Life Measurement, Inc.; p. 63, © Imagesource/Jupiterimages; p. 67, Courtesy William E. Prentice; p. 85, Rothwell, J. C., Traub, M. M., Day, B. L. Obeso, J. A. Thomas, P. K., & Marsden, C. D. (1982). "Manual motor performance in a deafferented man." *Brain*, 105, 515–542.; p. 88, Photos by Kelly Cole; pp. 101, 107, Courtesy Susan B. Hall; p. 142, © Bettmann/Corbis; p. 143, © Dynamic Graphics/JupiterImages; p. 146, © Royalty-Free/Corbis; p. 149, Library of Congress; pp. 150, 151, 153, © Royalty-Free/Corbisp. 162, Getty Images; p. 163, Bronwyn Kidd/Getty Images; p. 164, PhotoDisc/Getty Images; p. 67, Courtesy of the University of Evansville; p. 187, Dynamic Graphics/JupiterImages; p. 190, © The McGraw-Hill Companies, Inc./Gary He, photographer; p. 193, Courtesy of Palestra

Illustration Credits

Figure 5.1, From Seeley, RR, Stephens, TD, and Tate, P: *Anatomy and physiology*, ed. 8, New York: McGraw-Hill Higher Education, 2008; Figure 5.3, Kandel et al, *Principles of Neural Science* ed. 3, New York: Elsevier, 1991; Figure 5.4, From Rothwell, J. C., Traub, M. M., Day B. L., Obeso, J. A., Thomas, P. K., & Marsden, C. D. (1982). Manual motor performance in a deafferented man. *Brain*, 105, 515–542 by permission of Oxford University Press; Figures 5.5, 5.6, From Kandel et al, *Principles of Neural Science* ed. 4, New York: McGraw-Hill Medical, 2000. Figures 6.1, 6.2, 6.3, 6.4, 6.5, 6.6, 6.7, 6.8, 6.9, 6.10, 6.11, 6.12, 6.13 from Hall, SJ: Basic Biomechanics, ed. 6, New York: McGraw-Hill Higher Education, 2007. Figure 7.1, 7.2, 7.3, reprinted by permission of the National Athletic Trainers' Association. Figure 13.1, from Cavanaugh, GF: *American Business Values*, 3rd edition, Prentice Hall, 1990. Figure 14.1, Reprinted from American Journal of Preventive Medicine, Vol. 23:2, King, AC, et al., "Theoretical approaches to the promotion of physical activity: Forging a transdisciplinary paradigm," p. 2, 2002, with permission from Elsevier

Name Index

Subject Index